Until 120

URI RASKIN

Until 120

A BABY BOOMERS' SAGA OF LIFESTYLE CHANGE

URI RASKIN

GREEN TEA BOOKS
ATLANTA

LIBRARY OF CONGRESS CATALOGUE–IN–PUBLICATION–DATA

Raskin, Uri
Until 120: A Baby Boomer's Saga of Lifestyle Change
Includes bibliography references.
ISBN 978–0–9797585–0–8
LCC 2016903121

Cover Design by JSR All Productions
Cover Photo Creative Commons
Printed in the United States

In Loving

Memory of My Parents

From whose garden of values I grew!

I think the writer's mission is to explain human relationships, and you have to do it from your guts. Any writer, who is worth a damn, writes from inside out, from the bowels of his family. It is really frightening to go into the dark rooms of your past, and of other people's pasts. But you can't write unless you absorb the pain, and translate it, and your joy and your fear, to your readers. Other people feel things as deeply as writers, but they can't convey their emotions the same way. That's the writer's unique quality—and curse—and why writers have such a high suicide rate, a high insanity rate, a high rate of drunkenness, because we have to absorb this pain all the time.

Leon Uris
Jerusalem Post
December, 1994

Contents

	Preface	11
1.	Chanukah 1998	15
2.	Boomers	21
3.	Survival and Change	29
4.	Childhood	35
5.	Shame and Self–Esteem	45
6.	Addictions and Emotions	57
7.	Psyche—Soma	69
8.	Attitude	85
9.	Судьба	95
10.	Inner Child	105
11.	Reframing	119
12.	Catharsis	131
13.	Personality	145
14.	Character	161
15.	Relationships	175
16.	Divorce, Marriage, Love	185
17.	Doctored	199
18.	Big Parma	217
19.	Fat Lies	243
20.	Timeless Aging	267
21.	Inner Calm	281

22. Telomeres   299

23. 2070   311

Epilogue   331

Appendix: Frequently Asked Questions—FAQ   335

References   347

10

Preface

The purpose of a writer is to keep civilization from destroying itself.

Albert Camus

The man who writes about himself and his own time is the only man who writes about all people and about all time.

George Bernard Shaw

Every secret of a writer's soul, every experience of his life, every quality of his mind is written large in his works.

Virginia Woolf

Every author in some way portrays himself in his works, even if it be against his will.

Goethe

Ten years ago, I went to Hadassah Hospital in Jerusalem to visit a very good friend of mine who was scheduled to have bariatric surgery to cure his diabetes. However, because of complications caused by years of pancreatic abuse and tissue scarring from liver cancer surgery, he ended up having a very complicated gastric bypass.

Over the next months he was in and out of the hospital with a host of surgical complications. He had elected to have the band procedure simply as he put it because he did not think he would live through another attack of pancreatitis.

On one of my visits, he paid me what I consider one of the finest compliments I had ever received. He looked at me from his hospital bed and said, "You know you are the only person I know who had

11

a serious medical problem and consistently did anything about it. You changed your lifestyle and stuck with it after all these years."

Riding home that day on the bus his compliment gave me pause. Could there be something special about me? Did I do anything unique? And what about our mutual friends he was referring to? Why couldn't they have done the same as me?

True, I had reversed coronary artery disease, had a running head start on beating colon cancer and had dealt with a host of other problems. Upon reflection, however, I realized my friend was not referring to any specifics rather the overall changes I had made in my lifestyle which enabled me to succeed where others could not. Many people have told me they know what to do, but unlike Nike *they just can't do it.* The thought of putting it all down in a book entered my mind, but that is as far as it ever got.

A few months after that visit a co–worker, a young woman in her early 40's told me that she had just been diagnosed with breast cancer. Along with others at work she jokingly made fun about my style of living. At lunch, I only ate brown rice, lentils, and Shitake mushrooms seasoned with a host of Indian spices and downed my green tea. Never would I have a piece of birthday cake, share the occasional ordered in pizza or succumb to the "a little bite won't kill you" logic.

One day before her leave of absence she tearfully showed me her lunch. "See," she cried, "I am just like you now." Her lunch consisted of brown rice, the first whole wheat bread she had ever eaten in her life, several pieces of fruit and of course, a thermos of green tea. I later discovered she repeated those same words to our co–workers. Yet, when they individually related that to me I asked the pointed question. "Maybe you should think of making some lifestyle changes before you wind up in the same position as she is in?" Their answers were typical.

That night I resolved that I would put my story down in a book. After all, I had already published two novels and several short stories.[1] But just to tell my story had to be more than blueberries, tofu, beans and green tea. For years I unsuccessfully tried to persuade my friends and family to live a healthier lifestyle. They looked at me as if I was Chicken Little; the sky hadn't fallen in their lives yet, so why change.

There is an old saying in the South, "An expert is someone who lives out of town." To my friends, family, or anyone else for that matter, I knew I had to convincingly sound like an expert. So began my odyssey of research which weaved its way through more than a thousand peer–reviewed articles and over four hundred books. Still, I am not a physicist, physician, cardiologist, oncologist, philosopher, psychologist, theologian, nor was I born in India. I hear you asking yourselves, if he is none of those things, why on earth should I listen to what he says?

The 18th century philosopher and Kabbalist, Moshe Chaim Luzzatto, wrote in his classic work *The Path of the Just*, about a garden maze much like the famous one at Chatsworth, England. Rabbi Luzzatto explained that for amusement the nobility would wander in the maze, traversing its confusing and interlacing paths, trying to reach the colonnade in the middle.

Someone who is walking the maze cannot possibly know whether he is on the right path or not. Yet, those already standing on the colonnade by virtue of their having successfully completed the maze are in a position to assist one still in the maze, "This is the way . . . Walk as I say and you will reach the colonnade."

I have written *Until 120—A Baby Boomers' Saga of Lifestyle Change* standing on the entablature of the colonnade in order to help you negotiate the maze as I have done. Take my hand and together we will navigate the maze of lifestyle change.

1

Chanukah 1998

Brave and loyal followers! Long ago we resolved to serve neither the Romans nor anyone other than God Himself who alone is the true and just Lord of mankind. The time has now come that bids us prove our determination by our deeds we have never submitted to slavery, even when it brought no danger with it. We must not choose slavery now.

Elazar Ben Yair

It is not the delicate neurotic person who is prone to angina, but the robust, the vigorous in mind and body, the keen and ambitious man, the indicator of whose engine is always at full speed ahead.

Dr. William Osler, 1849–1919

Here are the facts. Coronary artery disease is the leading killer of men and women in Western civilization. In the course of a lifetime, one out of every two American men and one out of every three American women will have some form of the disease.

Dr. Caldwell B. Esselstyn Jr.

Chanukah commemorates the defeat of the Greeks by Judah Maccabee in the year 166 BCE. Schools in Israel are closed that week and my family always looked forward to spending a few days seeing the country. That year we stayed at a kibbutz guest house a few miles from Tiberius near Lake Kinneret, the Sea of Galilee.

The first morning I awoke with an atypical severe backache. I call it atypical because the pain was located in my upper back not the lower back. I attributed the pain to sleeping on a firmer mattress than I was accustomed to. Our plans for that day included hiking up to the archeological site of Gamla.

While the Roman conquest of Palestine tried to suppress the Jewish rebellion of 66 CE, Gamla was a strategic fortress located at the northern tip of Lake Kinneret. The rest of the Galilee had succumbed to the Roman legions; Gamla refused to surrender relying on its inaccessibility. As Josephus chronicled, "sloping down from a towering peak there is a spur like a shaggy neck behind which rises a symmetrical hump . . . cut off on the face and both sides by impassable ravines."[1]

How could I allow my back pain to spoil my family's holiday? My sons found a cast–off walking stick someone had left behind. So, like Moses, staff in hand, we set off to climb Gamla, but it went slow for me. Every so often I had to stop. Exertion bought on pain, not only to my back, but a pain that encapsulated my whole chest cavity.

Finally, we made it to the top, wandering among the ruins. Most everyone has heard of the valiant suicidal sacrifice made on Masada, but few know of the heroic defenders of Gamla. As Josephus records, "Despairing of escape and hemmed in every way, [the defenders] flung their wives, children and themselves too into the immensely deep ravine that yawned under the citadel . . . 4000 fell by Roman swords, but those who plunged to destruction proved to be over 5,000."[2]

My story actually starts not at Gamla, but twenty–one years earlier in the States. In November of 1978 I was a healthy 27 years old. The two previous years I had completed graduate school, married a college friend and was well on the first rung of what I hoped would be a successful career ladder. Then one morning I awoke with rectal bleeding. A barium enema later that day revealed ominous "shadows" lurking in my colon. A few days later a successful colonoscopy removed two hyperplasic non–malignant polyps from the sigmoid area of my colon.

I was just beginning life; the talk of colorectal cancer freaked me out. My doctor explained to me the good news, bad news. Yes, it was *highly* unusual to have colon polyps at my age, but he doubted I would ever die from it. Adding parenthetically that colorectal cancer was the number one killer of men over the age of forty.

He was more concerned, he said, over something he saw in my blood results. My cholesterol was 314 and my triglycerides were 346.[3] The doctor explained what he called the silent killer, heart disease. Coronary heart disease is called the silent killer because the first manifestation frequently is sudden death.

It seems funny to me now, but I left his office that day with the utmost faith in medicine. I believed in *Ben Casey, Dr. James Kildare* and *Marcus Welby, M.D.* To beat the shadow of cancer and the silent killer of heart disease all I had to do was have a colonoscopy every few years, use margarine, and remove the skin from chicken before I ate it. *The Bold Ones*, those men in white, were supposed to do the rest!

Ten years later, well into my second marriage, my family and I decided to immigrate to Israel. After a successful mid–level management career in the public, private and non–profit sectors, I was looking for a radical change. Burnout can come at any age.

We settled into a collective farming settlement, Moshav Mattiayhu. Similar in structure to a kibbutz, all work was assigned for the communal good. I grew grapes initially, but soon found myself managing hatchery egg laying and genetic experimentation poultry operations. Every day I walked at least two miles, up and back along the poultry runs, collecting eggs. I had not been that healthy since I played high school football.

Israel has a compulsory military draft. After settling in to farming life, in 1989 I reported to the induction center in Jerusalem. Luck, the Grace of God, and a high lottery number had kept me out of Vietnam. At the time Israel was battling the first *Intifada*. Our moshav was one of those infamous West Bank settlements you

17

always hear about in the news. Each night I slept with an army issue M–16 under my bed.

At thirty–eight years old I was far from Rambo; my army service would be doing guard duty on a settlement similar to the one in which I lived. To my shock, the army rejected me for medical reasons, 4–F. Of all things, my cholesterol was 330 and my triglycerides were over 600. The army doctor explained heart disease to me again for the second time in my life. She suggested I see my family doctor. My doctor sent me to a dietitian.

Nine years later we were at Gamla. The night after we returned home from vacation I walked to the synagogue for evening prayer services. On the way, I felt an excruciating pain in my chest. Immobilized, I stood in place a few minutes to catch my breath trying to decide if I should go to pray or return home. Praying is always a good idea, I thought. A couple of times I paused before finally getting to prayer services a few minutes late.

After services, I went to say hello to a friend's father who had just arrived from the states for a visit. He took one look at me and said, "You're having a heart attack . . . sit down!" My friends' father just happened to be a retired male nurse. I vaguely remember him saying something about pallor, but I rejected his suggestion to call an ambulance. I felt better, I assured him. Prayer does work.

The next morning I drove to the Hebrew University in Jerusalem. A neighbor of mine was working there as a researcher which gave him faculty privileges. The best perk for me was his library card. As faculty, books checked out of the university library had no return date. To me that was heaven. I always had a steady stream of books I borrowed on his card.

That morning the normal ten minute walk from the parking lot to the library took me nearly an hour. Every few steps I felt a stabbing pain in my chest. I can't recall now how many benches there were along the walk to the library, but I stopped to rest at every single one of them. In pain, I thought of the Simon and Garfunkel song, *Old Friends*. I sat on the end of the benches looking like a bookend.

Assuring myself it was nothing, I went straight to my doctor's office. He examined me, did an ECG, and just to rule things out, made me an appointment for a stress test later that afternoon. Likely it was a muscle sprain or some such thing, I told myself.

Well, it only took four minutes and thirteen seconds before the technician stopped the treadmill, telling me to wait outside. About ten minutes later he appeared handing me an envelope. He had called my doctor who wanted me to come early that evening to a clinic near his home with the results.

My doctor showed me two blips circled in red that worried him. I sat while he called a cardiologist he knew who recommended I come see him the next day at his hospital with the ECG. It wasn't a heart attack, but maybe I had a *slight* blockage.

I left with a prescription for nitro–glycerin spray and tablets to be used to abate the pain for what later I discover was called angina. For those of you who have never taken nitro–glycerin for angina pain allow me to describe what it feels like. Imagine someone holding a double barreled shot gun to your head and pulling both triggers at once. Got it?

The cardiologist explained to me "the results of the positive effort test show unstable angina." I always liked balloons since I was a kid. He described the procedure he recommended, a coronary angioplasty. He was going to insert something into my heart from my groin with a balloon attached. When the probe reached the blockage, he would blow up the balloon, then "poof" the artery would be cleared. *Sounded simple enough.*

In January of 1999, I had the angioplasty *without* the insertion of a stent. Above and in front of me were two large monitors which gave me a ring side seat for the main event. I mentioned to my doctor that my artery looked like the Amazon River pumping away. He pointed out to me a thin black line on the screen. "That," he

said, "was my right coronary artery which had a 100% stenosis."
Gulp!

Four days later, I was released. I had single vessel coronary artery
disease. That day I left the hospital with a refurbished heart. The
silent killer was no longer silent. Apprehensively, I started thinking
about those "shadows" lurking in my colon. I was only forty–eight
years old.

Twenty years had passed since my first colonoscopy. Heart
disease, colorectal cancer, it all sounded like a bad dream. But no
matter what I had done in the past to awake from that dream,
nothing worked. For the first time in my life, I was really scared of
dying!

2

Boomers

This was a decent godless people. Their only monument the asphalt road and a thousand lost golf balls.

T.S. Elliot

The more bombers the less room for doves of peace.

Nikita Khrushchev

Being president is like being a jackass in a hailstorm. There's nothing to do but to stand there and take it.

Lyndon B. Johnson

Yippies, Hippies, Yahoos, Black Panthers, lions and tigers alike–I would swap the whole damn zoo for the kind of young Americans I saw in Vietnam.

Spiro T. Agnew

I need to make a confession. This is not another of those books about someone who was diagnosed with stage four cancer, sent home for hospice care with only a few months to live, turned to alternative treatments, and miraculously is still alive twenty–years later or some such tale.

Until 120 is the story about an average person like you who received a medical wake–up call fifteen years earlier and did something most people do not do. I picked up the phone to answer the call so I would *not* get cancer, heart disease, diabetes, or any other disease of affluence as I aged.

My high school football coach used to say that the best offense is the best defense. I agree. Western medicine is offensive. (Pardon the pun) When you get sick, they rush in with a full arsenal of weapons to save the day; most of the time. Yet, Western medicine is like a SWAT team anxiously waiting for their call up with little skill at preventing a crime. And that aspect of Western medicine *is* truly a crime.

After my wake up call, I became proactive. Years earlier after my army physical exam, the dietitian I saw mapped out a nutrition plan for me which I mostly followed for nine years until my angioplasty. Unbelievably, in the hospital the new dietitian was giving me the same diet that put me in the hospital in the first place. Something intuitively seemed wrong to me.

One of my neighbors on my moshav was a Canadian doctor. A few days after the angioplasty, I asked him for advice on how I could prevent my heart clogging up again. I was told in the hospital, within four months after an angioplasty, 40% of the arteries will close up nullifying the procedure. Most people usually have to repeat the procedure every two to three years.

His advice: go on Amazon.com and buy a book called *Reversing Heart Disease* by Dr. Dean Ornish and treat it like a second Bible. Now when one Orthodox Jew tells another Orthodox Jew to treat a book as a second Bible, there enters a tone of heresy if you don't. Especially if the other person is a doctor giving you advise on coronary artery disease. So, with utmost piety and reverence, when the book arrived, I went through it as if it were a tome of Talmud, the fundamental work and the primary authority for all decisions of Jewish law redacted in the second century CE.

Since I brought up the Talmud, I guess it might be appropriate to discuss my further qualifications for writing *Until 120*. I am a practicing Orthodox Jew, faithfully following the Jewish traditions. In 2010–2011 the Gallup–Healthways Wellbeing Index was conducted by a 1,000 interviewers a day resulting in more than

676,000 people surveyed. Gallup measured the overall wellbeing of the American population using six indexes:

Life evaluation asking respondents if they felt they were thriving, suffering or struggling.
Emotional health based on levels of anger, stress, and depression, contrasted by happiness, enjoyment, and respect.
Physical health measured by illness, energy levels, and obesity.
Health behavior demonstrated in lifestyle habits like smoking, healthful eating, and exercise.
Work environment measured by job satisfaction, supervisors' treatment, and talent compatibility.
Basic access to health care, food, shelter and safety.

Very religious Jews, the survey results showed, had the highest wellbeing of *any* faith group in the United States. I am not advocating all that your problems will be solved if you convert to Judaism. But just maybe there are things inherent in our lifestyle, emphasis on character develpoment, Sabbath observance, or our steadfast belief in God, which have helped place very religious Jews at the top of wellbeing in America that you can benefit from.

The nation's first Baby Boomer is Kathleen Casey–Kirschling born in Baltimore, MD on January 1, 1946 at 12:00:01 a.m. Kathleen applied for Social Security benefits on October 15, 2007. *Until 120* is a book exclusively written for Baby Boomers irrespective of color, creed or religion. If you were born between 1946 and 1964, then the information contained is tailor made for you.

Most of the information in this book is applicable to people born after 1964. Boomers, though, are an aging population where we see our friends, loved ones and ourselves being afflicted by illness that can only be theoretical to a younger population. And almost all of us in the coming years will be faced with the decision of changing our lifestyles just to survive.

As Boomers, we knew no times of depression like our parents. Defining our own culture, we took advantage of the post World War Two technology explosion. It may seem funny now but the transistor radio was our Facebook connection to our world. Remember the Cuban missile crisis, the three K's: John, Bobby and Martin, Vietnam, Woodstock, the Beatles, Motown, and freedoms of all kinds? We don't need to remember Elvis because the King still lives! Those events in our lives in recent years are trading themselves for aging and end–of–life issues.

Collectively Baby Boomers were named *Time's* Man of the Year in 1966 as a generation under twenty–five. *Time Magazine* suggested that we would "infuse the future with a new sense of morality, a transcendent and contemporary ethic that could infinitely enrich the empty society," but our legacy will be an era of consumerism and self–indulgence.

In the early 1950's, Rollo May, an existential humanist author and psychotherapist, described the empty society which was the nest we were nurtured in:

> The clearest picture of empty life is the suburban man, who gets up at the same hour every weekday morning, takes the same train to work in the city, performs the same task in the office, lunches at the same place, leaves the same tip for the waitress each day, comes home on the same train each night, has 2.3 children, cultivates a little garden, spends a two–week vacation at the same shore every summer which he does not enjoy, goes to the same church every Christmas and Easter, and moves through a routine mechanical existence year after year until he finally retires at sixty–five and very soon thereafter dies of heart failure, possibly brought on by repressed hostility. I have always had a suspicion, however, that he dies of boredom.[1]

When I started my research, I believed in the traditional causes of illness: viruses, germs, genes, pesticides, toxins, etc. But early on, I kept discovering anomalies to that theory. Discovery commences with the awareness of anomaly, i.e., the recognition that nature somehow violated the paradigm–induced expectations that govern normal science.[2]

Allow me to share a few anomalies with you:

Case Western Reserve University discovered men who answered "yes" to the simple question "does your wife show you her love?" had substantially less angina even when they had high levels of other risk factors.[3]

Cold and distant mothers were found to be a recurring element in the background lives of many women with breast cancer.[4]

In a study of Israeli adult males, men who said they felt a lack of emotional support from their wives were far more likely to become heart attack victims.[5]

In the Harvard Grant Study, an astounding 91 percent of those who had reported that they did not have a close relationship with their mothers suffered serious medical crises by mid–life.[6]

100 percent of those in the Harvard Grant Study, who reported that both parents were cold and aloof, had serious medical problems by mid–life.[7]

The late psychologist Jeanne Achterberg could predict with 93% accuracy which cancer patients would completely recover, get worse or die, simply by examining their visualizations.[8]

The Johns Hopkins Medical School study found that the best predictor of who would get cancer decades later was the closeness of the father–son relationship earlier in life.[9]

In six studies of nearly 25,000 people the best predictor of cancer survival over the next decade was the answer people gave to the simple question: What do you think about your health?[10]

As many as half of the coronary disease cases cannot be linked to traditional risk factors of family history, smoking, high blood pressure, obesity, and inactivity.[11]

Of the 10 leading causes of death in the United States (heart disease, cancer, stroke, emphysema, accidents, pneumonia, diabetes, suicide, AIDS, and homicide), only three (emphysema, pneumonia, and AIDS) are not related to what we eat or drink, including alcohol.[12]

These findings and many others caused me to question exactly what do we mean by health. Most of us think of health as the absence of disease. But that definition just did not go along with the conclusions I was reaching. Health was becoming more of a verb than a noun to me. It has been estimated that it takes four to forty years for a cancer cell to grow into a dangerous tumor. And maybe a lifetime of eating saturated fats, the long–chain fatty acids that are found in meat and dairy products, until your arteries clog up as mine did. *Are we really healthy during those intervening years?*

Finally I found a definition of health more in accord with reality. But it was neither authored by a physician nor an august body like the World Health Organization. Rather a physicist, the late David Bohm, gave what I consider the best definition of health:

Good health is basically a manifestation of the overall creative intelligence working in concert with the body through various means that include exercise, diet, and relaxation, etc.[13]

What Bohm means by creative intelligence will be expanded at a later point in the book. For now let it suffice Bohm says: "in the free play of thought, creative intelligence responds to opposition and contradiction to new proposals . . . when something new is encountered which does not fit into what is already known; creative intelligence can put forth new sensory orders and structures that form into new perceptions."[14]

May 12, 2071 will mark my 120th birthday. I plan on being there to blow out the candles. Jews are always wishing each other to live until the age of 120. This golden goal was reached long go by our teacher, Moses. If fact, Jews are always talking about health. Our toast at get–togethers is, "*L'chaim*—To Life!" In Yiddish, we wish each other "*Zol zain tz u gizunt*—Let it just add to your health." "*Abi gizunt*—As long as you have your health." "*Zog a l'chaim*—Drink to Life."

My goal to live until the age of 120 is motivated by my desire to be included in the *Guinness Book of Records*. Scanning it, I couldn't think of any categories I could excel at. Life seemed to me to be a worthy pursuit. The longest documented human life span is that of Jeanne Calment of France who died in 1997 at the age of 122. Jiroemon Mimura of Japan was the longest documented male dying at the age of 116 years and 54 days. I want to beat Mimura's record. I already have a certified copy of my birth certificate in hand.

Life expectancy studies show that if you reach the age of 65 without a serious medical complication, the probability is that you will make it to age 84. The main lesson I learned from all of my research is that if you want achieve successful aging, living until the end in good health—*gizunt*—without the normal pains and illnesses, you have to heal the mind, the body and the soul.

The information contained in this book I believe can help you start to heal, as it has done for me, but the healing must be done by *you*. You can push your life passed 84 and maybe U*ntil* 120 as I am doing. *You are all invited to my birthday party!*

3

Survival and Change

Survival is a celebration of choosing life over death. We all know that we are going to die. We all die. But survival is saying: perhaps not today. In that sense, survivors don't defeat death; they come to terms with it.

Lawrence Gonzales[1]

Changes need to be based not of fear of dying but on joy of living.

Dr. Dean Ornish[2]

Survival is a privilege which entails obligations. I am forever asking myself what I can do for those who have not survived.

Simon Wiesenthal

If you do not change direction, you may end up where you are heading.

Lao Tzu

Early on I realized that in order to insure that cancer and heart disease would not be ever present in my life, I needed to change and become a survivor. Change and survival at first glance do not seem complimentary, but the more I learned about those concepts, the closer they came.

What better place to learn about survival than an army survival manual, I thought. One of the first books I bought was the *U.S. Army Field Manual FM21–76*. The manual was an eye opener. Of course it spelled out *flora* and *fauna* that a solider needed to be aware of; how to deal with an indigenous population; escaping capture and the all important shelter requirements.

Interspersed were jewels of sagely advice applicable to my particular situation. The manual stressed good health is essential to survival under any circumstances.[3] Your physical condition has much to do with your will to survive.[4] It is worth repeating: good health and physical condition are essential.

The manual also gave me direction. One of the first survival problems you must solve is determining where you are and in what direction you must go.[5] When I read that I thought of the Robert Frost poem, *Two Roads Diverged in a Yellow Wood.* At a crossroads in life we must choose direction. I knew I didn't want to travel the same path I had been on, but which way to go? The manual gave me sound advice. "The route that you select to travel depends upon the situation in which you find yourself. Experience has proved that *the most difficult route is frequently the safest.*"[6] [Emphasis added]

I am reminded of a story in the Talmud:

> Once Rabbi Joshua was walking along when he saw a little boy sitting at a fork in the road. He asked the boy, "Which is the road we take to town?" The boy answered him, "This is a short and long path, and this one is long and short." Rabbi Joshua went down short and long one. When he approached the town he discovered that it was surrounded with impassable gardens and orchards. Returning to the boy he said, "My son, did you not tell me this way was short?" He answered, "And did I not tell you it was also long?"[7]

The moral is that the seemingly longest route is often the shortest. As the army manual advised, the most difficult route is frequently the safest. *"I took the one less trodden on and that has made all the difference."*

What qualities help survivors to live against all odds while others unfortunately don't? It matters little whether you are lost at sea, stranded on a mountain, or trying to defeat cancer. There are common qualities to all survivors. Life's best survivors accept meaningful coincidences as part of the way life works[8] and react to disruptive change forced upon them as though it is a change they desired.[9]

Rambo is the first to die in a survival situation. People, who remain calm, devise a plan, get in touch with their body messages,[10] are flexible and adaptable,[11] take delight in small achievements,[12] possess the universal qualities of a survivor. And last but not least, survival psychologists have long observed that successful survivors pray, even when they don't believe in a god.[13]

"The more things change, the more they remain the same." I am sure you have heard this old saying. Those words of wisdom contain an explanation why most of us fail at attempts at changing our lifestyle, our eating habits, or a host of situations like marriages, careers, etc. In a book called *Change*[14] I gained an insight on how to make change successful.

The authors explain that what they called first order change is always doomed to failure because the system's structure itself has not under gone any fundamental change. First order change always appears to be based on common sense, but cannot generate from within itself the conditions for its own change.[15] *Monty Python* was famous for this when they would announce, "And now for something totally different" and repeat the same scene.

An example would be changing to a healthier diet like my dietitian advocated for me. Low fat cheese is no better than high fat cheese if in reality it is the cheese itself that is unhealthy. Was it prudent for me to leanly trim my steaks when it was the red meat that was causing all the problems? Nor are statements like "reducing the amount of sugar, refined foods, etc." Less of a bad thing is *still* bad.

31

Second order change usually appears weird, unexpected and uncommonsensical, like a quantum jump with a puzzling, paradoxical element in the process of change, but is successful because it changes the system itself while first order changes occur in systems which remain unchanged. Second order techniques deal with effects not with presumed causes: the crucial question is what? Not why?[16]

Most of us of no doubt believe that we are hard wired in our basic behaviors and it is impossible to change. The life we live does shape the brain we develop.[17] The more we act in unhealthy ways, the more we teach our brains that these bad habits and learned behaviors are essential to our survival,[18] the more entrenched they become.

As David Bohm says the mind has a strong tendency to cling to what it finds familiar and to defend itself against what threatens seriously to disturb its overall balance and equilibrium. Unless the perceived rewards are very great, the mind will not willingly explore its unconscious infrastructure of ideas but will prefer to continue in more familiar ways.[19]

What we don't know is that the brain is not static. Despite the fact that the majority of the neurons in our body are as old as we are, it has an incredible ability to change itself. Neuroplasticity is the ability of the brain to forge new neuronal connections, blaze new paths through the cortex, even new roles; in short the rewiring of the brain.[20]

The process involves three components: creating and strengthen connections, *synaptogenesis*; stimulating new neurons to grow, *neurogenesis*; and increasing the sheathing along the axonal lengths to enhance conduction speed of neuronal electrical impulses, *myelinogenesis*.[21] When properly understood, neuroplasticity teaches us that the brain can never be the whole story about our mental development.[22]

Changing our brains requires us to reframe the deceptive messages we have been sending it and engage in new, healthy behaviors. I am living proof that it is possible as you will see later on in the book when we discuss reframing your past. Now you are getting a glimpse of the mind–body connection. And as there is a mind–body connection, there is also a mind–body–soul connection.

When you put it all together, change sounds remarkably like repentance. What must the sinner do in order to be found worthy of repentance and redemption rather than merely attaining repentance of expiation? The repentant must undergo a complete transformation, a fundamental change in the quality of his life.[23] Repentance is about changing oneself; about knowing you have the ability to change no matter how deeply you are entrenched by a sin.

The crowning quality of repentance is turning away from any temptation to walk in the path of sin.[24] One of the cornerstone beliefs in Judaism is our ability to repent. An essential part is the confession. We declare to God the nature of our sin, our regret and embarrassment for our deeds and most important, our solemn promise never to repeat the sin again.[25] To me, that is also the essence of change.

How does one know if his repentance has been accepted, achieved a complete transformation of himself or he has changed an unwanted behavior? When a person confronts the same situation in which he previously sinned with the potential to sin again, but because of his desire to repent and not because of fear or lack of strength, he chooses to abstain from sinning,[26] then he has repented; he has changed.

I can't tell you how many times I was placed in that situation. Under stress, wandering in a convenience store, checking ingredients, looking for something to sooth me; rationalizing well it is only 10% fat, there is not that much sugar, or tomorrow will be a better day. But then came the repeated times when I would abruptly end my search, leaving the store as a penitent.

33

Until finally reflecting on success, a renewed health, that thin black line I once had, I didn't enter the convenience store. Oh, there are still stressful times in my life, but bananas, apples, a can of chick peas, and rice cakes have become my St. Bernard.

4

Childhood

Life would be infinitely happier if we could only be born at the age of eighty and gradually approach eighteen.

Mark Twain

The child explains the man as well as and often better than the man explains the child.

Jean Piaget[1]

The less of parents' work that has to be corrected, the quicker man moves ahead.

Harry Stack Sullivan[2]

All happy families resemble one another; each unhappy family is unhappy in its own way.

Leo Tolstoy

Growing up I remember my father being very critical of Dr. Benjamin Spock and Sigmund Freud for their blaming everything on parents. I have heard that criticism repeatedly in every walk of life. But around the same time as my angioplasty, I was being exposed to theories of childhood development in an effort to understand what was happening in the lives of my children. In our first few years, the ingredients of intellectual, emotional, and moral growth are laid down.[3] From that perspective I readily understood why most of the anomalies about health I was uncovering centered on the family crucible.

Please don't think I am against motherhood and apple pie. Well, maybe the apple pie if it is made with bleached white flour, refined sugar, margarine and canned apples, but definitely not motherhood.

In the post war period, American mothers found themselves standardizing and over adjusting children who later were expected to personify that very virile individuality which in the past has been one of the outstanding characteristics of the American. The resulting danger was that of creating, instead of individualism, a mass produced mask of individuality.[4]

By the time Boomers were being born, *Mom* had become a stereo typed caricature of existing contradictions which emerged from intense, rapid, and as yet unintegrated changes in American history. In truth, Mother became *Mom* only when Father became *Pop* under the impact of identical historical discontinuities.[5] *Mom* is a victim, not a victor.[6]

I have to admit that I was well into college before I understood the *Riddle of the Sphinx*. Not because I couldn't get the punch line like the joke what is black and white and red all over? No matter which newspaper I saw, none were red. Oh, READ, not red! Now I get it. With the sphinx I never actually heard the riddle. I was left thinking the riddle was why the sphinx had a smirky smile like that of the Mona Lisa. Then I finally saw the riddle in print: what goes on four legs in the morning, two legs at noon and three legs in the evening?

Naturally there seems to be a tendency to categorize the years of mankind. The *Mishnah*, the classical compendium of Jewish oral law which forms the basis of the Talmud,[7] is one such attempt:

At five–years–old a boy begins learning scripture; thirteen he is obligated in the commandments, by fifteen he commences the study of the Talmud; at eighteen he is ready for marriage, a thirty–year–old attains his full strength; at forty he gains understanding, at fifty he can give advice; at sixty he becomes a senior citizen; ripe old age happens at seventy; by eighty he gets a second wind; at ninety his frame becomes stooped and bent; and by one–hundred–years old with one foot in the grave, he is ready to pass over to the next world.

Contemporary times tend to focus more on a person before the age of six unlike the *Mishnah* which was only written down for the first time 1800 years ago. One categorization I discovered, that was original and vastly influential, was Eric H. Erickson's the Eight Ages of Man found in his classic work *Childhood and Society*.[8] Published in 1950, I feel this study represents Boomers probably more than it does later generations.

The Harvard Grant Study is part of the Study of Adult Development at Harvard Medical School, a 75–year longitudinal study of 268 physically and mentally healthy Harvard college sophomores from the classes of 1939–1944. The Grant study supported Erickson's hypothesis that the stages of life cycles must be passed through in sequence.[9]

Some modern scholars take the position that the way parents rear their children has no important effects on the way the children turn out[10] and are shaped and changed by experiences they have while they are growing up.[11]

I think that it is important to our healing all aspects, mind, body and soul, to understand how we have developed in stages over the years. I briefly summarize Erickson's *Eight Ages of Man*:

Stage 1—Basic Trust vs. Basic Mistrust (Infancy age 0–1): A child's basic identify forms at this stage as mothers create a sense of trust in their children. Trust implies a child's environment is predictable, a sameness and continuity of her life, where she not only learns to trust others, but herself as well. Thus, she is willing to let her mother out of her sight.

Stage 2—Autonomy vs. Shame and Doubt (Toddler age 1–2): The child's environment allows him to literally stand on his own two feet and must protect him against arbitrary experiences of shame and doubt. He is completely exposed at this stage whether he is ready or not to be visible. If encouraged by a world that looks at him, all goes well. If not, then shame and self–consciousness set in. And if he is shamed beyond endurance, he starts to express defiance.

Stage 3—Initiative vs. Guilt (Early Childhood age 2–6): As implied, the child begins to take the initiative in her life. She begins to manipulate her world to suit her; at no time is she more ready to explore and learn. She gains self–esteem by her success and learns guilt from her failures. Maybe this is the origin of a simmering rage that follows her throughout life and a precursor of psychosomatic disease.

Stage 4—Industry vs. Inferiority (Primary School age 6–12): Tools and tool–partners populate this stage. His exuberant imagination is tamed and harnessed to the laws of impersonal things—even the three R's. Recognition is achieved by production; a sense of industry is the tool–world. If family life has failed him in preparation, he develops a sense of inadequacy and inferiority.

Stage 5 Identity vs. Role Confusion (Adolescence age 12–18): Having hopefully gained a good relationship with the tool–world, childhood comes to an end. She is more concerned with other's opinions than her own self feelings. Here she connects the dots of the previous stages, which reveal her fated course of life. Peer environment helps color her prototype personality. Classically, she is a teenager.

Stage 6 Intimacy vs. Isolation (Young Adulthood age 19–40): The emerging adult is ready for intimacy, committing himself to affiliations and partnerships ripe with sacrifices and compromises. He is ever–tested; applying his skills to the betterment of the tool–world. But the territory is wrought with danger. Unsuccessful, he will seek distance, isolation, and avoidance of intimacy.

Stage 7 Generativity vs. Stagnation (Middle Adulthood age 40–65): The adult is concerned with turning over the fruits of her tool–work, guiding the next generation. No longer a benefit to society by procreation, she utilizes other avenues. If life's misfortunes were not kind to her, she stagnates. A search for meaning is especially important to the mature person at this stage in life.

Stage 8 Ego Integrity vs. Despair (Late Adulthood age 65 till death): Only one who has taken care of things and people; adapted himself to triumphs and disappointments; the originator of others or the generator of products and ideas—only in him may gradually ripen the fruit of the previous seven stages.[12] The lack of integrity is signified by fear of death. Despair comes with the feeling that the time is now short, too short for the attempt to start another life and to try out alternative roads to integrity.[13]

A child's development can best be described as a scavenger hunt, the purpose of which is to build a widget at the end. There are eight points along a designated route where you must stop to collect and assemble parts necessary to build the next level. You find that there are more than enough parts at each level to be gathered, but there is an uncompromising time limit that must be adhered to.

Each development line itself tends to unfold in a sequential, holarchical fashion: higher stages in each line tend to build upon or incorporate the earlier stages, no stage can be skipped, and stages emerge in an order that cannot be altered by environmental conditioning or social reinforcement.[14]

You soon discover that at each level are impediments, distractions, and unpredictable forces that influence your assembly. Suddenly, time is up. You needed twelve and a half percent of assembled parts to adequately succeed at the next level. A higher number makes success easier; with less it will be more difficult. Nevertheless, you must move on. *For better or worse, we are our hastily assembled widgets.*

Childhood is where we become who we will be for the rest of our lives. The family crucible is where we first learn about ourselves. And our destiny depends to a large extent on the health of our caretakers.[15] Parental efforts that create a good child unfortunately frequently produce an adult who is not able to cope well with life.[16]

A young child's environment directly and permanently influences the structure and eventual function of his brain.[17] In fact, almost every decision parents make boils down to a matter of our children's brain development.[18]

J.M. Barrie in his classic work *Peter Pan* illustrates a mother's influence on a child's brain development:

> Mrs. Darling first heard of Peter when she was tidying up her children's minds. It is the nightly custom of every good mother after her children are asleep to rummage in their minds and put things straight for the next morning, repacking into their proper places the many articles that have wandered during the day. . . . When you wake in the morning, the naughtiness and evil passions with which you went to bed have been folded up small and placed at the bottom of your mind; and on the top, beautifully aired, are spread out your prettier thoughts, ready for you to put on.

Unlike other creations, humans are thrust into their world without any inherent survival skills. We learn as we grow. Unskilled, we erect defensive structures to the best of our ability to tame our environment. Each stage of development sees a different world— with different needs, different tasks, different dilemmas, different problems and pathologies.[19]

The more we can trust our environment, the less need for protection. But stress at each development stage is ever present and may produce the building blocks for an assortment of diseases. Childhood traumas influence adult's health to a greater degree than traumatic experiences that have occurred in the last three years of a person's life.[20]

While it is clear that babies can have no conscious memory of pain, repeated painful experiences may have a lasting effect at a more subconscious level. Painful events may invoke a certain pattern of unconscious emotional responding that might influence mental development in some long term way.[21]

The key to healing the mind, body and soul I learned is the recognition and awareness of the defenses that one has developed as a protection against the pain of childhood deprivation, rejection, fear of death, and in identifying how they limit one's present day life.[22] Each level of self development has different types of defenses. The self, at every level, will attempt to defend itself against pain, disruption, and ultimate death, and will do so using whatever tools are present at each level.[23]

As a starting point, I must make an adjustment to Erickson's *Eight Ages of Man.* His developmental timeframe begins with birth and ends with death. In my opinion, there are at two other stages, one I will discuss now; the other, after death, in my next book.

Stage 0—*Prenatal* (conception till birth): Only in recent times has it become apparent that the womb's environment plays an important developmental role. Now we know that a child from six months *in utero* onward already remembers, hears, and even learns.[24] Our parents never knew other than the fetus was is the most protective environment possible.

An adult and to a lesser degree a child has had time to develop defenses. She can soften or deflect the impact of experience. An unborn child cannot. What affects her does so directly. That's why maternal emotions etch themselves so deeply on her psyche and why their tug remains so powerful later.[25] And definitely, what the father does profoundly effects the mother, which intern affects the developing child.[26]

Environment does not begin with birth, but begins much earlier with the circulatory system shared in utero with one's biological mother.[27] Evidence is accumulating that most stress responses are programmed in large measure by prenatal events.[28]

First taste buds emerge just eight weeks after conception. By thirteen weeks taste buds form throughout the mouth and are already communicating with their invading nerves.[29] Amniotic fluid is constantly changing over the course of pregnancy with the strong flavors in the mother's diet. The siring and wiring of neurons is critically dependent on maternal diet.[30]

A fetus's taste experience in the womb may bias his later behavior by influencing food preferences.[31] It has often been said that we are what we eat. Maybe it is more accurate to say we are what our mothers and fathers ate. Yes, fathers too. A father's diet can directly influence the epigenetic modifications, gene expression and health of his offspring.[32]

Dr. David Baker and his Medical Research Council Epidemiology Unit at Southampton University in England produced a very sound basis for the overall thesis that our health and our susceptibility to disease in later life are in large measure programmed before birth. Called the Baker Hypothesis, fetal origins research into the lifetime records of babies born in the early part of the 20th century show that the health enjoyed throughout our life is markedly affected by the conditions we experienced in the womb before we even enter this world.[33]

Intrauterine conditions program the development of cardio–vascular disease,[34] the risk of developing high blood pressure, or having a stroke later in life.[35] There is good evidence that adverse programming of the ovary, breast and prostate glands at some stage in fetal development can increase the risk of cancer of these tissues later in life.[36]

Hopefully, you are beginning to understand, as I did, that our problems and illness of today had origins much earlier in our lives. And that the contributing causes of disease are psychological and spiritual, not just physical.[37] Shame, anxiety, attitude, self–esteem, emotions, loneliness, loss, and abandonment are the causes of illness no less than viruses, germs, genes, pesticides, and toxins are.

This is the major difference in approach between Western medicine and Oriental medicine. Western medicine still looks at Robert Koch's germ theory as a paradigm of disease. Oriental diagnostic technique does not turn up a specific disease entity or precise cause, but renders an almost poetic, yet workable, description of the whole person. The question of cause and effect is always secondary to the overall pattern.[38]

I am not implying that we are the causes of our illnesses. There is no benefit in blaming ourselves for our illnesses, although the other side of the coin is that we often hesitate to take responsibility for our health.[39] To take responsibility for your health requires you to believe that you can.

As Dr. Herbert Benson, Professor of Medicine at Harvard Medical School and founder of the Mind/Body Medical Institute at Massachusetts General Hospital in Boston, says, "In my thirty years of practicing medicine, I've found no healing force more impressive or more universally accessible than the power of the individual to care for and cure him or herself."[40]

There is a discussion in the Talmud[41] whether on the advice of experts you can feed a sick person on Yom Kippur, the holiest day of the year when Jews are instructed to fast an entire night and day. But what if the sick person wants to eat while the doctors say that he does not need to? We listen to the sick person over the doctors' opinion. What is the reason? The Talmud says, *'The heart knows the bitterness of its soul.'*[42] Trust your inner physician and you can take responsibility for your health.

Rollo May recommended looking at illness as an opportunity:

> Illnesses, whether physical or psychological, [should] be taken not as periodic accidents which occur to our body, personality, or mind, but as nature's means of reeducating the whole person. The disease comes as a demand and an opportunity to rediscover the lost functions of myself. We may add that it is an actual clinical fact that some persons, viewing their illness as an opportunity for reeducation, become more healthy both psychologically and physically, more healthy as persons after a serious illness than before.[43]

5

Shame and Self–Esteem

Shame is a soul eating emotions.

Carl G. Jung

Shame is like everything else; live with it for long enough and it becomes part of the furniture.

Salman Rushdie

If we have good self–esteem, we will be careful not to damage ourselves, neither spiritually nor physically.

Rabbi Dr. Abraham Twerski[1]

Virtually all of us, deep inside, have a shamed based belief in the core that I am bad, unimportant, insignificant, unlovable, defective, incompetent, imperfect, inadequate of this sort that is controlling our life in a very negative way.

Margaret Paul[2]

Remember the 1955 hit song, *Ain't That a Shame* by Fats Domino? Shame is the philosopher's stone for understanding ourselves, our parents, our spouses, our children, our bosses, our co–workers, and everyone else we meet in daily life. As Erickson points out while discussing Stage 2—*Autonomy vs. Shame and Doubt*, shame is an emotion insufficiently studied because in our civilization it is so early and easily absorbed by guilt.[3]

Rabbi Joseph B. Soloveitchik was one of the twentieth century's outstanding Talmudists and seminal Jewish thinkers. Soloveitchik enlightens the existential link between shame and guilt. "Shame is due to a feeling of guilt, to an awareness of culpability, to the knowledge that I am not the one I should have been, that I failed to realize what was expected of me, that I lead a disappointing existence.[4] The feeling of guilt and the collapse of the usual mechanisms of self–defense result in shame."[5]

Rabbi Dr. Abraham Twerski, an eminent psychiatrist and descendant of the founders of the Chassidic movement, explains guilt should be defined as an unpleasant feeling for something one has done or failed to do; an unpleasant feeling that one is constitutionally bad.[6]

To Brené Brown, bestselling author and research professor at the University of Houston, "shame is the painful feeling or experience of believing that we are flawed and therefore unworthy of love and belonging.[7] Guilt = I did something bad. Shame = I am bad."[8]

Robert Firestone, author and clinical psychologist, clarifies shame as the emotion we feel when we see ourselves as inherently inferior or deficient in some way. Guilt is related to our behavior i.e. when we think we have done something wrong or when we fail to live up to our own ideals and values.[9]

Dr. Gabor Maté, a Canadian physician who specializes in addiction, says drugs do not make anyone into an addict any more than food makes a person into an overeater. "There has to be a preexisting [susceptibility].[10] I glimpsed shame in the eyes of my addicted patients in the Downtown Eastside [of Vancouver]."[11] Shame is the fitting name of that preexisting susceptibility.

In my opinion, shame is more than just a feeling that you are in some way inherently defective. Rather, it is the self–belief that there *is* truly something wrong with you. A belief you have nurtured and reinforced at every turn of your life by replaying the old recordings that were programmed when you were a child to the point that you hide from even yourself.

"Lonely man," Rabbi Soloveitchik says, "is protected against intrusion from the outside feelings of shame which prompt him to withdraw into seclusion whenever the arrogant *thou* tries to dispel the charm of being for oneself; shame expresses a state of insecurity."[12]

Erickson says doubt is the brother of shame.[13] Shame's sister, I believe, is low self–esteem. Our shame seems to come from what we do with the negative messages, negative affirmations, beliefs and rules we hear as we grow up. We hear these from our parents, parent figures, people in authority such as teachers and clergy.[14] What the shame–based mother was unable to find in her own mother she finds in her children. Since the child is there for the parent, there is no one to mirror the child's feelings and drives and to nurture the child's needs.[15]

Rabbi Dr. Twerski is also the best–selling author of more than sixty books. Over the years I have been privileged to hear him speak on many occasions both in the states and here in Israel. I remember once during a question and answer session someone asked him how he thought of so many different topics. Rabbi Dr. Twerski explained he only wrote one book, numerous times. In all his works he deals with the same idea—negative self–image.

"Whether patient or acquaintance," Rabbi Dr. Twerski says, "I have found low self–esteem to be universal, in every person I encounter; all seem to have feelings of inferiority.[16] People with low self–esteem are often fearful of entering relationships with other people, perhaps they anticipate rejection."[17]

The child has no materials out of which to build his self–image except those provided by his relationships with other people—primarily his parents. He estimates himself by the way these others treat him. He has no grounds for feeling important if they treat him as unimportant.[18]

J.M. Barrie again in *Peter Pan* makes a very cogent observation when he describes Peter Pan's reaction to Captain Hook's biting him:

> Not the pain of this but its unfairness was what dazed Peter. It made him helpless. He could only stare, horrified. Every child is

affected thus the first time he is mistreated unfairly. All he thinks he has the right to when he comes to you to be yours is fairness. After you have been unfair to him he will love you again, but he will never afterwards be quite the same boy. No one ever gets over the first unfairness; no one except Peter.

People with high self–esteem in effect carry with them a loving parent who is proud of their successes and tolerant of their failures. In contrast, people with low self–esteem carry the psychological burden of a harsh, disproving parent.[19]

I am a victim of shame. At certain points of my life, I would review my resume and letters of reference and wonder who they were referring to. When you are shamed, your world is built, no surrounded, by shaming jobs, shaming relationships, shaming people, and shaming events. *No one ever sees the real me.* King Arthur never dressed in so fine an armor. And eventually, we even lose sight of who we are to ourselves.

When you enjoy healthy self–esteem, you know yourself and you accept yourself with your limitations; you are not ashamed of your limitations but simply see them as a part of the reality of who you are, perhaps a boundary you're challenged to expand.[20]

Self–esteem has two components: a sense of competence and a feeling of self–worth;[21] the ability to see yourself as capable and competent, lovable and loving, unique and valuable.[22] Shame and self–esteem are diametrically opposite.

Ernest Becker, the Pulitzer Prize winning social anthropologist, said unlike the baboon that gluts himself only on food, man nourishes himself mostly on self–esteem.[23] Unfortunately, most of us are gluttonous baboons and severely under nourished humans. Self–esteem requires that a person be spiritual[24] and self–esteem is a basic spiritual food group.[25]

Up close and personal. I want to share with you an example from my life which clearly illustrates shame and its origins. I mentioned that a high lottery number was one of the things that kept me out of the Vietnam War. I entered college well before the lottery was created. A confession: I only became a ritually practicing observant Jew after I finished graduate school. Before then you might say that I was the late John Belushi's character from the movie *Animal House*.

After a couple of semesters of party, party and party, I came home for winter break with two Western Union telegrams patiently waiting for me. One was from the Dean of Students informing me that I was being placed on academic probation the returning semester. The other, my local draft board revoking my 2–S deferment and reclassifying me 1–A!

I did the math. To stay in school and not sing a chorus of "and it's one . . . two . . . three . . . what are we fighting for?" I had to make three A's the next semester. Our high school graduating song was *To Dream the Impossible Dream*, but I had never made three A's in my life. In fact, I was rejected by every college I applied to. I ~~failed~~ repeated the ninth grade; ADHD had not been invented yet. The only reason I was admitted to my university was because of an impassioned plea from my high school guidance counselor, begging to give me a provisional trial.

The first night back knowing in ten weeks I would be heading for rice–patty–land, I really tied one. Very late the next afternoon when I awoke, I staggered to registration. To my shock, all of the freshmen and sophomore IBM class cards had already been given out. In a panic, I grasped the fact I had to enroll in classes, any classes. Catalogue in hand, I stammered over to the Political Science station and asked what classes they had left.

The professor did not know me since although I was registered as a PoliSci major, I had never yet been to the department. The only classes left were junior–senior split level courses. In order to get one of those class cards I had to convince him I was a transfer student that semester. I walked away with three upper level classes in international relations.

Two days later I got a note from the head of the PoliSci department telling me to come ASAP to her office. My bluff was called. She checked my record; not only was I not a transfer student and on probation, she said, based on my high school record I would not succeed. Besides she added the bureaucratic regulation that I had to have taken the Intro PoliSci course as a prerequisite.

I felt like Arlo Guthrie at *Alice's Restaurant* explaining the two telegrams, my sincere desire not to come home from Vietnam in a body–bag, and I even threw in a brief soliloquy about the Gulf of Tonkin Resolutions. Ice cubes to Eskimos, she said it was my money and my time, and agreed with my level of patriotism. Her son was a conscientious objector.

Upper level classes were a breath of fresh air to me. Gone were the multiple choice tests; it was a world of classroom discussion based on the syllabus and the all important research paper. For all three classes, I had a total of sixteen books to read. Until then, I had never read a book cover to cover in my entire life. Five days a week I sequestered myself in the library. Surrounded by its quiet, I read my first, second, third . . . and sixteenth book and spun the *New York Times* microfilm to the tune of the *Iron Butterfly*.

I said I had never made three A's in my life. That was true. My only A was in Government my last year of high school. That is where I learned to do research. My paper was on the 1964 presidential election. Dozens of magazines and newspapers made their way onto a neat stack of index cards. Like a Las Vegas dealer, I shuffled the deck until I knew I could beat the house. I made an A$^+$ on my high school paper. And Vegas dealing was also my winning strategy that semester. Triple aces, I raked in the chips.

Usually after the semester I went home to work in my father's shirt factory. Most days I accompanied him mid–morning to the Coffee Shoppe in the Jefferson Hotel across from the courthouse. There gathered the daily ritual of store owners, politicians, lawyers, etc. I sat to the right of my father. One of the men at our table turned to my father and said that he saw in the local paper where I had made the Dean's List at college. *I beamed!*

My father not missing a beat said, "That's nothing, his brother made the Dean's List at Emory University Law School." "That," he added "was something to brag about." THAT'S NOTHING! Blood, sweat and tears reeled from my very being for ten weeks to get those A's. *That's shame with a capital "S".*

Couple this with the time I heard my mother explaining to my aunts when I was about nine or ten–years–old, that I was just not as smart as my brother and two sisters, etc, etc, etc. Perpetually on the Dean's List until I finished graduate school, self–esteem has always been ephemeral in my life. BTW, the Intro PoliSci course was the last class I took as an undergraduate.

Shame is ubiquitous. By now you're probably wondering if shame is the ghost stalking your life. No, it's not only me, I assure you. Below is a list of statements I have culled[26] from my readings that can help you decide. Read each question. After consideration, give each question a yes or no answer. If you feel that a question sometimes, occasionally or frequently applies to you, then answer yes. If more than a few apply, then you are a victim of shame.

> I experience anxiety whenever I anticipate doing anything new.
> I am a people pleaser (nice guy/sweetheart).
> I feel there is something wrong with me in my inner self,.
> I am a hoarder and I have trouble discarding anything.
> I feel inadequate as a man or woman.
> I feel guilty when I stand up for myself.
> I would rather give in to others than defend myself.
> I have trouble starting or finishing things.
> I continually criticize myself for being inadequate.
> I consider myself a terrible sinner and I'm going to hell.
> I am rigid and a perfectionist.

I feel I never measure up; never get anything right.

I feel like I really don't know what I want or how I feel.

I am driven to be a super achiever.

I really don't know who I am or what my values are.

I don't like being touched.

I am often engage in sex when I really don't want to.

I find myself compulsively eating, working, drinking, etc.

I feel ashamed when I get mad.

I rarely get mad, but when I do, I rage.

I fear other people's anger and will do anything to prevent it.

I am ashamed when I cry.

I almost never express my unpleasant emotions.

I have trouble sleeping most nights.

I believe that food and/or having sex are my greatest needs.

I basically distrust everyone, including myself.

I have been or am now married to an addict.

I am obsessive and controlling in my relationships.

I hate being alone and will do almost anything to avoid it.

I avoid conflict at all cost.

I rarely say no to suggestions; feeling it an order to be obeyed.

I have an over developed sense of responsibility.

I find it easier to be concerned with others than with myself.

I don't know how to resolve conflict.

I am either over powering or I withdraw.

I rarely ask for clarification of statements I don't understand.

I never felt close to one or both of my parents.

I ridicule others if they make a mistake.

I am fiercely competitive and a poor loser.

I attract and/or seek people who tend to be compulsive.

I feel alive when I am in the midst of a crisis.

I find it difficult to visit my parents.

I feel a lack of personal fulfillment in my life

I feel my life is empty.

I feel everyone takes advantage of me.

I feel it impossible to relax and just let go.

I know when things are going too good, the axe will fall.

I feel nothing matters anymore; what's the use.

I haven't accomplished anything I have set out to do.

I feel no one wants to hear what I have to say.

I really could use a hug!

Eleanor Roosevelt said no one can make you feel inferior without your consent. After much hard work, which I will discuss in an ensuing chapter, I gave myself permission to be who I was. I accepted my assets and my limitations. When my wife started a sentence with, "You're so stupid," I answered, "What I did may not have been what you expected but, no, I am not stupid." *I stopped giving people authorization to shame me.*

The defining moment came after I had published my second novel, *The Scribe*. I saw a review on a website called *Goodreads*. Someone wrote that the book wasn't quality fiction, but even so was an enjoyable read. My intention was not to win the National Book Award. All I had hoped for was that people would be affected in a positive way by reading my book. A few years earlier I would probably have given up writing after I read that review.

Soon I realized I was able to admit my mistakes to myself and others. At the time I was working in a laser factory on my moshav cutting steel. One morning I noticed the purple glow indicating the plasma reaction in the laser was very pale. Suddenly, the machine stopped cutting. The technician we called in Switzerland diagnosed the problem. The blower had blown itself. He had seen these effects in other machines. My company immediately ordered a replacement from Switzerland. The cost was $100,000 plus more than a week's lost production. There were no happy faces in the crowd.

I remembered that earlier in the day I had preformed the scheduled maintenance on the laser. I phoned Switzerland and asked what would occur if by mistake I used lighter weight oil in the blower? The answer came back that oil would seep into the laser tubes effecting the reaction.

That afternoon we disassembled the blower and the tubing and painstakingly cleaned the oil residue. Two days later we were back in production. I admitted to the owner of the company I had put in the wrong oil. The blower was fine, we cancelled the order. I thought I was going to get fired, but no one ever said anything to me about the mistake.

A few months later the Swiss technician was in Israel. He told me at the time, my boss was livid by my mistake. But when the Swiss technician told him that he was lucky I worked for him because no other person in the world would have ever confessed a mistake like that, he quickly calmed down. Shame is world–wide.

I make mistakes. We all do. But I know that if I try my best and despite precautions, mistakes happen, it does not mean there is something wrong with me. To put a stop to shame you have to start liking yourself. That may sound simple, but I think it is the hardest thing for a person to do. There is nothing wrong with a healthy dose of narcissism. As the poster says, "I am not junk because God doesn't make junk!"

Authenticity is the daily practice of letting go of who we think we're supposed to be and embracing who we are.[27] Get up in the morning and leave your armor at home. If you do then the scariest thing will happen. You are naked to the world; you broadcast your vulnerability. Bené Brown says, "To believe vulnerability is weakness is to believe that feeling is weakness.[28] Vulnerability is the core, the heart, the center, of meaningful human experiences."[29]

According to Bené Brown, vulnerability is the birthplace of love, belonging, joy, courage, empathy, and creativity; the source of hope, empathy, accountability, and authenticity. If we want greater clarity in our purpose or deeper and more meaningful spiritual lives, vulnerability is the path.[30]

Dr. Gabor Maté says when we flee our vulnerability; we lose our full capacity for feeling emotion.[31] Vulnerability is the core of all emotions and feelings. To feel is to be vulnerable.[32] Vulnerably only begins when we decide no longer to be shamed.

As a starting point to healing your shame, I strongly urge you to watch Dr. Bené Brown's two talks featured on TED.COM: *Listening to Shame*[33] and *The Power of Vulnerability*.[34] In fact, put the book down and go do it now. Consider it a homework assignment.

6

Addictions and Emotions

The heart lusts after delicious foods.

Rabbi Moshe Chain Luzzatto[1]

We become addicted to what makes us unconscious, so we don't feel the pain we create.

Dr. Dean Ornish[2]

We cannot heal what we don't feel.

Dr. Bernie Siegel[3]

Most of us have left home physically but very few of us have left home emotionally.

Susan Forward[4]

When I first read Dr. Gabor Maté's comment that drugs do not make anyone into an addict any more than food makes a person into an overeater in his book *In the Realm of Hungry Ghosts: Close Encounters with Addiction* I knew I was headed for a paradigm shift. Until then, everything I had learned about food and addictions was diametrically opposed to that idea.

Endorphins are chemicals produced in the brain that have rewarding effects similar to drugs such as morphine and heroin.[5] Elevation of endorphins appears to be an innate psychological mechanism to protect mammals and perhaps other animals against the emotional and physical dangers of terror and pain.[6] These are commonly referred to as the feeling good hormones. We feel good while endorphins are circulating through our system. Self–generated opiates, endogenous morphine, do in fact exist.[7]

The foods we eat stimulate these chemicals in our brains through a host of ways with one purpose: to make us feel good. Foods particularly hyper–palatable ones demonstrate similarities with addictive drugs.[8] Naloxone is an opiate blocker which stops heroin, morphine and other narcotics from affecting the brain. Check into a drug treatment center and Naloxone is probably what will be used to curb your addiction.

A funny thing happened on the way to the local supermarket. Naloxone was found to curb a desire for foods as well. On average, we consume 71 pounds of calorie sweeteners each year, which is 22 teaspoons of sugar, per person, per day.[9] Naloxone curbs the appeal of sugary snacks.[10] Meat has drug like qualities. As soon as meat touches your tongue opiates are released in the brain. Researchers in Scotland found that Naloxone cut the appetite for ham by 10 percent, salami by 25 percent and tuna by almost half.[11]

In the Talmud[12] there is a discussion of the laws pertaining to a mourner who has lost either one of his parents or another close relative. Certain restrictions apply during the mourning period. One example is bathing which is prohibited. Yet, surprisingly, eating meat is permitted. The Talmud asks why one is permitted and the other not. Washing does not relieve the anxiety of the mourner, while eating meat certainly does.

Chocolate is a drug! It stimulates the same part of the brain that morphine acts on. Chocolate also contains phenylethylamine, PEA, an amphetamine like compound although only about one tenth as much as is found in cheddar cheese or salami. It also harbors traces of compounds similar to tetrahydrocannabinol, THC—the active ingredient in marijuana.[13]

Up close and personal. Whenever I was damaged by my wife's shaming, the first thing I would do was to go out and buy a container of French Vanilla ice cream. I wasn't looking for self–

generated opiates or endogenous morphine. French Vanilla ice cream I realized much later was the closest thing to mother's milk I could get.

When my sons were breastfeeding, I never got over seeing them roll their eyes in the back of their heads full of warmth, security and contentment brought on by skin touching skin while they sucked milk. Not knowing any better at the time, I called it a narcotic high. Milk itself contains a natural morphine like substance called beta–casomorphine[14] which occurs when casein breaks apart during digestion.[15] Traces of morphine were found when analyzing cow's milk and human milk.[16]

Addicts, Erickson says, depend, as babies once did, on the incorporation by mouth or skin of substances which make them feel both physically satiated and emotionally restored. But they are not aware that they yearn to be babies again.[17] Don't let us kid ourselves; the foods we eat are designed with the most potent ingredient there is—the missed feeling of mother's caring touch.

I am not prone to conspiracy theories, although I would like to know who really did kill JFK. But it surely sounds to me if there is a conspiracy somewhere lurking in the aisles of our supermarket.

When it comes to food, we follow an eating script that has been written into the circuits of our brains.[18] Rewarding foods rewire our brains. We cannot control the responses to highly palatable foods because our brains have been changed by the foods we eat.[19]

Parallels between non–drug addictions like food, gambling, drug addictions and cravings, impair control over the behavior, tolerance, withdrawal, high rates of relapse; evidence natural rewards are capable of inducing plasticity in addiction–related circuitry.[20]

Orosensory self–stimulation refers to the cyclical process in which eating delicious foods tells the brain to make us want more of those foods.[21] Exorphins cause our brain to instruct us to eat more food and increase caloric consumption.[22]

Just as the transition from drug use to dependence is associated with a down regulation of brain reward circuitry and a concurrent enhancement of "anti–reward" circuitry, so does the transition to a food addiction appear to involve a "dark side."[23]

Although sugar alone trips the opiate machinery, the food industry has found that whipping a bit of fat accentuates its effects.[24] As Michael Moss says in his book, *Salt Sugar Fat: How the Food Giants Hooked Us*, "If sugar is the methamphetamine of processed food ingredients, then fat is the opiate."[25]

The transition of food to an industrial product has stripped away the nutritional value of food, most grains have become converted to starches, sugar in concentrated form, and many fats have been concentrated and hydrogenated which creates trans–fatty acids with very adverse effects on health.[26]

I told you I smelled a conspiracy somewhere. Food was beginning to look a lot like cigarettes to me. Karl Marx was wrong; religion is not the opium of the people—food is! Several years ago I worked as an armed security guard at a major supermarket chain in Israel. All day long my job was to watch people come in and out obviously looking for trouble makers and terrorists. But soon I embarked on studying the people who came into the store.

One of my many observations was that there was an imaginary addiction line approximately ten feet in front of the store where people stood for a few moments to quickly finish their last cigarette before entering. And it was this same line they hurried back to when they ended shopping to light up the long awaited next cigarette.

But smokers were not the only people who stood on that line. I noticed there were also mothers who stopped to give their children the ice cream, chocolate bars, cookies, candies, sodas, rolls, yogurts, cheese, Slim Jim's, etc that they had just purchased. And what was good for the children was always good for Mom. Men in fact usually were prone to ice cream, bread and salami sticks. In three years it was rare to see a *baguette* leave the store without having its corner torn off.

These same people could not have been starving because invariably they entered the store while eating something. The adjacent shopping center hosted burgers, ice cream, falafel, schwarma, pies, candy, pastries and breads of all kinds. The addiction line was steadfast; the same whether cigarettes or food. And no wonder; cigarette companies control the food industry. Philip Morris runs the largest food company in charge of icons like Cool Whip, Entenmann's, Oscar Mayer, Velveeta, Lunchables, Shake n' Bake, Macaroni & Cheese, Jell–O, Tang, Maxwell House, and the Post cereals: Raisin Bran, Grape–Nuts and Cocoa Pebbles.[27]

Dr. Maté, however, proved his point. Twenty percent of returning enlisted men in the Vietnam War met the criteria for the diagnosis of addiction. Yet, once home, use of drugs decreased to near or below pre–service levels. The remission rate of 95 percent was unheard of among narcotics addicts treated in the U.S.[28] Medical evidence has repeatedly shown that uploads like morphine prescribed for cancer pain, even for long periods of time, do not lead to addiction except for a minority of susceptible people.[29]

The dominate view has always been that if you take an addicting drug such as heroin or morphine, you will get hooked. In the late 1970's, Dr. Bruce Alexander, a psychology professor at Simon Fraser University in Vancouver Canada, conducted what has been called the Rat Park experiments. Alexander's thesis was that it was social conditions not opiates which were the addictive culprit.

Using a modified Skinner box that allowed self–administered drugs, he and his colleagues proved that rats consumed far more morphine under isolated conditions than they did in the socially housed Rat Park. What was true for rats is also true for humans.

Alexander went on to develop what he calls the Dislocation Theory of Addiction.[30] The three principles of his theory are:

> Psychosocial integration is an essential part of the human well–being
> and that dislocation, the sustained absence of psychosocial
> integration, is excruciatingly painful.[31]
> Globalization of the free market society produces a general
> breakdown of psychosocial integration, spreading dislocation.[32]
> Addictions are a way of adapting to sustained dislocation.[33]

By now the broader picture revealed itself to me. Reflecting back
on Erickson's Eight Stages of Man, a pattern of a dislocated
person's life, like a fractal, emerged. Basic trust happens only in a
predictable environment. A discouraging child's world sets shame.
Age six, guilt from failures dominates, yielding a rage which trails
throughout life and heralds psychosomatic disease. Ill prepared at
the tool–level, a sense of inadequacy and inferiority develops.
Unsuccessful at affiliations and partnerships, distance, isolation, and
a haunting avoidance of intimacy reign.

As Alexander says, "addiction is neither a disease nor a moral
failure, but a narrowly focused lifestyle that functions as a meager
substitute for people who desperately lack psychosocial
integration."[34] At the root of all of our cravings, addictions,
compulsions, and out–of–control behavior is our subconscious
choosing to use these behaviors to stay away from our inner
feelings of desperation.[35]

Nick, a forty–one year old heroin and crystal meth addict patient
of Dr. Maté, viscerally proves the point, "The reason I do drugs is
so I don't feel the fucking feelings I feel when I don't do drugs."[36]
Nick's explanation is ubiquitous. Allow me to quote two doctors
who encompass the worlds of heart disease and cancer.

> Dr. Dean Ornish: We become addicted to what makes us
> unconscious, so we don't feel the pain we create. The temporary
> pleasure is used to hide the chronic pain. Worse than that, we blunt
> the capacity to feel pain; we also diminish the capacity to feel
> pleasure, joy and love, both for ourselves and for others. When we

deal with the pain more directly, then we can increase our awareness and our joy rather than diminish it.[37]

Dr. Bernie Siegel: I have had many patients who developed a dependence on food, drugs, alcohol, or other addictive behaviors, and what I learned from them was that this was their response to a childhood in which they experienced indifference, rejection, or abuse—the opposite of love—from their parents. They sought to reward themselves in order to feel better, but these choices were self–destructive for they were only temporary fixes. People who choose a path of self–destruction don't live that way because of a lack of information. What they lack is inspiration and a sense of self–worth.[38]

Not all addictions are rooted in abuse or trauma, but Dr. Maté believes that they can all be traced back to painful experience. A hurt is at the center of all addictive behaviors. The wound may not be as deep and the ache not as excruciating, and it may even be entirely hidden—but it's there.[39] A recurring theme emerged in his interviews with addicts: the drug as an emotional anesthetic; as an antidote to a frightful feeling of emptiness; as a tonic against fatigue, boredom, alienation, and a sense of personal inadequacy; as a stress reliever and social lubricant.[40] Foods and drugs are inter–changeable as stress relievers and social lubricants.

An important point I learned: you do not have to inject, smoke, imbibe, eat, drink, swallow, or take in food or any other addictive substance to be lured, enticed, tempted, or ensnared by it. Cues, whether they are just thoughts, or seeing the substance, entrap us.

A group of former heroin addicts who were free for 10 years agreed to board a bus to 125th street in New York where they had previously bought their drugs. As soon as the bus reached the corner, the ex–addicts went into a state of drug withdrawal.[41]

Recent findings have helped demonstrate the interaction between the homeostatic and reward circuits of feeding behaviors, particularly the dopamine system. The D2 receptor function is critical for food motivation and brain signaling in obesity.[42] Usually, when enough food is consumed, physiological brain signals to terminate eating, however, this homeostatic regulation is steadily overridden by the omnipresence of food and food related cues causing eating extended beyond satiation.[43]

Activity in the brain is stimulated not only by food itself, but also by cues suggesting that food is nearby.[44] *The ubiquitous jar of candy on your desk.* How do you feel when you look at the gourmet magazine in the doctor's office? A cue triggers a dopamine–fueled urge; dopamine leads us to foods; eating foods leads us to opioid release; and the production of both dopamine and opioids stimulates further eating.[45] And the opioids produced by eating high sugar, high fat foods can relieve pain or stress and calm us down.[46]

Love and food are synonymous and interchangeable in the unconscious mind.[47] Rabbi Dr. Twerski says we may form a relationship with food to compensate for the absence of relationships with people. Relating to food is safe because food can never reject you.[48]

Dr. Mona Lisa Shultz is a medical intuitive who received her doctorates, an MD and a PhD in Behavioral Neuroscience, from Boston University's School of Medicine. Dr. Schultz says for a man, there is food and there is sex. For a woman, however, there is food–sex. Women have the same sensations similar to those they experience when they are in love and having sex.[49]

There are seven basic feelings: love, hate, hurt, anger, happiness, sadness and fear. To overcome dislocation, shame, childhood traumas, etc we numb those feelings. Repression is the way children numb out so they don't feel their emotions. Once an emotion is repressed, one feels numb. No one comes through childhood without being emotionally scarred to some extent.[50]

Psychological defenses in a normal person are extremely puzzling because at first glance they seem detrimental to survival.[51] Defenses that protect people from suffering emotional pain and anxiety when they were children later play destructive limiting roles in their adult lives. An individual's defense system acts to keep him insulated, mechanical, and removed from the deepest personal experiences.[52]

The defensive mechanisms we used as children to survive are not selective, but broadly based. If we numb hurt we also numb love, numb fear and happiness get numb. It's easy to numb out watching television, hunting for happiness in cyberspace on Facebook or chat rooms, drinking, smoking, doing drugs, or eating something full of fat, sugar, or salt that is instantly satisfying.[53]

By the time we are adults, we have become hostages to our emotions. Emotional hostages spend much of their lives in service to their emotions, or even in sacrificing their lives to their emotions, instead of their emotions being in the service of their lives.[54] But rather than feeling our emotions, we become them; we are swallowed up by these emotions.[55]

Our feelings are the way we perceive ourselves. They are our reaction to the world around us, the way we sense being alive. Without awareness of our feelings we have no awareness of life. Feelings are our most helpful link in our relationship with ourselves and the world around us.[56]

Emotions are also one of the keys to understanding illness. Our emotional experiences early in life may play a strong role in shaping our health later in life.[57] Symptoms are meant to draw the person's attention away from the hidden emotions.[58] All too often we end up merely numbing the pain, ignoring the symptoms and as a result, silencing the very voice that is trying to help us find a way out of the situation that underlies our present distress.[59]

Feelings of loneliness, worthlessness, despair and hopelessness are all translated into disease.[60] Emotional states are capable of inducing physical symptoms without physiological alteration of specific tissues.[61] Emotional influences, including nutrition, stress and emotions, can modify genes, without changing their basic blueprint.[62]

Repressed emotions are stored in the body—the unconscious mind—via the release of neuropeptide ligands and the memories are held in their receptors.[63] If we ignore our emotions or our memories from the past, our bodies will express them all the more forcefully.[64]

The late Candace Pert was an internationally recognized and a significant contributor to the emergence of Mind–Body Medicine as an area of legitimate scientific research. In her book *Molecules of Emotion,* her research has shown that when emotions are expressed, all systems are united and made whole. However, when emotions are repressed, denied not allowed to be whatever they maybe, our neural network pathways get blocked, stopping the flow of the vital feel–good unifying chemicals that run both our biology and our behavior.[65]

Immune cells make the same chemicals that we conceive of as controlling mood in the brain. So, immune cells not only control tissue integrity of the body but they also manufacture information chemicals that regulate mood or emotion.[66] The immune system acts as a pattern recognition system which communicates information across the body and stores it as memory.

The immunes system's failure to fight off disease may be related to the whole organism's internal lack, or confusion, of meaning. Indeed, if the meaning of the body is taken to be its intelligent, coordinated activity in health, then disease is a degeneration or breakdown in meaning.[67]

The ability to say no is essential for a healthy immune system, found in people who have developed enough intelligent self interest to meet their own needs first.[68] By now the threads I have been weaving in the fabric of health should start to become apparent. Saying "no" is a critical first step. *I rarely say no* is a common expression in shame. Remember the 1965 song by the Zombies? *"Tell her no, no, no, no, no, no, no, no, no, no, no, no, no, no, no, no, no."*

I think it prudent to repeat David Bohm's definition of health: good health is basically a manifestation of the overall creative intelligence working in concert with the body through various means that includes exercise, diet, and relaxation, etc. Developing creative intelligence is a precursor of wanting to meet our own needs. Most of us would much rather take care of the world and everyone else than ourselves.

Been in an airplane recently? The stewardess in explaining emergency procedures informs us that when the oxygen mask drops down, parents please place the mask on yourself first and then your children. I learned this lesson the hard way. *If we do not take care of ourselves first, then we really are in no condition to care for anyone else.*

7

Psyche—Soma

When psychologists speak of the unconscious, it is the body that they are talking about.

Dr. Franz M. Alexander

Who we are and what our lives consist of are the most common causes of psychosomatic symptoms.

Dr. John Sarno[1]

We develop a psychosomatic illness that justifies letting ourselves be cared for.

Rabbi Dr. Abraham Twerski[2]

When people are sick all the time, it is the moment to take a good look at the unconscious.

Dr. Arthur Janov[3]

In 18th century Hungary lived Rabbi Jungreis, the Righteous One of Tshenger. People thronged to him from every province of the country in order to receive recovery and salvation. Many stories are told of his exemplary personality and his great deeds.

One such story goes that after he had become a very rich man from the patients that Rabbi Jungreis had sent him, the Christian pharmacist in the village of Tshenger sold his pharmacy to another and moved to the capital city of Budapest. After some time, the two met in the capital city. The first pharmacist inquired of the second how his business was doing.

He was primarily curious to know how successful he had been in cooperating with Rabbi Jungreis and the patients who brought him their prescriptions. The second pharmacist whined that he was barely eking out a living and was on the verge of declaring bankruptcy.

"Could it be," asked the pharmacist from Budapest, "that Rabbi Jungreis is still living in the village and that sick people are still coming to him?" "Yes," answered the second pharmacist, "nothing has changed. People still inundate him from every province of the country. After he hears what a sick person has to say, without an examination he writes a prescription and sends them to buy the medicine at my pharmacy. But nearly every type of medicine that the saintly Rabbi prescribes is missing from my pharmacy."

"You are such a foolish man," the pharmacist from Budapest sighed, "that's exactly the way it was when I was there. I gave them some other type of medication—whatever I had in stock. Do you really think it was the medicine that led to the patients' recovery?"

Rabbi Jungreis and the pharmacist knew what most doctors know. The mind has an incredible power to control the body, both in its illness and in its cure. In modern terminology it is called the placebo effect derived from the Latin *placebo*—I shall please.

Perhaps the most famous illustration of the placebo effect was the case of Mr. Wright, *nom de plume,* who in 1957 was diagnosed with terminal lymph node cancer that had spread throughout his chest, neck, abdomen, and groin. Hospitalized, unfortunately he was given only a few days to live. Mr. Wright had heard of a horse serum, Krebiozen, that scientists had discovered was effective in treating cancer. Cajoling his doctors, he received an injection of Krebiozen on a Friday and miraculously by Monday his tumors had "melted like snowballs on a hot stove."

Discharged, Mr. Wright resumed life as normal until a few months later he read that his life saving horse serum had been proven ineffective in curing cancer. His cancer returned with a vengeance.

In a valiant effort to save his life, Mr. Wright's doctors told him to disregard the report and they backed up their words by giving him "a new super–refined double strength" Krebiozen treatment, which in reality was only a saline solution. Again, his tumors melted.

Unfortunately, two months later Mr. Wright read a "definitive report" describing Krebiozen as a worthless, quack remedy. Two days later, Mr. Wright was dead.

A Biblical[4] example of a placebo is recorded when the Israelites spoke against God and Moses complaining that they were lead into the wilderness with a lack of food and water. God sent burning snakes against the people with multitudes dying. As an antidote, Moses, made a copper snake and placed it on top of a pole. If someone who was bitten would stare at the snake and he would live.

The Talmud[5] asks if the copper snake really had the ability to restore life. Rather, the Talmud answers the people were healed because they looked heavenward with their hearts focused on God. In another passage of the Talmud,[6] we see that the copper snake accompanied the Israelites until the time of King Hezekiah when out of desperation he finally crushed the copper serpent because the people no longer looked to God as the cure believing the snake was the agent of relief.

The Talmud[7] tells of another example of a placebo. One day Rabbi Judah the Patriarch suffered from an eye illness and his doctor suggested that he put an ointment into his eye. Rabbi Judah told the doctor he would not be able endure that procedure. The doctor offered to put the ointment on the outside of the eye, but still Rabbi Judah said no. So in the end the doctor poured the ointment into a tube and placed it under his head and Rabbi Judah was healed.

Placebos are drugs or treatments that have no pharmacological properties of their own. Actually until the mid–Twentieth Century, all medical treatments probably could be classified as placebos. Most of what doctors had in their little black bags until then were ineffective treatments.

Modern day pharmacological drugs in order to obtain approval must go through expensive, rigorous years of testing. But the bottom line is reached when the treatment has proven more effective than a placebo. *Think about that for a moment. More effective than nothing!* Big Pharma not always tests drugs against a placebo. With improved or modified medications they only have to prove their effectiveness against the preexisting drugs. How are we, the consumer, to know if the newer drug is even better than nothing?

New drugs always seem most effective early in their career, losing some of their therapeutic potency with the passage of time.[8] The most striking feature of many of the most recently introduced drugs is that there is considerable doubt whether they do any good at all.[9]

In 1950 at a New York hospital, a doctor gave women suffering from nausea and vomiting of pregnancy a drug that they were told would eliminate the problem. In reality, they were given Ipecac, an emetic—a substance used to induce vomiting in cases of accidental poisoning. Surprisingly, the nausea and vomiting disappeared after taking the Ipecac.[10]

Doctors at a VA hospital in Texas did a pilot study comparing knee arthroscopy surgery for arthritis with three other types of operations: scraping out the knee joint, washing out the knee joint or just simply doing nothing; merely anesthetizing the patient, making three cuts in the knee as if they had operated. Two years after the surgery, all three treatments were equally effective; with the "do nothing" group reporting the same amount of pain relief as the real operations.[11]

Even how we perceive something determines the placebo effect. Dr. Bernie Siegel tells of an oncologist who noticed that the chemotherapy drugs used in a protocol named after the first letter of each drug spelled EPOH. He turned the letters around to become HOPE and more of his patients responded to therapy.[12]

The placebo effect is not confined only to medicine. In the mid–1920's the Hawthorne Works of Western Electric Company located in Chicago experimented with changing illumination to increase production, but they discovered that even by *reducing* the foot candle amount to light obtained from moonlight, the efficiency remained unimpaired. This series of studies concluded that the introduction of any change might lead to behavioral effects greater than the effects that might be predicted.[13]

Dr. Herbert Benson, Professor of Medicine at Harvard Medical School and founder of the Mind–Body Medical Institute at Massachusetts General Hospital in Boston, describes the placebo effect as having three components: the belief of the patient, the beliefs of the medical practitioner and the relationship between the patient and the practitioner.[14]

This relationship is so closely entwined that when a physician predicts a patient's improvement, we cannot say whether the doctor is giving a sophisticated prognosis or whether the patient's improvement is based in part upon the optimism engendered by the physicians' prophecy.[15] Placebos have a real not an imaginary effect. They are more than 50% effective as pain medications and their effect can be blocked by drugs such as Naloxone.

Who are the people influenced by placebos? It seems likely that they are patients who are provided with the means to redress some emotional instability. They may be depressed people, who need some hope, hostile people who need to channel their energies in a productive direction, or repressed suffers who are given a way to touch their inner selves.[16] In short, just about everyone in my opinion.

Just how prevalent is the use of placebos in the practice of medicine? Researchers at the University of Chicago published a study in the *Journal of General Internal Medicine* which revealed that 45% of the doctors surveyed said that they had used a placebo during their clinical practice.[17] A study published in *Family Medicine* concluded that more than half of family physicians surveyed use placebo treatments for patient care.[18] Placebo use is common in primary care in the United Kingdom.[19] A study of Danish general practitioners found that 48% had prescribed a placebo at least 10 times during the previous year.[20]

An Israeli study published in the *British Medical Journal*[21] surveyed 31 inpatient medical and surgical departments at two large hospitals and various community clinics in the Jerusalem area. Their findings were quite comprehensive choosing only senior physicians and nurses from the departments.

The authors wrote in the study, "When we planned the study we assumed that the use of placebo was not widespread and would not exceed 10%." However, among the respondents, 60% used placebos; 62% prescribed a placebo as often as once a month; 68% told patients they were receiving actual medication; 28% considered placebos were a diagnostic tool; and 94% found placebos generally effective. "Our finding that placebo prescribing is a widespread practice cannot be doubted."

A conclusion in a study published in the *Journal of General Internal Medicine*[22] showed that a growing number of physicians believe in a mind–body connection which may explain doctors use of placebos. The study said, "Our physician respondents generally believed that placebos have therapeutic effects and do not help differentiate between psychogenic versus organic symptoms."

In the same *Family Medicine* study cited above, doctors did not view the mind and body as distinct entities but largely endorsed the power of patient expectation to influence both psychological and physical health.

So, how far can the mind–body connection go in understanding the nature of illness? The short answer is a very long way. Dr. Georg Groddeck was a 19th–20th century physician and writer regarded as a pioneer of psychosomatic medicine. He took the position that the unconscious is the formative principle of all normal and abnormal bodily processes. Organic diseases ultimately have a psychological nature, since they express unconscious conflicts.[23]

The belief that a disease or illness involves the mind and body is called psychosomatic. A person's mental health influenced by stress, anxiety, and other factors tremendously affect physical diseases. Major studies indicate that approximately 75 percent of visits to the family physician are either for illness that will ultimately get better without treatment or for disorders related to anxiety, stress or unknown origins probably caused by "psychosocial" factors.[24] Most standard medical textbooks attribute anywhere from 50 to 80 percent of all diseases to psychosomatic or stress related origins.[25]

Previously, I said that I believed the key to healing the mind, body and soul was the recognition and awareness of our childhood defenses and in identifying how they limit one's present day life. Since the time of Freud, the repressed unconscious has been depicted as an iceberg lurking in our lives waiting for that Titanic collision when it surfaces to sink us.

I think that image is totally wrong and misleading. Our repressed unconscious in truth is more like a volcano, exerting tremendous pressure on our daily lives; fissures wreaking havoc until the volcano erupts into major illnesses. The fissures are the physical symptoms we experience as first warnings:

Dr. Mona Lisa Schulz: physical symptoms let us know when our emotional life is not working well, what we need to change and what's working fine.[26]

Dr. John Sarno: my patient's physical symptoms were the direct result of the strong feelings repressed in the unconscious.[27] Physical symptoms are intended to divert attention from emotions in the unconscious so that they will not become overt and thereby known to the conscious mind.[28]

Shivani Goodman, PhD: symptoms are messages from the body telling you that what you are thinking, feeling and doing is making you sick. It is the body's way of telling you that it is time to make changes.[29]

Dr. Mimi Guarneri: suppressed emotions, or ones we are unconscious of, don't just simmer on the back burner indefinitely; they eventually manifest themselves on a physical level and are reflected in our bodies as physical symptoms.[30]

Eric Erickson: a psychosomatic crisis is an emotional crisis to the extent to which the sick individual is responding specifically to the latent crises in the significant people around him.[31]

Dr. Stanislav Goff: when we start experiencing symptoms of a disorder that is emotional rather that organic in nature, it is important to realize that this is not the beginning of a disease but the emergence into our consciousness of material that was previously buried in the unconscious parts of our being.[32]

Dr. Charles Whitfield: Physical illness may also develop through disallowed or repressed grieving.[33]

Peter Levine, PhD: the cumulative consequences of suppressing impulses take its toll in the form of back pain, headaches, high blood pressure, heart disease and gastrointestinal disorders.[34]

Rabbi Yisroel Salanter: As long as an emotional force is hidden in its root, it will remain concealed from man's understanding. Moreover, it will continue to influence his actions, for he is not aware of its existence.[35]

I know it may sound counterintuitive that emotions can cause physically manifested symptoms and illnesses. Our physical health is intimately connected with our patterns of thinking and feeling about ourselves and also with the quality of our relationships with other people and the world.[36]

Take as an example the phenomena of pseudocyesis—false pregnancy; the mistaken belief of a woman that she is pregnant. She may exhibit some or all of the symptoms of pregnancy: nausea, backache, weight gain, swollen belly, enlarged nipples, fetal movement and even craving for pickles and ice cream. The brain can trigger the release of estrogen and prolactin. She has everything but the fetus to really be pregnant. Researchers believe that the emotional stress of infertility, child sexual abuse, problematic marital relations are some of the causes of pseudocyesis.

Up close and personal. Several years ago one of my sons decided during winter break that he'd had enough of high school and was due a sabbatical. A Big–Brother of his helped him get a job with a gardener. For several weeks he worked long hard hours "tilling the soil" as we say. Then one morning he awoke with a persistent cough. Our family doctor said it could be the beginnings of a virus even though his sinuses were clear and his throat was normal. But the cough lingered all day and all night. His every waking moment was spent coughing.

Doctors prescribed a cascade of antibiotics to no avail. After a few weeks we turned to a major hospital in Tel Aviv where he was subjected to a cycle of tests. We waited outside a conference room one morning for the conclusion of the specialists. Their diagnosis: a bacterial infection. Even after three weeks of Star Wars types of antibiotics, they held firm that given time, the treatment would stop the coughing.

In desperation, we turned our back on our chosen health care provider and decided to pay privately. A teenager with a non–stop day and night cough can wear even the best parents down. At a different hospital in Jerusalem, with checkbooks in hand, we started another round of testing. Many samples, scopes, tubes and reports later, we had a different diagnosis: a fungal infection with classic symptoms similar to Blastomycosis.

Blastomycosis is relatively rare but potentially lethal fungal disease predominantly of the lungs caused by the dimorphic fungus *Blastomyces dermatitidis* endemic to the regions surrounding the lakes and waterways of central North America including Ontario Canada.[37] Although we were in Israel, the etiology fit. Infection is acquired by via inhaling aerosolized spores (conidia) from disturbed contaminated soil with a low pH, especially soil that is enriched with organic debris such as decaying vegetation, rotting wood and animal excreta (high nitrogen content).[38] My son, after all, was working as a gardener.

Inhalation therapy at the hospital brought no relief; it had been an expensive second opinion. Nine weeks of raspy, persistent, unshakable, relentless, enduring coughing. We went back to the hospital unconsciously seeking some sort of guarantee on money we spent. Then while sitting in the office, the young staff doctor said he noticed something unusual and asked our son to wait outside.

He began asking us those time–honored questions about our son's life which long ago had been sacrificed in order to achieve the 12 minute patient encounter. We explained that he had quit school and until the coughing worked long hours as a gardener. With a characteristic nod of satisfaction, he explained that the triggers of his coughing were reversed. What appeared to be causation was opposite to what it should be. I learned much later that Dr. John Sarno believes that on a more individual basis, physical triggers are one of the most common catalysts of the psychosomatic process.[39]

What he explained to us was that our son had a psychogenic cough; a chronic dry cough that defied all explanation and resisted all the usual standard treatments. He called our son back in to the office and after speaking to him about the job, school and in general his life, convinced him to return to school while continuing the lidocaine inhalation at home until the coughing stopped.

He returned to school and within a few days, he came home *without* the cough. If you ask him today what finally worked, he will tell you it was the home inhalation. Of course that was only a placebo. What had caused the cough was the *Catch 22* he had placed himself in. He couldn't admit that it was a mistake to quit school nor could he quit the gardener because he felt it would let his friend down after all the trouble he had gone through to get him the job.

What about the Blastomycosis? As I will explain in a later chapter, I worked for several years as a therapist specializing in a person's unconscious. From what I gleaned during that time I believe the unconscious is much more than what most people think it is. In my opinion, since the mission statement of the unconscious is protecting us from our past in a way that it believes is best; it *chooses* wisely its course of action. I realize that I have no scientific basis for attributing agency to consciousness, but nonetheless I judge it to be true.

To be plausible, the unconscious picks symptoms to express, protecting us from our *Catch 22* dilemmas of life. It chose the symptoms of blastomycosis because my son worked with the soil. Almost as if the unconsciousness searched *Wikipedia* looking for something that would work. Automobile accidents, falls, physical abuse, and repetitive motion in the work place, according to Dr. Sarno, are examples of physical triggers that often result in chronic pain syndromes.[40]

You might well ask in the case of my son was his unconscious cagey enough to fool two sets of specialists at two different hospitals; one thinking it was a bacterial infection while the second was convinced it was fungal? Called the symptom imperative by Dr. Sarno: If the psyche has induced a physical symptom (such as back pain) or an emotional symptom (such as depression), which is then temporarily relieved in some fashion without dealing with the underlying emotional dynamic, the psyche will simply create another symptom to take its place.[41]

Dr. Sarno has spent his career successfully treating chronic disorders with just words. In his seminars, he explains to his patients the crucial idea that the mind–body disorder is a defense, an avoidance strategy designed to turn away attention from frightening repressed feelings.[42] "No matter how we react to life's pressures consciously, another world of reactions exists in the unconscious.[43] It's clear that symptoms are meant to draw a person's attention away from hidden emotions; that exposing the undercover operation and thereby ending it; the pain would disappear, as indeed it does.[44] Awareness, insight, knowledge and information are the magic medicines that cure this disorder—and nothing else."[45]

For Dr. Sarno the primary importance is each patient's psychological history: marital status; children, if married; place of birth and the quality of life during childhood and adolescence, with particular reference to personalities of parents and relationships with them; the ages and health of parents now; relationships with siblings; education and occupational history.[46]

Unconscious anger generated in the mind of a boy or girl of ten will be alive and equally intense when they are forty as on the day it occurred.[47] To the pain and anger generated in childhood, we now add the emotions arising from the conflict between the residual child–primitive in all of us and the pressures imposed by life—personal relationship, job, social obligations, and so on.[48]

Up close and personal: Very recently my son had another battle with the unconscious. One day while working in a hotel, he was picking up a large couch with his boss when suddenly he was seized with a sharp pain in his back. A CT scan at the emergency room showed a herniated disc, L5S1. Unable to work, he quit the hotel. His pain progressively grew worse by the day. A few months later an MRI confirmed a lumbosacral disc protrusion, L5S1.

After several weeks the back pain was so bad that my son needed a broom stick to help him walk. His doctor prescribed physical therapy as a remedy. But after a month my son put an end to the therapy. Each session instead of being a panacea, made the pain worse. That's when he started on pain medications.

Over the next year he took everything: Tramadex® Arcoxia® Oxycontin® Lirica® and finally morphine in the form of a Fentanl®75 mg patch. Three times the pain was so depilating that he went to the emergency room for an IV of pain killers. Nothing ameliorated the pain, not even acupuncture!

In desperation, we turned to one of Israel's best spine specialists. He ordered two new MRIs of the entire spinal column. The MRIs confirmed the L5S1 disc problem. However, the specialist explained that L5S1 could not be causing the pain in his lower back and his legs. Surgery was not an option because it might do more damage than good. The specialist gave a referral to a neurologist.

At this point I mentioned to my son's primary care physician his psychogenic cough story. I told the doctor that I believed his back pain was psychosomatic in origin. I explained to the doctor a study I read in the *New England Journal of Medicine*.[49]

MRIs were performed on 96 asymptomatic people and were read independently by two neuro–radiologists. Thirty–six percent had normal discs at all levels. Yet, 52 percent had a bulge in at least one level; 27 percent had a protrusion; 1 percent had an extrusion; 38 percent had an abnormality of more than one inverted disc.

The authors conclusion was, "given the high prevalence of these findings and of back pain, the discovery by MRI'S of bulges or protrusions in people with low back pain may be frequently coincidental."

The doctor filed the information away in his mind. Months later he told me he had consulted with a psychiatric specialist about my son's case. However unlikely, he admitted that I might be right in my assessment.

A subsequent EMG showed no distal neuropathy pointing instead to the L5S1 disc problem. Back to the spine specialist; he saw the pain my son was having with the slightest maneuvering and suggested a wheel chair might be advisable. He also recommended at this point a complete full–body bone scan and another referral to a neurologist who ordered an MRI of the brain just to rule out ALS and multiple sclerosis.

Seven months in a wheel chair, endless normal ultrasounds, CTs, MRIs, EMGs and bone scans, finally in anguish we headed to a pain clinic in Jerusalem. The doctor spent more than a half hour reviewing *all* of the tests. We had gone seeking an epidural, a shot of cortisone, a magic wand, anything to alleviate the misery our son had endured for nearly two years.

From all the evidence, the pain specialist explained, there was no procedure indicated that would help. At that point I discussed with him the psychogenic coughing story. He recommended returning to a neurologist to seek out a possible neurologic cause despite the fact that the brain MRIs and EMGs were normal. His diagnosis: PTSD.

Unexpectedly, the next morning the pain specialist phoned me. He said that it is normally not the case with patients that they will accept a non–physical cause for pain. But since I seemed to be understanding he wanted to explain that his recommendation for the neurologist was unnecessary. He only wrote that as a matter of protocol. A neurologist at that point, he explained, would usually recommend to the patient that a visit to a psychiatrist might be prudent.

Then we discussed the diagnosis: PTSD. He preferred Post Traumatic Stress Disorder to labeling it psychosomatic. His experience confirmed what Dr. John Sarno understood. The more intense or threatening the unconscious feelings are, the more severe the psychosomatic reactions are likely to be.[50]

After seven months in a wheel chair, it took a month of intense physical therapy to rebuild my son's atrophied muscles, but my son returned to his normal life again, totally free from all pain. Chronic back pain is another example of the unconscious mind causing physical pain. *The miracle cure ended up being an anti–depressant.*

William James was a 19th century physician, philosopher and psychologist. More than a century ago James said, "We have revealed to us whole systems of underground life, in the shape of memories of a painful sort which lead to a parasitic existence, buried outside of the primary fields of pains, convulsions, paralyses of feeling and emotion, and the whole possession of symptoms of hysteric diseases of the body and of mind. Alter or abolish by suggestion these subconscious memories and the patient immediately gets well."[51]

8

Attitude

The greatest discovery of my generation is that human beings can alter their lives by altering their attitudes

William James

Tracht gut, s'veht zein gut: Think positively and positive things will happen.

Rabbi Schner Zalman Schneerson

Our perception of the event is more important than the event itself.

Alfred Adler

Attitudes are more important than facts.

Dr. Karl Menninger

In the time of King Solomon, a rabbi approaching Jerusalem passed by a stone quarry. Soon he came upon some workers. "And what is your labor today?" he asked the first man he saw. The man paused a moment wiping the sweat dripping from his face with a piece of rag; his eyes bloodshot from the sun. Squinting, he looked at the rabbi, astounded by his question. "Isn't it obvious," he cried. "From sunup to sundown I toil in the heat, banging and chiseling these endless stones."

The rabbi walked a few paces more until he encountered another worker. "And what is your labor today?" he asked the second man. The man lifted his head, his face glistening in the sun, his eyes shown fiery contentment. "Can't you see, my dear Rabbi," the man replied, "The King has given me the honor and privilege of hewing out these precious stones he will use to finally complete his father's dream—the building of our Holy Temple where God's presence will reside!"

More than anyone Dr. Norman Vincent Peale promoted attitude as an important factor in our lives. His *Power of Positive Thinking* has guided generations in believing that "if you think in negative terms, you will get negative results. If you think in positive terms you will achieve positive results."[1] Science has confirmed that attitude can influence a variety of situations from experiments in the laboratory to our health. Experimenters obtain results in accordance with their knowledge of what the results would be.[2]

Dr. Jon Kabat–Zinn, Emeritus Professor of Medicine at the University of Massachusetts Medical School, says that our physical health is intimately connected with our patterns of thinking and feelings about ourselves and also with the quality of our relationships with other people and the world.[3] Self–efficacy, he states, is the belief in your ability to make things happen, even when you might have to face new, unpredictable, and stressful occurrences. A strong sense of self–efficacy is the best and most consistent predictor of positive health outcomes.[4]

I already pointed out one of the anomalies I encountered was that in six studies of nearly 25,000 people "the best predictor of survival over the next decade was the answer people gave to the simple question: What do you think about your health?"

Dr. Larry Dossey is a physician and an author who has become known for asserting the importance for healing of prayer and spirituality. He commented that in this study the predictive power of the answer to this question exceeded other factors such as physical symptoms, extensive exams, and laboratory tests or behaviors such as cigarette smoking.[5]

Cardiologist Dr. Mimi Guarneri says with heart disease, in particular, research has shown that optimism has been associated with a lowered risk of dying. In one study, patients who described themselves as highly optimistic had lower risks of all–cause death and lower rates of cardiovascular death than those with high levels of pessimism.[6]

Dr. Robert Rosenthal's research at Harvard has shown that expectation in an educational setting can determine outcomes. In his book, *Pygmalion in the Classroom,* he cites the case of a substitute teacher who was assigned mid–year a problematic underachieving class. To everyone's surprise, by year's end, her class was tops in achievement and performance.

In a conversation with the teacher, the principal tried to ascertain how she achieved her results. The teacher explained that she wasn't fooled by his not telling her that the class was the highest level in the school. Puzzled, the principle enquired further. She admitted she accidentally found the note he left with the students' names and IQ scores in the desk the first day of class: 135, 136, 140, and 147 etc. "Those weren't their IQ scores," the principle said, "Those were their locker numbers!"

Rosenthal points out that this substitute teacher was not an exception. Children who are expected by their teachers to gain intellectually in fact do show greater intellectual gains after one year than do children in whom such gains are not expected.[7] When a child's IQ test examiner expected superior performance, the total IQ earned was 7.5 points higher on average than when the child's examiner expected inferior results.[8]

His research has also shown that there is a type of relationship between prophecy and subsequent events in which the prophecy is not incidental but instrumental in its own fulfillment.[9] In medicine, Rosenthal says, we have too many examples before our eyes of situations considered irreversible and which became that way because this diagnosis had been given.[10]

Intention, purpose, goals, aims, targets and plans are all types of attitude to some degree. Lynn Mc Taggart in her book, *The Intention*

Experiment: Using Thoughts to Change Your Life and the World, describes the work of Robert Jahn, founder of the Princeton Engineering Anomalies Research Lab, and Brenda Dunne. Over the course of more than 2.5 million trials they decisively demonstrated that human intention can influence electronic devices in a specific direction.[11]

More interestingly, Mc Taggart describes an experiment by Helmut Schmidt that determined someone's intention could change a machine's recording tape output after it had been run. "It wasn't that his participants had changed a tape after it had been created," Mc Taggart explained, "their influence had reached 'back in time' and influenced the machine's output at the moment that it was first recorded. They changed the output of the machine in the same way that they might have if they had been present at the time it was being recorded. They did not change the past from what it was; they influenced the past when it was unfolding as the present so that it became what it was."[12]

The late Karl Pribram was a professor of neuropsychology at Georgetown and Stanford University; famous for his holographic model of the brain in which the mind is a probabilistic quantum process and not a thing. Mc Taggart believes that as Pribram proposed future intention might influence one neuron being fired and not another setting off a chain of chemical and hormonal events that may or may not result in disease. In fact, even the diagnosis itself might influence the future course of the disease and so should be approached with caution.[13]

Positive thoughts even have a profound effect on behavior and genes, but only when they are in harmony with subconscious programming. And negative effects have an equally powerful negative effect.[14] As Dr. Bernie Siegel says "perception affects our health; and most often, the way we perceive is our choice."[15] I mentioned that it is counterproductive to blame ourselves for ill health and disease. But we would be negligent if we fail to take responsibility for our own health.

Dr. Jill Bolte Taylor is a Harvard–trained and published neuroanatomist who experienced a severe hemorrhage in the left hemisphere of her brain in 1996. In her book, *My Stroke of Insight: A Brain Scientist's Personal Journey*, she defines *response–ability* as the ability to choose how we respond to stimulation coming in through our sensory systems at any moment in time.[16]

Viktor Frankl, the founder of Logotherapy, explains in his book, *Man's Search for Meaning*, "when we are no longer able to change a situation—just think of an incurable disease such as an inoperable cancer—we are challenged to change ourselves."[17]

"Principally," Rabbi Joseph Soloveitchik says, "it lies within man's power to determine the framework of cause and effect within which he lives and acts."[18] I believe that the challenge to change ourselves, our attitudes, taking response–ability, becoming proactive in our lives and especially our health grants us the restoration ability to heal ourselves.

Now I believe is an appropriate time to expand on what exactly physicist David Bohm meant in his definition of health by creative intelligence. Remember Bohm said that good health is basically a manifestation of the overall creative intelligence working in concert with the body through various means that include exercise, diet, and relaxation, etc.

Bohm says that the Latin *mederi* meaning "to cure"' (the root of the modern medicine) is based on a root meaning "to measure." This reflects the view that physical health is to be regarded as the outcome of a state of right inward measure in all parts and processes of the body.[19] As a person grows older, through infection, allergies, containments, misadventure, and the processes of aging, considerable "misinformation" or irrelevant information accumulates in the system.[20] Misinformation interferes with the right inward measurement. And indeed diseases like cancer are really caused by misinformation in the structure of the DNA.

Information plays a primordial role our world, our lives and our very existence. According to Bohm, information contained within the quantum potential will determine the outcome of a quantum process. The quantum wave carries information, Bohm says, and is therefore *potentially* active everywhere, but is *actually* active only when and where this information enters into the energy of the particle.[21] A case in point: a radio wave. The wave exists everywhere but is only active when its form enters into the electrical energy of a radio.

There are three ways, Bohm explains, of dealing with the problem of misinformation in the body: first, avoiding the introduction of misinformation in the first place by keeping away from infection, toxins, good sanitation and a careful diet. Second, it may be possible to correct or remove misinformation through various kinds of medical intervention. Third, but more significantly, involves the body itself.[22]

The human body possesses an immune system which is capable of clearing up misinformation in a natural way. This is indeed the body's main mode of dealing with misinformation. Bohm points out the fact that drugs are of little use fighting AIDS or other diseases which destroy the immune system. It can be compared to a kind of intelligence that responds to higher levels usually associated with thoughts and feelings. It is well known that depressive stress, thoughts, anxiety, etc inhibit the immune systems activity.[23]

It is not my purpose to fully discuss Bohm's theory of implicate and explicate orders except to say his assertion that the tangible reality of our everyday lives is really kind of an illusion. He called this deeper level of reality implicate (enfolded) order and our own level of existence as explicate (unfolded) order.[24] Bohm postulated that all information was present in some invisible domain or higher reality (implicate order) but active information (creative intelligence) could be called up at time of need, when it would be necessary and meaningful.[25]

Bohn uses the example of a hologram to characterize implicate order; each region of a photographic plate in which a hologram is observable contains within it the whole three–dimensional image, which can be viewed from a range of perspectives. When you break a holographic glass plate, instead of seeing pieces of the image in each shard and sliver, you see the whole image in each separate piece!

David Bohm says, "You could therefore say that everything is enfolded in this whole or even in each part and that it then unfolds. I call this implicate order, the enfolded order, and then this unfolds into an explicate order. The implicate order is enfolded order. It unfolds into the explicate order in which everything is separated."[26]

The response to this movement is an unfoldment of creative intelligence which originates in the depths of implicate order. When something new is proposed in the free play of thought,[a change in attitude] creative intelligence responds to the opposition and contradictions; something new that does not fit into what is already known, creative intelligence puts forth new sensory orders and perceptions and structures that form new perceptions.[27]

"It should be clear that creative intelligence cannot be grasped by the intellect in any form and it will necessarily elude all such attempts to capture it in this way.[28] The implicate order does not rule out God," Bohm states, "nor does it say there is a God. But it would say that there is a creative intelligence underlying the whole, which might have as one of the essentials that which was meant by the word God."[29]

Using Bohm's model, tapping into creative intelligence is in essence the function of the immune system. The search engine for the immune system is a task of creative intelligence connecting to the implicate order, whether directly or indirectly I cannot say.

Unbelievable, yes, maybe until you piece together all of the information I have been spreading out. There definitely is something more that reductionist physical forces at work. Pause for a moment and consider wireless internet.

As with the body, Bohm says, society attempts to deal with misinformation by trying to prevent it from entering its fabric or attempting to cure it with some form of therapy. To some extent psychotherapy and group therapies can help clear up individual misinformation which may go back to early childhood or start in a later phase of life.[30]

After I first read and then re–read Bohm's ideas, I started to formulate in mind what health was and what I needed to do restore health to my mind, body and soul. As with mathematics, physics and cosmology, the more elegant and simple a theory is, the more likely it is to be true. After all the books, articles, videos, etc I have digested over the past 15 years since my angioplasty, using David Bohm's definition as a base, I have come up with what I call the *Information Theory of Health*.

In order to achieve and restore health, you must correct the MIS–information in all aspects of your life (MIS is an acronym for Mistaken Information Sent). Life comprises not only the mind, body and soul, but our personalities, our relationships, our beliefs. That's the essence of the Information Theory of Health: correcting the MIS–information in your mind, body and soul. My theory fits well with Occam's razor: the simplest explanation to the problem of health. Bohm said good health is a manifestation of the overall creative intelligence working in concert with the body through various means that include exercise, diet, and relaxation, etc.

Health is not just the body as I have shown. If we correct MIS–information in our body by exercise, diet, and relaxation; reframe the MIS–information deposited during our early childhood and our current life; ponder the MIS–information that makes existential questions rhetorical— What is the meaning of life? Why do we live? Why were we put here? What do we live for? Is there life after death? What is God? — and finally answer them, then I believe that creative intelligence will enter in to the picture and accomplish the restoration of *good health* to every one of us.

To reiterate, Socrates said there is no illness of the body apart from the mind. Dr. John Sarno believes awareness, insight, knowledge and information are the magic medicines that cure mind–body disorders—and nothing else.

And finally as William James prophetically said a century ago, "alter or abolish by suggestion these subconscious memories and the patient immediately gets well." In the next chapter I will put in plain words how I learned to accomplish James's cure.

9

Судьба

Guided Imagery is the oldest and most ubiquitous form of medicine.

Dr. Martin Rossman[1]

One of the greatest gifts mankind has received is the elucidation of the working of the unconscious mind.

Rabbi Dr. Abraham Twerski[2]

The subconscious mind is a programmable "hard drive" into which our life experiences are downloaded.

Bruce Lipton, PhD[3]

The healing routine begins with deep relaxation.

Shivani Goodman, PhD[4]

A movie from our past that was a hilarious political commentary on the Cold War chill we Boomers felt in 1966 was *The Russian are Coming, The Russians are Coming.* It hosted a star–studded cast: Alan Arkin, Carl Reiner, Eva Marie Saint, Brian Keith, Jonathan Winters, and Theodore Bikel.

I still heartily laugh when I think of the scene where the Russian submarine commander was trying to convince the townspeople that it was a crazy idea to think that given the animosity between the two countries, they were Russian. Obviously, he explained, they were Norwegians on a NATO mission. Little did I know at the time how fortuitous the title of that movie would be in my life?

As the new millennium turned, I had left the chicken runs on my moshav to work in the Old City of Jerusalem. A year had passed since my angioplasty and in addition to my new heart; I was looking for a new life. Much later I was to realize it wasn't a new life I sought, but to regain a life that should have been but never was.

I worked for an internationally known Jewish outreach and educational organization located directly opposite the Western Wall in the Old City of Jerusalem. My job was the coordinator of their Executive Learning Program. I had the responsibility of developing tailor-made educational programs for the organizations key financial supporters and partners who came to study in Jerusalem from all over the world. In essence, I functioned as their spiritual *concierge* while they studied in the Holy City.

The organization boasted the *crème de la crème* of internationally known rabbis as their teachers. In the three years I worked there I absorbed a cornucopia of information on Jewish philosophy, ethics, ritual, tradition, science, cosmology and mystical understandings. Privilege is the only word that comes to my mind to describe time spent there.

A lucky few in life feel destiny when they encounter new people, places and situations. Working a stone's throw from where the Holy Jewish Temples stood, in a city sacred to the three predominate world religions; destiny paved the stone streets I walked on to reach work every day.

I must admit that one of satisfactions of my job was fielding the impressions people had after their time spent one-on-one with our rabbis. They were challenged, inspired, contemplative, amazed, tested, encouraged, stimulated, moved, pensive, and astounded to say the least. But I noticed that when they spent time with one particular rabbi everyone who encountered him had the same reaction. Afterward they were *changed* in obvious spiritual ways.

I did not have as much interplay with this particular rabbi as I did the others on a daily basis. All I knew was that to a man, most all of our local rabbis wanted their people to send time with him while they were learning at our ELC. But soon our lives would cross in a most profound way.

Rabbi Efim Svirsky at the time was the Educational Director of the Russian Program at our organization. Born in Moscow in the era of the Iron Curtain, his father was famous dissident writer, one of the first to shake the foundations of the Communist Party. Ultimately, he immigrated with his family, first to France, finally settling in Canada.

He graduated from the Canadian College of Massage and Hydrotherapy, took post graduate courses in manual medicine at the University of Michigan Medical School and was the first Cranial Sacral Therapy instructor in Canada. After a highly successful career as a chronic stress and pain therapist in Toronto, he and his family immigrated to Israel.

Since his move to Jerusalem, Rabbi Svirsky has touched the lives of hundreds of thousands through his weekly radio show broadcast to more than a million Russian Jews in Israel and Russia. And he is also popular from his numerous television appearances in Israel and Russia.

Rabbi Svirsky is the author of well–known Russian language books including: *Without Dialog–Abyss; Freedom and Choice; Torah and Psychology* and *Transformation: A Journey of Psycho/Spiritual Healing.* His English work, *Connection: Emotional and Spiritual Growth Through Experiencing God's Presence* is the culmination of his twenty years of developing and refining his unique spiritual and emotional growth system.

One day while talking to a colleague I discovered that Rabbi Svirsky had just completed a training session with a few young rabbis of our organization in his Torah–based system of psychological/spiritual counseling. For years he had taught in Russian but now he was beginning to teach his unique ideas in English. I jumped at the chance!

Our class was made up of rabbis and young rabbinical students seeking tools that would assist them in working in communities around the world where they would be assigned. More importantly, all were seeking to broaden their personal and spiritual growth. As a staff member I was able to wiggle in.

Rabbi Svirsky's philosophy is based on the premise that there is a lot of misinformation circulating among both secular Jews and surprisingly even among those who had grown up in religious homes about who God really is and exactly what Judaism truly entails. He explained to us many times that this misinformation not only confuses people in a religious sense; it also serves as an insidious, underlying cause of many of our emotional problems. (Misinformation—you can understand why a light went on in my mind when I first encountered David Bohm several years later.)

Primarily the intended purpose of the training was to give us the skills to counsel people as qualified psycho–spiritual therapists. Rabbi Svirsky was fond of saying that in his experience, a therapist can only take a client as far as he or she has gone. We would need more than learning skills and techniques; we had to explore the depths of our *own* souls. And after a few weeks of initial instruction that was exactly what we started doing.

Over the years, Rabbi Svirsky has developed a series of sixty exercises that became the basis of his book *Connections* with four stated goals: integrating a person's feeling of the presence of God in their life with special emphasis on the emotional level; developing and expanding ones spiritual and emotional resources; working on basic feelings such as love and freedom; and focusing on different aspects of a person's personality in order to give foundations of working on emotional blocks.

In *Connections,* he put down in writing what he had given over to us in our training, sharing a new way of interpreting the story of Adam and Eve in the garden. "Adam was right," Rabbi Svirsky writes, "that he had to eat from the tree to redirect negative energy into positive energy. That was his task. What was wrong was only his timing. According to the Jewish oral tradition, God told Adam, 'Don't eat of the Tree of Knowledge of Good and Evil *yet*. You are too young.' The ban was not forever. The oral tradition tells us that Adam was supposed to wait until the Sabbath, when he would have been more mature. At this point, God would have allowed him to eat from the Tree of Knowledge and Good and Evil, and nothing would have happened."[5]

This problem, Rabbi Svirsky explains, is still relevant today. *Information is not neutral*. Very often, when people receive information too early, it can destroy them. For this reason, we guard our children from knowing about horrific crimes and perversions. One day they will likely find out about them, but, at a young age, this information can harm them. This damage is what happened to the first man Adam. He underestimated that the knowledge of evil could harm him and that he might not be able to withstand it.[6] *I was becoming possessed by the concept of information.*

After weeks of lectures and the various exercises, Rabbi Svirsky began instructing us on the techniques of Progressive Muscular Relaxation originated by a physician named Edmond Jacobson in the 1930's, a pioneer in muscle physiology at Harvard, Cornell and the University of Chicago. A form of deep relaxation, Rabbi Svirsky explained, was required for developing our ability to concentrate; increasing our sensitivity; enabling our brain to work in different modes; and opening gateways to our sequestered subconscious.

Rabbi Eliyahu Dessler, the renowned 20th century teacher and master of Jewish ethics, asked the following question: How does one exert influence on the subconscious? His answer: one of the most effective ways is the use of imagination. Thoughts and logical arguments may have difficulty in penetrating the subconscious, but images can reach down and affect its springs of action.[7]

The use of imagination to successfully navigate the unconscious is called guided imagery. The leading Jewish practitioners of *Mussar*, the branch of rabbinical literature that focuses on self–perfection and correct behavior, over the centuries called it *tziurei halev*. They understood that the key to both our personalities and experiences lies in imagination.

The mind ultimately cannot differentiate between the neural holograms the brain uses to experience reality and the ones it conjures up while imagining reality. For the unconscious mind, there is no difference between an actual experience and a similar experience created solely by imagination.

Rabbi Dessler defined the practice of *Mussar* as returning knowledge into the heart. Stated another way, allowing the knowledge of the conscious mind to penetrate the subconscious achieved by use of the imagination. Vivid imagery combined with reflection can make a lasting impression.[8]

And indeed, Rabbi Eliyahu Lopian, one of the most prominent 20th century rabbis of the *Mussar* movement, agreed defining *Mussar* as "making the heart feel what the intellect understands."[9]

Guided Imagery is one of simplest and oldest techniques known for teaching people to use their mind's imagination via relaxation to create deep states which promote well–being by creating harmony between the mind, body and soul. It is a relaxation technique aimed at easing stress and promoting a sense of peace and tranquility at a stressful or difficult time in someone's life.

Under the right conditions of learning to relax, a person can discover ways to promote problem solving, let go of painful emotions stored in your body, and disengage those thoughts and beliefs that interfere with daily life. Dr. Martin Rossman, an author who raised awareness about the power of mind/body self–healing in the health professions, says, "Imagery is the language of the unconscious, and healing is an unconscious process."[10]

Many physicians have begun to put aside their skepticism and encourage the use of guided imagery to enhance their patient outcomes. Research has shown that guided imagery gives you the ability to lower levels of muscle tension; shift internal states and fine tune the immune system, strengthen your natural abilities to engage in your own healing process. Through guided imagery many disease states such as cancer can be fought and driven out of the body.

In the 1970s, Dr. O. Carl Simonton, chief of Radiation Therapy at Travis Air Force base in Fairfield, California at the time, and psychotherapist Stephanie Matthews–Simonton, devised a program—today known as the Simonton method—that utilizes guided imagery to help cancer patients. Patients picture their white blood cells attacking their cancer cells, sometimes in scenes that resembled the popular video game *Pac Man*. Simonton found that the more vivid the images his patients used the better the process worked.

Dr. Bernie Siegel helps his cancer patients remove their disease in a loving way, such as by visualizing God's light melting a tumor that appears as a block of ice.[11] The late Dr. Simonton said relaxation and mental imagery are among the most valuable tools found to help patients learn to believe in their ability to recover from cancer.[12]

I can personally attest to the truth of guide imagery use in cancer. Much to the disbelief of a young friend's surgeon, I helped her shrink her malignant breast tumors with guided imagery. Also, years ago an elderly friend underwent chemotherapy for her cancer. I worked with her prior to her treatments; visualization aimed at lessening pain and side effects. She remarked to me that everyone in the after–treatment room was sick and in pain. No one could understand how an old woman such as herself could just walk out symptomless.

Progressive muscle relaxation training and guided imagery were both associated with improvements in anticipatory and post–chemotherapy nausea and vomiting and in the quality of life of patients with breast cancer.[13] In a study reported in *Complementary Therapies Clinical Practice*, strategies like guided imagery and progressive muscle relaxation are useful in treating cancer pain for some patients. Many reported a clinically significant change in pain with the interventions.[14]

Dr. V.S. Ramachandran, Professor of Neurosciences at the University of California San Diego, explains that it seems extraordinary even to contemplate the possibility that you could use a visual illusion to eliminate pain. "Bear in mind," he says, "that pain itself is an illusion—constructed entirely in your brain like any other sensory experience."[15]

Mind–body imagery for 'meaning–making' as experienced in a study of Alaska breast cancer patients was a potent skill for supporting optimal patient recovery.[16] A pilot study showed that relaxation guided imagery is a promising treatment for Parkinson's disease.[17] The list seems endless.

In fact, Sigmund Freud once successfully used guided imagery to treat a 14 year old boy with a tic. And in all the twenty–five volumes of Freud's published writings, this was the only successfully completed treatment mentioned and also the only time he used imagery as a therapeutic technique.[18]

According to Dr. Herbert Benson, neurological research reveals that before we consciously color the world around us with our thinking and acquired beliefs, brain mechanisms marl our perceptions, forming opinions and assigning emotional values.

Before we even have a chance to mull over the presence of new sights or sounds, regions of our brain react by assigning an initial but influential value to it. These automatic attitudes, emotional blocks, make us incapable of utter objectivity or neutrality, in more profound ways than we've ever suspected.[19]

How does the brain develop these automatic attitudes? From the MIS–information acquired during our childhoods. To power automatic attitudes requires us to expend a tremendous amount of psychic–energy each day. Rabbi Dr. Twerski points out that our energies are not limitless. Whatever energies we expend keeping things bottled up in the subconscious mind are not available to us for other purposes.[20]

To interject sustainability in to our psyche; to correct the MIS–information in all aspects our lives, Dr. Bernie Siegel maintains guided imagery can help you do anything. He advises to use it to see yourself becoming the person you want to be and doing the things you want to do. This is a powerful way to give your body whatever it needs to be well.[21] Guided imagery is where we turn next.

BTW, the name of this chapter, Судьба, means destiny in Russian!

10

Inner Child

Inner child healing is the only way to empower ourselves to stop living life in reaction to the past.

Robert Burney

Inner child work has amazing healing potential.

Bernie S. Siegel, MD

I believe that the principles and techniques in inner child healing can have an important application in helping to ameliorate all illness and suffering.

Charles L. Whitfield, MD

The inner child holds the key to intimacy in relationships, physical energy, and well–being.

Lucia Capacchione, PhD

Then he grew quiet and not only ceased weeping but even held his breath and became all attention. It was as though he were listening not to an audible voice but to the voice of his soul, to the current of thoughts arising within him.

"What is it you want?" was the first clear conception capable of expression in words that he heard.

"What do you want? What do you want?" he repeated to himself.

"What do I want? To live and not to suffer," he answered.

And again he listened with such concentrated attention that even his pain did not distract him.

"To live? How?" asked his inner voice.

"Why, to live as I used to—well and pleasantly."

"As you lived before, well and pleasantly?" the voice repeated.

And in imagination he began to recall the best moments of his pleasant life. But strange to say none of those best moments of his pleasant life now seemed at all what they had then seemed—none of them except the first recollections of childhood. There, in childhood, there had been something really pleasant with which it would be possible to live if it could return. But the child who had experienced that happiness existed no longer; it was like a reminiscence of somebody else . . .

And the further he departed from childhood and the nearer he came to the present the more worthless and doubtful were the joys . . .

Latterly during the loneliness in which he found himself as he lay facing the back of the sofa, a loneliness in the midst of a populous town and surrounded by numerous acquaintances and relations but that yet could not have been more complete anywhere—either at the bottom of the sea or under the earth—that terrible loneliness Ivan Ilych had lived only in memories of the past. Pictures of his past rose before him one after another. They always began with what was nearest in time and then went back to what was most remote—to his childhood —and rested there. If he thought of the stewed prunes that had been offered him that day, his mind went back to the raw shriveled French plums of his childhood, their peculiar flavor and the flow of saliva when he sucked their stones, and along with the memory of that taste came a whole series of memories of those days: his nurse, his brother, and their toys . . .

Then again together with that chain of memories another series passed through his mind—of how his illness had progressed and grown worse. There also the further back he looked the more life there had been. There had been more of what was good in life and more of life itself . . .

Without a doubt, *The Death of Ivan Ilych*, written in 1886 by Lev Nikolayevich Tolstoy is one of the most profound existential stories ever put to paper. Ivan Ilych is everyman: *his life had been most simple and most ordinary and therefore most terrible . . . he was what he remained for the rest of his life: a capable, cheerful, good natured, and sociable man, though strict in the fulfillment of what he considered to be his duty. And he considered his duty to be what was so considered by those in authority.* Yet, in his final hours, racked by the pains of a disease that would defeat him, his only refuge were his childhood memories.

Rabbi Dr. Abraham Twerski in his book[1] *Generation to Generation: Personal Recollections of a Chassidic Legacy* tells the story of a patient, Morris, in his fifties who was battling the extreme pain of cancer reoccurrence after surgery. Understandably depressed, he lost his appetite. This former pillar of his community no longer went to his business or to his community meetings.

Morris had been referred to Rabbi Dr. Twerski in an attempt to ease his pain utilizing hypnosis. Efforts at pain reduction were unsuccessful, but Morris began relating an event from his childhood: riding a bike at 13, his bar mitzvah present, on a country road. Rabbi Dr. Twerski repeated the childhood regressions and soon Morris's appetite returned after an absence of many weeks and he started going to his office a few times a week.

He re–experienced many enjoyable events from his past; a loving grandfather who he would accompany to the synagogue on Friday night; boat rides and baseball games with his father; trips to Israel and family vacations. Most often were the long bike rides, alone or with friends. Childhood memories regained his life, giving him precious time instead of pain until he died peacefully.

Alfred Adler was an Austrian medical doctor, psychotherapist, and founder of the school of individual psychology. Adler said by looking back through childhood memories we are able to uncover the prototype—the core of the lifestyle—better than any other method.[2]

Dr. Kenneth Pelletier, a Clinical Professor of Medicine at the University of Arizona's College of Medicine, says the ability to reflect upon and consciously reconstruct an early life experience and thereby more fully comprehend it marks one of the most striking personal strategies in attaining optimal health. By this strategy we are able to contact the part of ourselves that some schools of psychotherapy refer to as the inner child. It is that aspect of our person that remains emotionally immature, in both the negative and positive aspects of immaturity, despite the fact that the body grows taller, ages, and becomes an adult.[3]

Everyone has within them an inner child. And if our nurturing process has been normal, our inner child develops and matures along with us through each stage of our life. We enjoy the agility of youth together while eventually sharing the morning pains and graying temples of middle age as we both drift into our golden years. That's if our childhood was normal.

But if, on the other hand, our developmental years were trapped within the confines of a shamed dysfunctional life, our inner child's growth is stifled; a flower that never blooms. As a result, while we grow biologically in years, our inner child is left behind. A spell is cast, dooming our inner child to remain forever a child; a hostage within us, as Nobel laureate Doris Lessing titled her 1987 book, *Prisons We Choose to Live Inside*. And it is the inner child's eternal struggle to be free that scripts the tragic events of the lives we live.

No matter how dysfunctional your childhood might have been, you have the free will to choose whether you respond to life as your inner child or as an adult should. It is possible to actually contact, reclaim and nurture your inner child, discover its needs and in effect reparent it, reintegrating you and your inner child as a whole.

John Bradshaw, author, counselor, theologian, who popularized such ideas as the wounded inner child and the dysfunctional family, says in order to reconnect with the wounded and hurt child, we have to go back and re–experience the emotions that were blocked.[4]

Reclaiming your inner child involves going back through your developmental stages and finishing your unfinished business.[5] Three things are striking about inner child work Bradshaw concludes: the speed with which people change, the depth of that change, and the power and creativity that results.

Alice Miller was a Swiss psychologist noted for her books on parental child abuse. She wrote that every childhood's adverse experiences remain hidden and locked in darkness and the key to our understanding of the life that follows is hidden away with them.[6] If we identify our overwhelming childhood experiences and become comfortable with them, we can remain more rational and loving in face of adult stresses.[7]

According to Rabbi Joseph Soloveitchik, some people lose their inner child as they mature. They stop dreaming and hoping, becoming very practical, pragmatic, and utilitarian. But in some people, no matter how mature they are, a little boy remains. From time to time, the old man somehow retraces his steps and turns into a little boy, a dreamer with imagination, who searches around the corner for a miracle.[8]

In my opinion, Rabbi Soloveitchik also teaches a very forceful lesson on the potentials of a person with an intact inner child. Commenting on the Biblical verse, *these are the lives of Sarah*,[9] he explains, "that Sarah at twenty was mature and fully developed both intellectually and emotionally. The adult in Sarah did not destroy the child. Maturity did not do away with childhood. And in the deep recesses of her personality always resided an innocent child. Abraham, like Sarah, was a child all his life."[10] Sarah and Abraham never lost touch with their inner child which, I believe, enabled them to give birth to monotheism to the betterment of humanity.

Inner child healing is a psychological tool based on the idea that however grown up you imagine you are, there exists within you a part that is completely innocent and childlike. Your inner child's learned responses to events in your life set the subconscious patterns that follow you each day. If developmentally your inner child could not understand these events, then it probably misinterpreted the meanings, creating MIS–information. Some events could have been beyond your inner child's capability to render any interpretation at all.

Jean Piaget was a Swiss developmental psychologist known for his epistemological studies with children. Piaget explained when the child has forgotten something or understood it imperfectly he fills in the gap by inventing in all good faith. If he is questioned on what he has heard he stops inventing, but left alone will believe the inventions he has made up. Romancing or conscious and deliberate invention is thus connected with an unconscious distortion of the facts by a whole chain of intervening stages.[11]

The more wounded the selfhood, the more the protective side of our subconscious must take over and make choices that are based solely on the immediate protection of selfhood of the person.[12] And if you think that you have put all that behind you, that is called suppression; a conscious act on your part in contrast to repression which in unconscious.

However you define it, the net result is the same. Outwardly you still are able to function but until these issues are resolved, you will never find it possible to be completely at peace with yourself. Defenses that were erected by the vulnerable child to protect him or herself against toxic environments may become more detrimental than the original trauma.[13]

Most people are content to stay the same. "After all, life's been good. I have no old wounds to open anyway. I had a loving childhood." The Roman poet Horace rhetorically asked: "why do you hasten to remove anything which hurts your eye while if something affects your soul you postpone the cure until next year?"

M. Scott Peck was an American psychiatrist and best-selling author of the book, *The Road Less Traveled*. Among the myriad of lies people often tell themselves, Peck says, two of the most common, potent and destructive are "We really loved our children" and "Our parents really loved us."[14]

"Mothers may love their children," Nancy Friday, an author who writes on the topics of female sexuality and liberation, says, "but they sometimes do not like them. The same woman who may be willing to put her body between her child and a runaway truck will often resent the day-to-day sacrifice the child unknowingly demands of her time, sexuality and self-development.[15] Our job as adults is to understand the past, learn its lessons, and then let it go. Blaming mother is just a negative way of clinging to her still."[16] The same applies to fathers.

Inner child work gives a new adult perspective with which you can learn to reevaluate those unresolved or repressed events of your life and finally put them away where they will cause no difficulty. The amazing thing about inner child work is that you don't have to embark on a psychoanalytic archeological expedition. Once you have dealt with some of these events, the others seem to fall into their place like dominoes. If you don't, then stress, anger, addiction, compulsive behavior, co–dependency, cancer, heart disease, apathy, depression, shame, loneliness, emotional imprisonment will haunt your life.

But these are not the only problems. The numbing caused by childhood MIS–information prevents very crucial spiritual growth. The inner child is the part of you that is most closely linked to God, as we saw with Abraham and Sarah. Inner child work can help lead you to an immediate, personal relationship with God, in a theistic sense; the deepest healing of all!

The time I spent in Jerusalem working for the Jewish outreach organization enabled me to avail myself of many outstanding lectures from some of Judaism's greatest rabbis. One such event was the weekly lecture lead by the late Rabbi Shlomo Wolbe, a multifaceted 20th century rabbi and author of the modern *Mussar* classic, *Alei Shur.*

Anticipating Freud, *Mussar's* philosophy of self–perfection, behavior, personality and character trait correction believed the subconscious mind has to be moved by severe introspection before ethical and religious conduct become second nature.

An element of one of Rabbi Wolbe's talks[17] illustrates the benefit of *Mussar's* inner work:

Let me return to the subject we have been speaking about: your internal world. There is no doubt that the whole world today looks only at external appearances. This is the case not only for the general population as a whole, but also for individuals. Every individual points themselves totally externally, reading, searching, and trying to find out what is going on outside them.

If you were connected to your internal world you would be happy to find yourself alone for a half hour. You would think about yourself and where you are in life, you would think about your good and bad qualities and what has to be fixed, and you would think about how you live your life and fulfill the commandments. You would do an accounting of your soul.

You could reach a deeper recognition of yourself and discover your real duties in life. Even more than that, you might draw yourself closer to spirituality, to God, and to love of every other person during that one half hour. You could accomplish all those things in one half hour.

The inner child is the ultimate connection to your internal world. Rabbi Svirsky's program qualified us to help others connect with their inner child. Remember his philosophy is that you can only take another person as far as you have been yourself. The sessions we had during our training were always in a group. But when we started exploring our internal world, opening up our unconscious, displaying it publically the first time without an initial period of time for own personal digestion, attrition started to take its toll.

As only Mark Twain can put it, "everyone is a moon and has a dark side which he never shows to anybody." Those of us who remained I feel fully understood a statement I read many years ago by Carl Jung, a prolific writer and Swiss psychiatrist who founded analytical psychology, in his book *Memories, Dreams, Reflections*. "As far as we can discern, the sole purpose of human existence is to kindle a light in the darkness of mere being."

Alice Miller writes that you do not need a regular therapist to do inner child work. You need an enlightened witness; someone who does not regard the emotions of an adult as haphazard but sees them as the logical fruits, sometimes poisonous fruits, of a misguided process of insemination.[18]

Enlightened witnesses have the courage to face up to their own histories and thereby to gain their own autonomy rather than seeing to offset their own repressed feelings of ineffectuality by exercising power over their patients.[19] With the help of an enlightened witness, our early emotions will stand revealed, take on meaning for us, and hence be available for us to work on.[20]

"Perhaps wounded healers are effective because they are more able to empathize with wounds of the patient," Irving Yalom, an American existential psychiatrist and emeritus professor of psychiatry at Stanford University says, "perhaps it is because they participate more deeply and personally in the healing process."[21]

A famous parable given by the 19th century Chassidic master, Rabbi Chaim of Sanz personifies a wounded healer. The Nobel Laureate S. Y. Agnon[22] tells the following version of the parable:

> A man had been walking about in a forest for several days, not knowing the right way out. Suddenly he saw a man approaching him. His heart was filled with joy. "Now I shall certainly find out which is the right way," he thought to himself. When they neared one another, he asked the man, "Brother, tell me which is the right way. I have been wandering about in this forest for several days." Said the other to him, "Brother, I do not know the way out either. For I too have been wandering about here for many, many days. But this I can tell you: do not take the way I have been taking, for that will lead you astray. And now let us look for a new way together."

Up close and personal. A few years prior to my angioplasty, a social worker recommended to gain insight in the lives of my sons, I read a book, *I Don't Want to Talk About It: Overcoming the Secret Legacy of Male Depression* by Terrence Real, a contemporary psychotherapist specializing in men's issues, mainly depression and relationships. I

113

read the book twice, but I confessed I did not see my sons anywhere in the book. I re–read the book a third time after my experiences with Rabbi Svirsky and finally realized it wasn't my sons the social worker had seen in the book; it was me.

By the time I read the following passage, I had already learned the hard way what it took to turn a wounded man into a wounded healer and in turn a healed father. Real wrote:

> A depressed man's tendency to exude pain often does more than simply impede his capacity for intimacy. It may render him psychologically dangerous. Too often, the wounded boy grows up to be a wounded man, inflicting upon those closest to him the very distress he refuses to acknowledge within himself. Depression in men, unless it is dealt with tends to be passed on.[23]

Allow me to describe my first encounter with my inner child. Our first chanced meeting came after having achieved a state of focused awareness during deep relaxation early on in Rabbi Svirsky's training. Since that time, we have spent many enlightened moments renewing our acquaintance, together flipping the pages of my childhood memory. And so too are the times we've considered the crossings our paths have taken during my lifetime and the tolls they exacted on my relationships.

One of the crucial discoveries in inner child work is the self–recognition that we suffer from psychic numbing. The suppressions our inner child is forced to make for his survival effectively dislocate our ability to feel. In psychiatry this lack of feeling is referred to as alexithymia. While readily shedding tears at end of sad movies, griping novels and life's beautiful moments, we fail to see these are merely expressions of emotions.

Feelings are not emotions. And unless we unshackle our feelings, we will forever remain frozen by their control. When we become distanced from our feelings, a lot of valuable information about what is taking place in your current life is lost; replaced by MIS–information.

While my father lay dying in a hospital from the complications of a successful operation, I stood by his side till the end. A well–like popular man, a steady stream of visitors entered his room offering my mother and me their comforting prayers. Stoically I handed out tissues while explaining the latest futile attempts to prolong his life. Everyone to a man commented how bravely I was taking it and the strength I exhibited.

Looking back, I had no courage, being depressingly numb to my surroundings. Like the story of the *Emperor's New Clothes*, I awaited my inner child to scream, "Look at the King! Look at the King!" But the King remained silent and the reality of my father dying set in only after it was already too late. No wonder many years later I was still in desperate need of closure. And the totality of my life's events, were they any less in need of closure?

But how does one so numb begin to feel? Inner child work is appropriately called grief therapy. Resolution requires release and without grief there can be no release. Until we agonize over the loss of what our childhoods could have been, start shedding the tears of innocence stored within our very souls, and recognize the unintended tragic realities our caregivers used to nurture us, our inner child will never set our feelings free.

As I slowly concentrated on my breathing, Rabbi Svirsky had me focus on the areas of my body that were beginning to relax. He brought me into my parent's living room. About age five, I stood alone in the empty room. On one wall hung my aunt's Venetian needlepoint; on another was the faded print of a nymph streaking through a white wood. And before me was our recently upholstered couch, a victorious trophy of my mother's inner child.

Rabbi Svirsky asked what feelings I sensed about the room. A fight had just taken place, I said. "Was I sure?" he prompted. "Yes," I assured him. Like the heaviness of the air at a battlefield, I felt the lingering of my parents. I went further back, just a few moments, until I was there in the room while my parents acted out the tattered script that had been their life.

"I'm curious," Rabbi Svirsky asked, "how do you feel at this moment?"

"I feel like I don't exist; that I don't matter to anyone. They are screaming at each other and they don't see I'm in the room. Or do they even care? How could they act like that in front of me? Don't they realize how it makes me feel?"

"Tell them that," he encouraged. "You're there now. Say what you want to say."

At that moment my inner child and I were united, gleaning mutual strength. "STOP!" I yelled. All the might in that one word unleashed itself as silence fell upon that room. Then slowly both my parents took notice of me. I still cannot get over the feeling at seeing them so young. My mother wore a cream dress with printed roses and an appropriate amount of red lipstick for the times.

Looking at my father, I realized it was a Saturday afternoon. He wore no shirt, his chest displaying a clipper ship tattoo he'd gotten when his inner child ran away to sail the seas.

"How can you fight like this?" I asked. My father smirked, saying that my friend's parents fight as well. He had been drinking; my father's self–prescription for treating chronic covert depression.

"That's supposed to make me feel better? I don't care about anyone else but us," I answered.

I could see the alcohol had already bleached my father's blue eyes, but I struck a chord in my mother. She just stared, as if she was unable to recognize me. Or was it disbelief at what I had said?

In that room, the center of my inner child's world, I explained the damaging effects of their years of disagreements, fights and dysfunctional traumas. The story would have been tragic enough had it stopped there, I said, but it didn't. The same one act plays they had rehearsed and performed in my childhood had been revived for yet another seasons run with my own children. My father was numb, but my mother cried.

There I stood, a hybrid personality of me and my inner child, shielding myself from their pleas of ignorance. The fact that if they had known, then things would have been different brought no comfort to me. Then they fell, my first tears of grief.

I told Rabbi Svirsky I cried for my childhood that had died before it lived. I should have had a different childhood; I cried for that. I felt sorry for my mother having to feel what she now felt, but I was empowered by the strength it had given me. And my father just sat stagnant; a man who never realized he really did indeed make it in life, having died waiting for someone to shout for him, "Look at the King!"

11

Reframing

If a problem can't be solved within the frame it was conceived, the solution lies in reframing the problem.

Brian McGreevy

For any single thing of importance, there are multiple reasons.

M. Scott Peck

My life has been filled with terrible misfortunes, most of which have never happened.

Mark Twain

The real voyage of discovery consists not in seeking new landscapes, but in having new eyes.

Marcel Proust

In the *Preface* I mentioned my research entailed reading a thousand peer–reviewed articles. Of all the articles, one stood out as the mother of paradigm shifts for health: The 'Adverse Childhood Experiences and Risk Premature Mortality Study' which was published in the *American Journal of Preventive Medicine*.[1]

Until I read that study, I thought that the Fetal Origins–Baker Hypothesis was the groundbreaking shift for me which encouraged my adding Stage 0—Prenatal to Erickson's *Eight Ages of Man*. David Baker said of his theory that the old model of adult degenerative disease was based on the interaction between genes and an adverse environment in adult life. The new model that is developing will

include programming by the environment in fetal and infant life."[2]
Psychological events in the mother can change the physical
structure of the fetus she is carrying in her womb.[3]

Fetal Origins studies, as I mentioned earlier, confirmed adult
lifestyles factors that are influenced by prenatal nutrition:

> contribute to more atherogenic lipid profiles in later life;[4]
> intrauterine environment influences the subsequent development of
> adult diseases;[5] intrauterine origin of communicable diseases;[6] fetal
> undernutrition programs later coronary heart disease;[7] intrauterine
> growth restriction is associated with an increased propensity to
> develop adult onset disease;[8] exposure to Holocaust conditions in
> early life may be associated with a higher level of obesity,
> dyslipidemia, diabetes, hypertension, cardiovascular morbidity,
> malignancy and peptic diseases in adulthood;[9] adverse programming
> of the ovary, breast and prostate gland [at the time of] fetal
> development can increase the risk of cancer of these tissues later in
> life.[10]

The 'Adverse Childhood Experiences (ACE) and Risk of Premature
Mortality Study'[11] was collaborative effort of the Centers of Disease
Control (CDC) in Atlanta and Kaiser Permanente's San Diego
Health Appraisal Clinic which served an adult population of more
than 50,000. All health plan members who completed a standard
medical exam in two time periods during 1995–1996 were mailed a
health behavior and ACE questionnaire. The overall response rate
was 68%.

The study found that adverse childhood experiences, ACE, *are
associated with an increased risk of premature death.* Now before you jump
to the conclusion that sure, the study was probably conducted in an
inner city ghetto, the questionnaire non–respondents were generally
younger, nonwhite and less educated. In fact, 75% who responded
were white and college educated while 80% stated they had no
current problems with finances.

Reframing

The study looked at two areas of ACE occurring during the first 18 years of life: *childhood abuse* comprising emotional, physical, sexual abuse and *household dysfunction* broken down in five categories: substance abuse, mental illness, domestic violence, incarceration and paternal separation or divorce.

Questions of emotional abuse were focused on how often parents or other adults in the house swear at you, insult you, put you down, or act in a way that made you afraid that you might be physically harmed.

Physical abuse concerned the frequency you were pushed, grabbed, slapped, had something thrown at you or if you were hit so hard that you had marks or were injured. I'll leave to your imagination the graphic questions about sexual abuse. Household dysfunctional questions concentrated on if household members were problem drinkers, alcoholics, street drug users, mentally ill, jailed, separated or divorced, and if mothers were treated violently.

An ACE score was given reflecting how many positive answers you gave in each of the eight categories. Of the respondents age 65 or below, 60.1% had at least one positive answer in the eight categories. 26.8% had an ACE score of 3–8. The higher the ace score the more likely you were to develop one of the five leading causes of death. Respondents who had an ACE score of six or more were likely *to die nearly 20 years earlier* on average than those with a 0 ACE score.

The study's conclusion was that adverse childhood experiences are common and these health consequences are often hidden from clinicians and health professionals. To me it is sad that so much in the way of preventive medicine has been sacrificed to achieve the 12 minute patient encounter. What if all intake forms doctors and hospitals used included ACE questions? ACE could give a wealth of information to assist medical practitioners assessing potential health problems.

The doctor is at a disadvantage, Dr. Arthur Janov, an American psychotherapist and the creator of Primal Therapy, writes he can see hypertension before him. What he cannot see is a six–month–old infant crying it out in a crib, all terrified, nor a child of five all bottled up by critical, tyrannical parents. [12]

In my opinion the ACE score is probably more valuable than knowing a genotype. Genes don't cause anything unless acted on by an environment that flips their epigenetic switch. However, adverse childhood experiences wreak constant havoc in our lives!

Based on my experience working with people during my association with Rabbi Svirsky and the information I have gleaned over the past few years, I think that both theories, Fetal Origins–Baker Hypothesis and Adverse Childhood Experiences have common ground. Maternal nutrition and fetal weights are not the only prenatal influences on illness later in adult life.

Adverse childhood experiences affect our health not only after we are born, but in utero as well. Dr. Stanislav Goff, a psychiatrist and one of the founders of the field of transpersonal psychology, says that reports of embryonic and fetal experiences suggest that it is possible to experience not only gross disturbances during this period, but also mother's feelings: her emotional shocks, her anxiety attacks, her outbursts of hate or aggression, her depression, her sexual arousal, as well as her feelings of relaxation, satisfaction, happiness and love. [13]

Feelings are absorbed from the mother and the father and the unborn child cannot distinguish between feelings directed toward him and feelings directed towards others. [14] Babies can form memories before birth; babies do carry memories out of the womb that last for weeks, if not longer. Though these earlier memories are inaccessible to conscious recall, they undoubtedly influence the way babies perceive and react to the world after birth, and thereby shape much of the important learning that takes place in the early months of life. [15]

Reframing

Even the skeptics' skeptic, the late Carl Sagan wrote, "At age three, my son Nicholas was asked for his earliest event he could recall and replied in a hushed tone while staring into a middle distance, "it was red, and I was very cold." He was born by Caesarean section. It is probably unlikely, but I wonder whether this could just possibly be a true birth memory."[16]

My inner child work with people also included taking clients back before birth to experience memories of the womb. Many times my request to go back to the earliest memory preceded birth. Whether in utero or at the age of five, I was able to help my clients reframe their childhood memories.

The Talmud relates the following story:

Once there was an incidence involving a certain man who traveled from the upper Galilee to work for someone in the south for three years. On the eve of Yom Kippur, the man sought to travel home. He said to his employer, "Give me my wages so I can go and provide for my wife and children." His employer confessed, "I have no money." The man offered an alternative. "Give me produce and I will sell it."

Again the employer said, "I have none." Back and forth they parried. "Give me land." "…I have none." "…give me pillows and cushions." "…I have none." Seeing that there was no resolution in sight, the man slung his personal effects over his shoulder and returned home crestfallen.

After the festival, the employer took the man's wages in his hand along with three donkeys laden with various sweet delicacies and traveled north to the man's home. After they had dined, he paid the man his wages. Curious, the employer asked, "When you said give me my wages and I answered I have no money, what did think?"

"I thought perhaps underpriced goods came your way and you used my wages to buy them." "When you said to me give me livestock and I said to you I have none, what did you think?" "Maybe you did have livestock but they were leased to others at the time."

"And when I said to you I have no produce?" "I thought you had not yet taken the Biblical tithe."

Finally he asked, "And when I said I have no pillows or cushions?" "I thought maybe you had consecrated all your wealth to Heaven." The employer shouted, "All of what you suspected of me was true!" [17]

Changing contexts generates imagination and creativity as well as new energy. When applied to problem solving, it is often called reframing.[18] Reframing is a way of changing the frame in which a person perceives events in order to change meaning.[19] Reframing challenges the mind, opening the way to let go of old conditioning so that we can wake up to the moment.[20] Reframing is a specific way of contacting the portion or part—for lack of a better word—of the person that is causing a certain behavior to occur, or that is preventing a certain other behavior from occurring.[21]

In order to recover your health, peace of mind, and effectiveness, you need to inquire into your own past history, learn to reframe it, and then look at it in a new more realistic way.[22] Reframing helps to reinterpret and to restructure life events with an adult perception.[23]

Reframing is the treatment of choice for *any* psychosomatic symptom.[24] The reframing format differs radically from the usual techniques in psychotherapy, because in this format the therapist is merely a consultant [an enlightened witness]; the client is actually her own therapist and she takes responsibility for accessing and eliciting her own responses.[25]

An article that appeared in the *Journal of Pain Research* brings to light the effectiveness of reframing in resolving the MIS–information and treatment of PTSD:

Up to 80% of patients with severe posttraumatic stress disorder are suffering from "unexplained" chronic pain. Pain disorders in traumatized persons often have in common that they are not sufficiently explained by a structural somatic injury. This fact could mislead an observer to rush to the conclusion that the pain reported by a patient is of "virtual" origin. In order to be able to understand this type of pain disorder, one must differentiate between the somatic injury that triggers pain and the neuroperceptive process of perceiving pain. [26]

"We consider that the psychotherapeutically desirable step of reframing is strongly supported by our model," the study said. "For patients, it is therapeutically very meaningful to conceive trauma–associated sequelae as a 'normal' reaction to an extremely 'abnormal' event. If a patient arrives at an understanding that their situation is not the result of personal failure but is rather an expected consequence of excessive auto–protective strategies of the nervous system, this can open the way to a vital reassessment of their suffering."

Without a doubt based on my experience working with people, reframing a childhood memory can create a new history, giving the unconscious an adult frame of reference upon which to act. I have seen the results in the people I have helped. I have seen the difference in myself.

After meeting my inner child with Rabbi Svirsky, I started carrying a first grade picture of me in my shirt pocket. For nearly two years before I reacted to my wife, my children, my boss, my coworkers or the many people in the streets that cluttered my day, I would take out the photo and looking at it, would decide if my response was going to be his or mine with my newly gained adult perspective.

Using the magic of guided imagery I have helped people reframe the MIS–informed feelings that occur in their lives: love, hate, hurt, anger, happiness, sadness, fear and abandonment; reframing the loss of a loved one to achieve closure. I know that reframing these feelings promote health.

When my friend ten years ago said I was the only one he knew that had a serious medical problem and consistently did anything about it, reframing was the reason. I spent the needed amount of time going back through my childhood, reliving, rescripting and reframing my experiences until I had reparented parity with my inner child. *That is the difference that makes a difference.* And if you desire good health–*gizunt*–reframing your past can make the difference in your life as well. *It is never too late to have a happy childhood!*

Up close and personal. The next chapter will I assure provide an in depth understanding of inner child work, the effects of reframing and how I came to set my goal not only achieving good health–*gizunt*, but really wanting to live until 120. The chapter consists only of an unedited transcript between Rabbi Svirsky and me in one of our critical sessions.

But before then I want to end this chapter with sharing my own understanding of how the therapeutic process of healing should occur. Abraham Maslow was an American psychologist best known for creating a hierarchy of fulfilling innate human needs in priority. Probably his most famous saying was "if all you have in your tool box is a hammer; then you tend to treat everything as a nail." My view is not based on any particular school of therapy basically because my training was not specific; rather it was eclectic.

My forte is writing fiction. To conclude, I dip my quill and offer you my outlook on good therapy:

What makes this case study interesting is the universal nature of the life experiences of the client. Even before the client was born his life was already being influenced. Birth and prenatal experiences help form the foundations of human personality. Everything we become or hope to become, our relationships with ourselves, our parents, our families and our friends, are influenced by what happens to us during these two critical periods.

Reframing

Prior to Dumbo T. Elephant's birth, his mother, Mrs. Jumbo, was not very happy. All the other circus animals had given birth to their offspring. One can only imagine how Mrs. Jumbo felt as she watched the others. Feelings are absorbed from the mother; the unborn child cannot distinguish between feelings directed towards him and feeling directed toward others.

Unfortunately, Dumbo was born with an abnormality: his rather large ears. Despite Mrs. Jumbo's sheltering him from the cruelty of adolescence, Dumbo's self–esteem suffered greatly. Shamed, Dumbo knew no other world. Large ears were normal to his life; he vainly tried to understand the ridicule he received.

Then one day Dumbo's childhood reached its tragic turning point. As the band played a child pointed and laughed at Dumbo's big ears. Firmly entrenched within his defense mechanisms, Dumbo tried to take the child's comments in stride, but suddenly Dumbo stumbled. First he stepped on his right ear, then on his left ear and finally he fell flat on his face. All the children laughed. Then the boy shouted, "What a clumsy elephant!"

Mrs. Jumbo finally reached her tipping point. She picked up the boy with her trunk while he screamed for help. The keeper chained Mrs. Jumbo's leg and led her away to a small cage. "Don't take her away," cried Dumbo. "It was all . . . my . . . fault!"

Abandoned, full of self–pity and shame, Dumbo soon reached a state where he was confused about who he really was. Desperately trying to fit in anywhere life's regularity would shelter him; he got a job as a clown. Dumbo's performance was terrific. "Hooray!" shouted the clowns. "You were wonderful!"

But the damage to his self–esteem had taken its toll. Dumbo didn't feel wonderful. He missed his mother and he didn't want to be a clown. Dumbo had reached bottom. When the need arises, a solution appears. The next day Timothy, the circus mouse, found Dumbo looking sad.

"Don't be unhappy," he said. "I will be your friend. I will find a way to help you!" Timothy knew the value of friendship. He attached himself to Dumbo by esteem, respect and affection and listened empathically as he poured his heart out. Timothy's being empathic communicated to Dumbo that he was not alone. And feeling understood, people often explore themselves more deeply. Even a schizophrenic ceases to be schizophrenic when he meets someone by whom he feels valued.

Above all Timothy was genuine, not a phony playing a role. He was warm to Dumbo, showing his concern and caring by his compassionate tone of voice and sympathetic looks. At a crucial time in their conversation, Timothy shared his own personal feelings and experiences with Dumbo on how he felt growing up so short in such a tall world.

Timothy appreciated the value of feeling safe and secure when dealing with traumatic experiences. He took benefit of the proximity of the woods where he and Dumbo sat working out a solution to his problems. Timothy progressively relaxed the muscles in Dumbo's body. For Timothy also understood the effect the relaxation response has on people's healing ability, both physical and mental.

When Dumbo was relaxed enough, Timothy used the magic of guided imagery to conduct Dumbo to a time where he and his family were back on the Serengeti, away from the circus. Dumbo frolicked with his mother and father; gone were the worries of the day. The best of life was now to enjoy. A refreshed, reframed Dumbo slowly withdrew from his relaxed state.

"Those big ears must be good for something!" Timothy laughed. Attitude is probably the most important aspect in problem solving; our perceptions of the events in our lives are more important than the event itself. And when we are no longer able to alter a situation, we are challenged to change ourselves.

"Maybe I can teach you to fly with them!" Timothy was a master at the art of reframing: the ability to put commonplace situations in new frames that are more useful. Dumbo flapped his ears hard, jumped and fell flat on the ground. "I'll never be able to fly." Clever Timothy decided that until Dumbo's self–confidence was restored, he would rely on the power of the placebo effect. He gave Dumbo a magic feather. And suddenly Dumbo was flying!

At a later time when Timothy felt Dumbo was ready, he revealed to him that he no longer needed the magic feather. "The magic was always within you, Dumbo," Timothy explained. "You only needed to recognize your own strengths and abilities." Timothy had given Dumbo the force of presence and vibrancy that emanates from self–confidence and self–efficacy.

We all know the rest of the story. "I knew you would be a star someday," Mrs. Jumbo cried. "Yes, but I couldn't have done it without my friend, Timothy," said Dumbo. Timothy just smiled!

12

Catharsis

Catharsis is the purification of emotions through art or any extreme change in emotion that results in a spiritual renewal and restoration.

Wikipedia

One ought to write when one leaves a piece of one's own flesh in the ink pot each time one dips one's pen.

Leo Tolstoy

Every man has reminiscences which he would not tell to everyone but only to his friends. He has other matters in his mind which he would not reveal even to his friends, but only to himself in secret. But there are other things which a man is afraid to tell even to himself, and every decent man has a number of such things stored away in his mind.

Fyodor Dostoevsky

Session Transcript

After a few minutes of progressive muscular relaxation, the session begins.

R. *Svirsky:* Where do you feel God's Presence? Where do you feel it inside of you? How do you feel it inside of you right now? Say, "I feel as if . . . I feel like . . ." Describe it.

Uri: I feel like I have a pain in here in my—stomach.

R. *Svirsky:* I understand. But when you think about God being here—

131

Uri: I feel like I'm connecting. I feel good. I feel like a relationship with God.

R. Svirsky: Good. Where is this good feeling most in the body?

Uri: Every place but my stomach.

R. Svirsky: Ok. You said you feel pain in the stomach. So talk to this part now. What is it? "What are you?" Just ask the pain, "Why are you there?"

Uri: "Why are you there?"

R. Svirsky: Let this pain speak to you.

Uri: I'm not getting an answer.

R. Svirsky: Ok . . . Very nice. So ask yourself, "Where am I blocking the answer?"

Uri: The pain is getting bigger. It's going up to here now in my chest.

R. Svirsky: Right. So ask this part, "Why are you blocking the answer?"

Uri: "Why are you blocking the answer?"

R. Svirsky: And what does it say?

Uri: It says it's blocking to protect me.

R. Svirsky: Yes . . . Of course. So ask the block, what would happen if you're not going to block. Just ask it, "What are you protecting me from?

Uri: "What are you protecting me from?"

R. Svirsky: Right. What does he say?

Uri: I don't think he wants to tell me.

R. Svirsky: Of course, what would happen if it told you?

Uri: I guess I'd be able to challenge it.

R. Svirsky: Right. So tell it, "We're not going to remove anything we need." Or, "We're not going to remove anything without giving you something better." Just calm it down...did you tell it to this part? Say it. Say, "I have the right to know." Would you like to know why you have pain in the stomach? So tell it. Say it out loud so I can also hear.

Uri: "What are you, pain in my stomach?"

R. Svirsky: Right. So what's the answer?

Uri: No answer. It just intensified.

R. Svirsky: So ask this part, the block; did it accept what you just said?

Uri: No. It's fighting back.

R. Svirsky: What is it saying to you? How is it fighting back?

Uri: It's fighting back by the pain . . . Almost like I can see a face that's refusing to talk to me. That's ignoring me . . . Giving me pain.

R. Svirsky: Right. That's some part of you that's pretending to ignore you and give you pain. So ask it, "For some reason it's important for you to . . ." What? Ask it.

Uri: "For some reason it's important for you to act like this. Why?"

R. Svirsky: Ok. What does it say?

Uri: It just won't talk to me.

R. Svirsky: So you won't talk to yourself, right? So ask it, "Why won't you talk to me?" See . . . this part cannot not talk to you. There is another block that's not allowing you to get it, because this is part of you. And the parts have to listen to you, to what you say. So say, "Where's an additional block that allows it to act independently."

Uri: "Where's another block like this?" I feel like tightness in the back of my neck.

R. Svirsky: Very good. So talk to the back of the neck. Ask, "what are you?'

Uri: "What are you?"

R. Svirsky: What's the tightness say?

Uri: I feel like a hand pinching me.

R. Svirsky: Right. So ask the hand, "What are you?"

Uri: "Why are you pinching me?"

R. Svirsky: What does it say?

Uri: An image of my mother's coming up, that's all.

R. Svirsky: Right. Ok—Very good. So ask yourself, "What does it have to do with my mother." Just ask.

Uri: "What does it have to do with my mother?"

R. Svirsky: From this image comes the answer.

Uri: I don't have an answer. I just see the image of my mother more.

R. Svirsky: So look at your mother. What kind of emotions this image evokes?

Uri: Without emotions.

R. Svirsky: So talk to her. Say, "What do you have to do with the tension in the back of my neck?"

Uri: "What do you have to do with the tension in the back of my neck?"

R. Svirsky: All right. So be the mother . . .

Uri: A thought popped in my mind that's, I guess from my mother, that she wants to make sure I do the right thing.

R. Svirsky: What does it mean to do the right thing, when it comes from your mother?

Uri: I don't know. She was always saying things like that.

R. Svirsky: Right. Saying, "You should do the right thing?" So tell her the right thing is to find out...

Uri: "The right thing is to find out why I'm having this block."

R. Svirsky: Okay. What's happening with the tension in the neck?

Uri: I don't have the tension in the neck, but my stomach's intensifying again. I feel like it's running away back down to my stomach because I'm starting to get somewhere.

R. Svirsky: Yes . . . Of course. So say, "What would happen if I would find out what this tension and pain is all about? What would happen?"

Uri: "What would happen if I found out about this tension and pain? What is it afraid of? . . . That I wouldn't need it anymore.

R. Svirsky: Say, "But you're part of me . . ." Talk to this part.

Uri: "You're part of me."

R. Svirsky: Right. "I need all my parts."

Uri: "I need all my parts."

R. Svirsky: "That means you will change, but I will still need you."

Uri: That means you will change, but I will still need you . . . Now I feel the pain in the back of my neck again.

R. Svirsky: All right. So talk to the pain in the back of the neck. Say, "Why are you there?"

Uri: Why are you there? . . .

R. Svirsky: Ok. What's happening?

Uri: Doesn't answer.

R. Svirsky: Ok. So where's the block of this block?

Uri: It's like its playing games with me.

R. Svirsky: So it's like you're playing games with yourself. Say, "I'm playing games with myself."

Uri: "I'm playing games with myself," because it went from my stomach to the back of my neck, and now I feel it here, in the chest.

R. Svirsky: All right. So talk to the chest.

Uri: I'm not getting anywhere.

R. Svirsky: So ask the chest. Say, "Why are you allowing all these things to happen?"

Uri: Why are you allowing all these things to happen? . . .

R. Svirsky: What does the chest say?

Uri: "Because I'm scared."

R. Svirsky: Ask the block what kind of fear that is in the chest.

Uri: "I don't want to find out why I have these blocks."

R. Svirsky: Ask the chest, "What do you think will happen if you find out why?"

Uri: What do you think will happen if you find out why? . . .

R. Svirsky: What's the chest say?

Uri: "I'm afraid to think of what would happen if I don't have them."

R. Svirsky: So what's this? Are you too much used to those things?"

Uri: Yeah. I feel that I feel comfortable now.

R. Svirsky: Yeah. What's this part that feels comfortable now? Say, "Tell me about yourself." Ask this part.

Uri: I don't get hurt . . . I don't feel pain . . . So if they all go away, then I'll feel hurt and pain.

R. Svirsky: Uh huh . . . Okay. So talk to the chest more. Find out about this. How old is this part? Say, "How old are you?"

Uri: How old are you? . . . I just felt like I was 13 years old. Nothing specific, but I just feel like I'm 13.

R. Svirsky: What's going on with this 13–year old? Ask him, "What is it that hurts you. Or what is it that did hurt you?"

Uri: What is it that hurt you? . . . I'm younger. Maybe like 10. Yeah.

R. Svirsky: And what's happening there?

Uri: My mother left the house. She ran away.

R. Svirsky: Why is that? Did she have some problems with the father?

Uri: Yeah. She said she was leaving and just disappeared.

R. Svirsky: How did the 10–year old feel?

Uri: He didn't feel.

R. Svirsky: Ok. How did you manage not to feel?

Uri: Maybe in a way I was glad.

R. Svirsky: Why were you glad?

Uri: I think it had more to do with the fact that I could wrap my father around my finger and get things I wanted now that my mother was out of the house. He was more apt to buy me things and give me things.

R. Svirsky: Alright . . . Where is this feeling sitting? "I can get away with things. I can wrap my father . . ." Where is it sitting?

Uri: Where is it in my body?

R. Svirsky: Yes.

Uri: In my stomach.

R. Svirsky: Oh, in the stomach! I can manipulate my father. What kind of feeling is it in the stomach?

Uri: It's a cold pain. In other words, it's the same pain, but when I think about it, I feel cold inside my stomach.

R. Svirsky: So ask the cold part, "If it's such a good feeling, to manipulate my father and wrap him to do whatever I want, why it is called pain?"

Uri: Because I'm the one who's having to put the effort into making the relationship.

R. Svirsky: Alright. And why is it painful?

Uri: Because I don't want to have to be able to manipulate him. I want him to be able to care for me.

R. Svirsky: Yeah. And why is it cold?

Uri: I guess because I don't feel bad about it.

R. Svirsky: All right. So what is the feeling—the coldness?

Uri: That my mother's not there.

R. Svirsky: And where does it sit, you said?

Uri: In my stomach.

R. Svirsky: Is that a pleasant feeling or not a pleasant feeling, this cold pain?

Uri: It's not pleasant.

R. Svirsky: So ask this 10–year–old, "How do I release it?" "What did you do to not feel this?"

Uri: He started missing his mother. It was short–lived with the father's attention.

R. Svirsky: And where is this feeling of missing the mother?

Uri: All the feeling's in the stomach.

R. Svirsky: And as he feels the mother, how's it feel in the stomach?

Uri: When he feels the mother, it gets warmer.

R. Svirsky: No. I'm saying, when he misses the mother.

Uri: He gets warmer.

R. Svirsky: Why is that?

Uri: I guess he's feeling the warmth of his mother.

R. Svirsky: Ask the warmer feeling . . . "Why do you feel warmer?"

Uri: Why do you feel warmer? . . .

R. Svirsky: What does it say?

Uri: The thought popped in my mind that it's the feeling of being inside the womb. That warm feeling in the womb.

R. Svirsky: So, when he thinks about mother . . .?

Uri: He thinks about that warmth and security.

R. Svirsky: That was not there. It was missing. How's this feeling of missing manifest in the body?

Uri: I have a pain in my collarbone area now.

R. Svirsky: Ask. "Is that what it is?" Ask the pain.

Uri: I think so.

R. Svirsky: So, look at the boy, the 10–year old boy, and let's go to the 13–year old boy. What happened when he was 13?

Uri: I'm still 10 and I moved to where my mother was coming back. That thought just popped in my head.

R. Svirsky: How long was she not there?

Uri: 6 months . . . 7 months.

R. Svirsky: We'll go back to 10 in a second. But I just want to look at the 13–year old. What happened to the 13–year old?

Uri: My bar mitzvah.

R. Svirsky: What happened there?

Uri: I didn't want to have one.

R. Svirsky: Why not?

Uri: I don't know.

R. Svirsky: Ask the 13–year old.

Uri: . . . He says it's because we didn't believe in any of it.

R. Svirsky: So it felt hypocritical to him?

Uri: Yeah.

R. Svirsky: Did he have a bar mitzvah?

Uri: Oh yeah.

R. Svirsky: So, where are these hypocritical feelings sitting? Being a hypocrite, this kind of feeling, where's it sitting inside?

Uri: I still have it in the same place, my stomach.

R. Svirsky: The same place. You stuff it all there, huh?

Uri: Yeah.

R. Svirsky: Remember, the 13 said he was comfortable. Was he comfortable with eating? What were your eating habits at that time?

Uri: I started gaining weight then. I'd been very thin until then.

R. Svirsky: Why did the 13 start gaining weight?

Uri: I just started gaining weight then. He doesn't answer.

R. Svirsky: Does he know?

Uri: No.

R. Svirsky: How does the eating make him feel?

Uri: He only ate when he was full of anxiety; when his parents would yell at each other.

R. Svirsky: How's it make him feel when he feels this anxiousness?

Uri: Anesthetized.

R. Svirsky: But before he eats, how's he feel? There's a feeling . . . When the parents begin to yell.

Uri: Like an addiction.

R. Svirsky: Right. But before he starts eating, the parents are just beginning to yell . . . Just be there . . . 13–year old. You can hear that they're beginning to yell. There's an unpleasant feeling that immediately comes up. Where is this feeling? Notice it.

Uri: It's a feeling that I'm the reason my mother's in pain.

R. Svirsky: Right. Uh—huh. First of all, where's this feeling in the body?

Uri: It never left the stomach.

R. Svirsky: Ok. It's in the stomach. You feel this pain now?

Uri: Yes.

R. Svirsky: So ask, "Why am I the reason for my mother's pain?"

Uri: Because that last image I had when I was 10 was sitting in a hotel lobby and my mother's meeting with my father and I'm there. And the conditions of her coming back, and she kept telling me the only reason she's coming back is because of me.

R. Svirsky: And so now when they're beginning to fight and she's in pain, you feel guilty.

Uri: She's back because of me.

R. Svirsky: Is that what it is . . . what do you say?

Uri: After this time, I changed. I started making a life of my own outside the house.

R. Svirsky: After what age? 10?

Uri: No, after 13. I cared what my parents thought. I never did anything . . . when I got in trouble I didn't want them to find out about it, because I didn't want to hurt them, but I started being . . . a very typical problem child.

R. Svirsky: Which means what?

Uri: I got in trouble all the time.

R. Svirsky: Ok, but remember, let's go back to this feeling of guilt. The 13–year old . . .

Uri: I did away with the guilt for a while. I just didn't think about it, I didn't care. I went about my own life.

R. Svirsky: "I want my own life because of . . ." What?

Uri: There's no life in the house.

R. Svirsky: There's no life in the house, right? And how does the food affect this 13–year old? He had this terrible feeling in the stomach, that "I'm the cause of my mother's pain?" So what does the food do?

Uri: It would keep me from having to think about it.

R. Svirsky: Yeah. See . . . Alright. Wonderful! So now that we've looked at some of these issues, talk to the chest. Say, "Would you rather deal with that right now?" Remember the chest? So let's deal with that. What's the chest say?

Uri: I don't feel anything now. It just all went away.

R. Svirsky: Very good. What about the neck, back of the neck?

Uri: It's all gone. I feel a little tightness.

R. Svirsky: So ask the tightness, "What are you?"

Uri: What are you? . . .

R. Svirsky: So what's the tightness say?

Uri: He said it's my mother hanging on.

R. Svirsky: Your mother hanging on? How is she hanging on there?

Uri: Hanging on.

R. Svirsky: Right. So ask her why she's hanging on.

Uri: "Why are you hanging on?"

R. Svirsky: Right.

Uri: She won't let go. She doesn't want to let go.

R. Svirsky: So ask her why she wouldn't want to let go.

Uri: She doesn't answer.

R. Svirsky: Be the mother, hanging onto your neck.

Uri: She only came back for me. And if I'm not going to be there, what was the reason for coming back?

R. Svirsky: I understand . . . Alright. So let's go back to the 10–year old. The mother is leaving . . . Go back to the 10–year old . . . 5 . . . 4 . . . 3 . . . 2 . . . 1, mother is leaving. So I want you to do something right now. Bring yourself there as an adult. And tell them, saying, "I come from your future, and I want to give you a wonderful present." Tell him about God. Tell him that God loves him. And he's going to be ok . . . Good. How does that make him feel?

Uri: I think real fine.

R. Svirsky: Good. Can he feel God's Presence, the 10–year old?

Uri: I think he can.

R. Svirsky: You ask him.

Uri: "Do you feel God's Presence?" . . . He says he feels my presence there. That must be because God sent me.

R. Svirsky: Of course. But say, "I want you to feel inside of you God's Presence." Say it to the little kid.

Uri: That's what he can't feel. He didn't have mercy for his mother.

R. Svirsky: You see. How would he need to have mercy for his mother?

Uri: He could have begged to go with her.

R. Svirsky: Ok. Ask him, "Would you choose to do that now?"

Uri: Yeah.

R. Svirsky: So do it.

Uri: Do what?

R. Svirsky: Beg her to go with her . . . and what does the mother say?

Uri: She can't take me.

R. Svirsky: How's that make him feel?

Uri: Good. Because she said if she could, she would.

R. Svirsky: Very good. So how does that make him feel?

Uri: It makes him feel fine.

R. Svirsky: Good. So let him feel God's presence. Can he feel them?

Uri: Yes.

R. Svirsky: Good. Now let him feel how he would feel different about the relationship with his father if he felt the presence of God.

Uri: It makes him feel good.

R. Svirsky: How does it feel in your stomach now that he's making the decisions?

Uri: There's no pain in the stomach, but now he feels fat.

R. Svirsky: So now we can release this fat and use food only for health and nothing else. But I want before we finish this, I want you to go back to this hotel room, where there was a condition. Come there with God . . . And when mother says that she's only coming back because of you. Be there with God. What would you answer?

Uri: Don't come back just for me.

R. Svirsky: That's it. Tell it to her.

Uri: "Don't come back just for me."

R. Svirsky: Ok. What's the mother say?

Uri: She says that means, "I won't come back."

R. Svirsky: Ok. Again, be with God. What would you say to her?

Uri: But I want you to come back.

R. Svirsky: And what does she say?

Uri: She'll come back.

R. Svirsky: Say, "But I don't accept the conditions that it's only for me." What's she say?

Uri: "I'll come back anyway."

R. Svirsky: Good. How's the boy feel?

Uri: He feels fine.

R. Svirsky: So tell him, "You are completely released from this."

Uri: You are completely released from this . . .

R. Svirsky: "It's no longer your responsibility if she comes back."

Uri: It's no longer your responsibility if she comes back.

R. Svirsky: She's adult. She made a decision. This was her decision. How does he feel?

Uri: He's happy about it all.

R. Svirsky: Good. Go to the 13–year old now. Tell him, "You're released from all responsibility of feeling pain that she didn't come back because of you . . ."

Uri: You're released from all responsibility of feeling pain that she didn't come back because of you . . .

R. Svirsky: Give him the same feeling of God. How does he feel?

Uri: He wishes he could do everything different.

R. Svirsky: Say, "You can now." Say, "I'm coming to you from the future and you can. God is with you, right now, right here." How is it?

Uri: He hears it.

R. Svirsky: Let him feel like God's right there in the stomach . . . how's that feel?

Uri: Fine.

R. Svirsky: So let's make an agreement with the 13–year old and the 10–year old, that if he ever feels this anxiety coming up and he knows this feeling in the stomach, then he will signal you so that you can hear his anxiety and realize that what he really needs is another dosage of God's being here and now, right? And the food, we'll leave only for survival, only for the healthy purposes of biological survival. Is that ok with him?

143

Uri: The 13–year old is saying to me, going back, "But we see how you are. You feel anxiety over your kids, or your wife, and the first thing you do is eat something, so don't come telling us what to do if you're not going to do it either."

R. Svirsky: Great. So say, "We'll work together, guys. You taught me how to do it and I kept doing it. So now, you're going to tell me, and I'm also going to tell myself, that when I begin to feel the same feelings of anxiety in my stomach, that the way is to put God in there. So let's do it. I want you think about that anxiety, whether it's kids or wife, right now, being adult. And feel where this feeling of anxiety is. Think about God's presence, right here, right now. Wonderful! And put those feelings in there . . . God's presence. What does it do?

Uri: It takes away the anxiety.

R. Svirsky: That's it. . . So tell me. What signal are you going to give to yourself to remind you that this anxiety is coming . . . To bring God in as an adult now?

Uri: I'm going to see God standing there in front of me, the same way that I was in front of the 13–year old and the 10–year old.

R. Svirsky: Very good. Anything you want to tell me, ask me before we finish.

Uri: Just thank you.

R. Svirsky: You're very welcome. So every day you'll feel healthier and healthier, and you'll feel that you're doing this exercise and you're becoming more and more proficient with this exercise, and therefore you leave food only for biological survival. That's what food is good for. And every time you say the blessing before you eat the food, think about God and realize that this food, which has the blessing of God, will go for the blessing, which is biological survival. So the blessings will also help you to remember that, right? Okay. On the count of 5 . . . be fully aware . . . 1 . . . slowly coming . . . 2 . . . 3 . . . 4 . . . and . . . 5.

End of Session!

13

Personality

Personality is ripe when a man has made the truth his own.

Soren Kierkegaard

Don't take on a new personality; it doesn't work.

Richard Nixon

We continue to shape our personalities all our life. If we knew ourselves perfectly we should die.

Albert Camus

People's personalities like buildings have various facades, some are pleasant to view, some not.

Francois de la Rochefoucauld

In 1921 Carl Jung published his monumental work, *Psychological Types*, based on his clinical observations, introspection and anecdotal evidence rather than empirical study. Yet, it has weathered the time as a basic foundation on individual personality types. Jung built his theory on a two-step process. Man can be said to be generally two descriptive types: introverted or extroverted.

In addition, there is a certain characterization of those types due to the fact that most differentiated functions play the principal role in an individual's adaptation or orientation to life: sensation, intuition, feeling, and thinking.

These four functions coupled with introversion and extroversion creates a total of eight personality types:

Extroverted—Sensation	Introverted—Sensation
Extroverted—Intuition	Introverted—Intuition
Extroverted—Feeling	Introverted—Feeling
Extroverted—Thinking	Introverted—Thinking

Katharine Briggs and Isabel Myers further developed Jung's theories by adding the categories of Judging and Perceiving resulting in the following alphabet soup:

ISTJ, ESTP, INFJ, ENFP, ISTP, ESTJ, INFP, ENFJ
ISFJ, ESFP, INTJ, ENTP, ISFP, ESFJ, INTP, ENTJ

I was first introduced to personality types while I worked for the Jewish outreach organization. As my job was to marry the perfect teachers for our influential donors who came to study in Jerusalem, we utilized personality profiles quite a bit to insure an accurate matching of talent to need.

I also learned a great deal about myself once I took personality tests as a way of discovering who I really was. I am the poster child for the personality type–INFP as I will soon explain. About the same time my mother passed away. While back in the states for her funeral, my sister and I sorted through the house. Reflecting on the remnants of who my mother was in life, I had an epiphany that forever changed my life.

The combination of inner child work, the childhood reframing I had accomplished, and understanding what type of personality I had, suddenly I came to the realization that a life long journey thinking that I was a cast–graven image of my father; an outgoing, successful businessman, community leader, a politician who knew politicians starting with his shaking hands with Theodore Roosevelt as a boy of 12 and attested by invitations to Lyndon Johnston and

Jimmy Carter's presidential inaugurals on our den wall, had been wrong all these years. I was not like my father; I was in truth a clone of my mother.

She was a quiet, modest and unassuming woman, always there to help at every community function, deeply religious, the volunteers' volunteer verified by her being honored by the local hospital ladies auxiliary for her many years service as a Pink Lady, and the towns' Betty Crocker.

This new insight helped me explain why despite the successes I had achieved, demonstrated in the family tradition by plaques and citations hung on my own wall, I always felt it was someone else's life I had lived. I hear you asking what has all this have to do with health. The *Code of Jewish Law* states that one who desires to preserve his health must learn about his psychological reactions and control them.[1] A person's personality is often the key to learning about your reactions.

One of the most thought provoking sentences I read in my research was in a book called *The Self Healing Personality* by Dr. Howard Friedman. "A self–healing personality is a personality that lives a life appropriate for that person."[2] Or as William Shakespeare penned in *Hamlet,* act 1, scene 3 Polonius' advice to Laertes, "This above all: to thine own self be true, and it must follow, as the night the day. Thou canst not then be false to any man." And I will add to the bard's words by saying and not be false to your own self.

All too often we live lives that are not appropriate; that do not fit the personalities we have. I remember in collage taking a career interest test. The results revealed my high preference for actuarial, accounting, business and the lowest score on the helping professions. I decided to change my major to business. But after only one semester of accounting, economics, and finance, I literally ran back to the social science building for a safe haven. INFPs career choices are in the arts, teaching, counseling, religion, writers, social–workers, musicians and composers but definitely not a CPA.

When I answered the questions to the interest test, I later realized those *infamous little voices* told me how to answer: "you'll be a lawyer like your brother," "a doctor in the family will make us proud," "I want you to have all the things we never had growing up," "you can't support a family majoring in drama," "Jews go to therapy, they don't become therapists," etc.

If you have never taken a personality test, I urge you to search online for one. They are free and can be an eye opener for you as it was for me. My personality type INFP—introverted, intuitive, feeling, and perceiving:

> INFPs are quiet, creative, sensitive and perceptive souls who often strike others as shy, reserved and cool and have a rare capacity for deep caring and commitment, both to the people and causes they idealize.
>
> INFPs guide their behavior by a strong inner sense of values, rather than by conventional logic and reason. Forced to cope with this facts–and–figures 'real' world we inhabit, INFPs may appear to have been imported from another galaxy! They gravitate toward creative or human service careers which allow them to use their instinctive sense of empathy and remarkable communication skills.
>
> Strongly religious, spiritual or philosophical people, INFPs may see the purpose of their lives as an inner journey, quest or personal unfolding. More practical or rational types may tend to discredit the INFPs sources or understanding as mystical.
>
> The search for a soul mate is a preoccupation for many INFPs, who must balance their need for privacy and peace with their yearning for human connection. If there seems to be an air of sadness in the INFPs spirit, blame it on this type's longing for the perfect in all things.

The last sentence, *longing for the perfect in all things*, was the most telling for me. Longing for the perfect does not mean being a perfectionist; which I certainly am not. Nor is it a diagnosis of OCD. I think it is what Friedman meant by personality that lives a life not appropriate for the person; walking the yellow brick road, searching for utopia, yet hitching your horse perpetually to the wrong wagon; trying to live life with the opposite of a self–healing personality. When you live in opposition to a self–healing personality, stress dominates life.

In the 1950s cardiologists Meyer Friedman and Ray Rosenman conducted studies on the relationship between stress and heart disease. In doing so, they extended personality types specifically to heart disease. They broke down heart patients into a dichotomy of Type A and Type B. Friedman and Rosenman estimated that people with a Type A personality had double the risk of coronary heart disease than otherwise healthy individuals. The types are generally described as:

Type A: aggressive, competitive, constant sense of time, urgency, impatience, constant striving for ill–defined goals, vigorous, abrupt patterns of speech and movement,[3] seen as angry, tense, fast, and in control.[4]

Type B: laid back, relaxed, unaggressive, easy going, readily satisfied and not driven by ambition,[5] a balanced, moderate human being who can feel and express emotion without being driven and without losing himself in uncontrolled emotional outbreaks.[6]

Type A is the proverbial multitasking workaholic with a short–fused anger and hostility that can be triggered by the small stuff. Type A sweats the small stuff all the time. The amazing thing is all the years I thought I was like my father, I acted like I was a Type A person even though I knew inside I was not; definitely not a "life appropriate for the person."

In the states my jobs were in various levels of management with its attendant stress. I used to joke with people that my job was only to make a decision when no one else would. Sometimes the pressure to make that decision would be enough to turn coal into diamonds.

After the epiphany of being like my mother, I understood that my Myers–Briggs personality type of INFP was really associated with Type B and I began to change my real life accordingly. Careers of Type B are usually writers, counselors, therapists, actors, artisans, etc. And Type B's do not sweat the small stuff; we don't sweat anything. We live by definition a life of low level stress. It's a world of not winning but how you play the game!

Heart disease is not the only illness attributed to personality. Soon Type C for cancer materialized:

Type C: compliance with the wishes of others and a lack of assertiveness, avoidance of conflict or behavior that might offend others, a calm, outwardly rational and unemotional approach to life, obeying conventional norms of behavior and maintaining the appearance of niceness, stoicism and self–sacrifice, feelings of helplessness and hopefulness;[7] suppression of strong negative emotions, particularly anger, while struggling to maintain a strong happy facade.[8]

Linking cancer to personality is not a new idea. In the second century, Galen thought that melancholic women were predisposed to breast cancer.[9] In 1676 Dr. Richard Wiseman, King James 1st physician and surgeon said "depression and melancholy triggers the onset of cancer."

Dr. Richard Guy an English physician documented in 1759, "people who experience trouble and grief, who sit still and allow depression, leave themselves open to the possibility of cancer." In the 1890's the British physician Herbert Snow observed that a surprisingly high proportion of cancer patients he saw had lived difficult lives and had recently had experienced a traumatic event.[10]

People who survive cancer have different psychological profiles from those who do not.[11] In one study relying only on personality profiles, psychologist Bruno Klopfer correctly predicted nineteen out of twenty–four times which patients would have fast–growing cancers and which would have cancers that grew slowly.[12] In another study, researchers were able to predict the presence of cancer in up to 94% of the cases judging psychological factors alone.[13]

Robert Sapolsky, the author of *Why Don't Zebras Get Ulcers*, writes, "The cancer prone personality we're told is one of repression—emotions held inside, particularly those of anger. This is a picture of an introverted, respectful individual with a strong desire to please—conforming and compliant. Hold those emotions inside and increase the likelihood that out will come cancer."[14]

Dr. Larry LeShan explains that the basic emotional pattern of cancer patients:

> involves a childhood or adolescence marked by feelings of isolation; centered on the period during which a meaningful relationship is discovered allowing the individual to enjoy a sense of acceptance by others and to find a meaning to his life; when the loss of that relationship occurs, the conviction that life holds no more hope becomes paramount.[15]

LeShan in his book, *Cancer As A Turning Point*, asserts the presence of cancer is usually an indication that there is something else wrong in the life of the patient.[16] The cancer was not seen as something new in their lives, only as the latest and final example of basic hopelessness that had long been a part of their existence.[17]

The single thing that emerged most clearly to LeShan was that there had been a loss of hope in ever achieving a way of life that would give real and deep satisfaction that would provide a solid *raison d'être*, the kind of meaning that makes us glad to get out of bed in the morning and glad to go to bed at night.[18] Over the years,

LeShan found this pattern of loss of hope in 70 to 80 percent of his cancer patients and in only 10 percent of the control group.[19]

In his book, *The Psychology of Cancer,* Dr. Peter Lambley explains cancer people did not feel as close to their parents as did other people.[20] Four areas of psychological relevance were consistently found in cancer–prone people: a disturbance in family background, a disturbance in parent–child relationships, a disturbance in interpersonal relationships, and a disturbance in coping behavior.[21]

Cancer sufferers, Lambley writes, frequently had a limited ability to express their emotions both as children and as they grew older.[22] "Retrospective studies have reinforced the idea that cancer victims hold their feelings in too much and helped us to see that this, coupled with a feeling of helplessness and hopefulness seems to be a mark of general cancer proneness."[23]

The late Dr. David Servan–Schreiber points out in his book, *Anti–Cancer: A New Way of Life,* that those exhibiting Type C personality are often people who rightly or wrongly never felt welcome in their childhood. Their parents may have been violent or irascible, or simply cold, distant, and demanding. Often these children receive little encouragement and develop vulnerability and weakness. Rarely angry, they become really nice people as adults, always helping others, saints.

"They avoid conflict," he continues, "and put their needs and aspirations on the back burner, sometimes for the rest of their lives. In order to safeguard the emotional security that they so value, they may overinvest in a single aspect of their lives: their profession, their marriage, or their children. When this investment is suddenly threatened or lost, the childhood grief returns, arousing feelings of helplessness, despair, and abandonment."[24]

According to Dr. Bernie Siegel's experience, there are three kinds of cancer patients: 15–20% at some level of consciousness wish to die and will do so no matter how excellent their treatment, 60–70% passively cooperate with whatever the physicians say, and 15–20% are the exceptional patients.[25] It is a telling commentary that Dr.

Siegel asks four questions as a way of understanding the cancer in relation to his patients: Do you want to live to be a hundred? What happened to you in the year or two before your illness? What does this illness mean to you? Why do you need this illness?[26]

Lack of emotional outlet is a common theme in the histories of cancer patients. Dr. Howard Friedman quotes from a study done in Tecumseh, Michigan in early 1970's. People were asked to imagine that their husband, wife, sweetheart, yelled in anger or blew up at them for something that was not their fault. The questioners asked: "Would you get angry or annoyed and show it? Or would you get angry and annoyed and keep it in or not get angry at all?" Persons who said that they would hold in their anger were two and a half times more likely to die than those who expressed their anger with their mate from all mortality not just cancer or heart disease.[27]

If there is a Type A, Type B and a Type C, is there also a Type D? Yes, Type D was developed in the Netherlands by Johan Denollet, a medical psychologist at Tilburg University. The letter D stands for distressed. Utilizing 14 questions, the DS14 is a brief, psycho–metrically sound measure of negative affectivity and social inhibition.

Negative affectivity (NA) refers to the tendency to experience negative emotions across time situations. High–Negative affectivity individuals experience more feelings of dysphoria, anxiety, and irritability; have a negative view of self; and scan the world for signs of impending trouble. Social inhibition (SI) refers to the tendency to inhibit the expression of emotions—behaviors in social interactions to avoid disapproval by others. High–Social inhibition individuals tend to feel inhibited, tense, and insecure when with others.[28]

Type D personality is a vulnerability factor for general psychological distress that affects mental and physical health status; associated with disease–promoting mechanisms in apparently healthy individuals;[29] related to a twofold risk of metabolic syndrome and unhealthy lifestyle, independent of socio–

demographic, cardiovascular and lifestyle factors;[30] a prognostic factor for the development of cancer in men with established cardiovascular disease;[31] associated with more than a four–fold risk of a diagnosis of PTSD;[32] and associated with a reduction in health–related behaviors and low perceived social support.[33]

Type D coronary heart disease patients had a four–fold risk of death;[34] cardiovascular disease Type D's had a two to fivefold increased risk of adverse prognosis.[35]

Alphabet soup is not the only way to view personality. The basic Myers–Briggs types have been organized in a set of basic personality domains, Big–5 typology, by P.T. Costa and R. R. McCrae: extraversion, openness, agreeableness, conscientiousness, and emotional stability represented as neuroticism.[36]

Extraversion includes sociability, activity, dominance, and the tendency to experience positive emotions; *Openness* is seen in imaginativeness, aesthetic sensitivity, depth of feeling, curiosity, and need for variety; *Agreeableness* encompasses sympathy, trust, cooperation and altruism. *Conscientiousness* includes organization, persistence, scrupulousness, and need for achievement. *Emotional stability/Neuroticism* includes the predisposition to experience negative effects such as anxiety, anger, and depression, and other cognitive and behavioral manifestations of emotional instability.[37]

My own personality type, INFP, correlates with the Big–5 typology in that *I* and *P* negatively compare to with extraversion and conscientiousness respectively and the *F* and *N* connect positively with agreeableness and openness. I recognize that I "balance my need for privacy and peace with a yearning for human connection." But there is still a large part of me that understands King David's lament, "O that I had the wings of a dove! I would fly away, and find rest."[38] Conscientiousness has been, for me, a newly learned trait in my quest to take charge of my health and live *Until 120*. But if I had to choose, I would rather innately be agreeable and open, which are much harder to acquire, than being extraverted and conscientiousness.

While I found the Typology of A—B—C—D most prevalent in studies dealing cancer, metabolic syndrome and heart disease, the Big–5 typology featured itself prominently in the longevity studies of centenarians. Evidence suggests various personality traits are significant predictors of longevity; that personality is linked to a number of quality of life measures; personality assessment may play a role in prognosticating and improving quality of life in old age.[39]

In the Georgia Centenarian Study, centenarians who showed a special combination of traits i.e., low levels of emotional stability, high competence, and high extraversion were notable as exceptional survivors.[40] The Tokyo Centenarian Study found higher conscientiousness and extraversion in female centenarians in reconfirming the importance of these two behavior–related personality traits.[41]

The New England Centenarian Study found personality factors and more specifically low neuroticism and high extraversion may be important for achieving extreme old age.[42] The Long Life Family Study found personality factors and more specifically low neuroticism and high extraversion may be important for achieving extreme old age.[43]

We all wonder about our mental status as we age. Will we succumb to dementia or Alzheimer's? The Georgia Centenarian Study found:

> High levels of emotional stability, extraversion, openness, and conscientiousness with high levels of engaged lifestyle were more likely to show relatively high mental status scores, whereas participants with low levels of emotional stability, extraversion, openness, agreeableness, and conscientiousness with low levels of engaged lifestyle were more likely to show relatively low mental status scores. Only if centenarians exhibited high levels of emotional

stability, extraversion, conscientiousness, openness, was engaged lifestyle associated with higher mental status functioning.[44]

Dietary intake is additionally associated with the Big–5 typology traits. The Helsinki Birth Cohort Study[45] concluded emotional stability–neuroticism, extraversion, openness, agreeableness, and conscientiousness are linked with resilience, meaning adaptability in challenging situations. Resilient people usually comply with favorable health behaviors. Openness in men was associated with higher vegetable and lower confectionery and chocolate intakes. In women, neuroticism was associated with lower fish and vegetable and higher soft drink intakes.

Extraversion in women was associated with higher meat intakes, openness with higher vegetable and fruit intakes. Agreeableness was associated with a lower soft drink and conscientiousness with a higher fruit intake in women. Comparing resilient and non–resilient subjects, the study found resilience in women to be associated with higher intakes of vegetables, fruits, and dietary fiber.[46]

There is a silk thread weaving its way through the fabric of information about personality in this chapter. Allow me to unravel the strands to help you get a clearer understanding:

Dr. Carl Simonton: I'm okay and you're okay. Heart attack: I'm okay and you're not okay. Cancer: You're okay and I'm not okay.

Shivani Goodman, PhD: There is a disease–prone personality and that people with this personality have one thing in common: they do not feel deeply loved or lovable, which causes feelings of insecurity.[47]

Dr. T. Berri Brazelton: Many of the most important personality traits, such as the capacities for relating to others: trust and intimacy, empathy, creative and logical thinking, are largely determined by how we were nurtured as a child.[48]

Dr. Charles Whitfield: I believe that nearly all of our unhealthy and destructive aspects of our personality are due to a combination of being wounded and our attachment to our false self.[49]

Dr. Gabor Maté: The overwhelming need of a child to avoid pain and conflict is responsible for the personality trait or coping style that later predisposes the adult to disease.[50]

Dr. Karen Horney: Hopelessness is an ultimate product of unresolved conflicts with its deepest root in despair of ever being wholehearted and undivided.[51]

Dr. Judith Herman: A secure connection with caring people is the foundation of personality development.[52]

Martin Seligman, PhD: personality is only partly genetic; at least half of personality is not inherited. The other half comes from what you do and from what happens to you.[53]

Dr. Howard Friedman: Personality is a synthesis of biological tendencies, family environment and the culture and subcultures in which we develop.[54]

Dr. Bernie Siegel: As we grow an intricate weaving together of chance, genetic, and experiential input into the brain shapes what we call our personality with its habits, likes, dislikes, and patterns of response.[55]

Julie Harris, PhD: children are born with certain characteristics. Their genes predispose them to develop a certain kind of personality, but the environment can change them.[56]

In a study published in the *Journal of Personality*, Dr. Howard Friedman concluded that beyond the substantial evidence that well–adjusted, socially stable, and well–integrated people are at significantly lower risk for disease, the past decade has provided significant evidence that a conscientious, dependable personality, in stable psychosocial environments, is a key predictor and may be a central underlying causal factor. "This is not because there is a disease–prone personality with simple, direct links to ill health," Freidman says, "but rather primarily because certain people wind up with unhealthy habits and behaviors, unbalanced socio–emotional and psycho–physiological styles, and environments not conducive to good health."[57]

I steadfastly believe that to understand our personality, our illnesses, our unhealthy habits and behaviors, and our lives in general we need to add two more letters to the bowl of alphabet soup we have been cooking. All personality theories only taste the soup once it has been cooked. We need to examine the recipe and where possible change the ingredients:

Type E: Early childhood adversity as demonstrated by the CDC and Kaiser Permanente Adverse Childhood Experiences Study and Inner Child work.

Type F: Fetal origins hypothesis. In utero environment influences the development of diseases later in life by not only undernutrition, but embryo awareness of what is ongoing it its environment outside the womb.

The ancients believed man's actions were fated and fixed in the heavens; the stars and the planets exerting transcendental forces. Even today while most of do not believe in astrology, we muse ourselves with our daily astrological reading. Jewish sages also believed the stars and planets held power over the physical world with one major exception. Astrological readings were merely a snapshot of fate not its ongoing movie. *A man can change his stars!*

An existential dialogue is recorded in Genesis:[58] Abraham's lamenting to God that all his life's efforts will come to naught because he has no progeny. God took Abraham outside his tent and told him to "gaze toward the heavens and count the stars." The medieval French Biblical commentator Rashi explains, based on a *Midrashic* interpretation, God told Abraham to put aside his own personal astrological calculations as to whether he was predestined to be childless. Zodiacs can change; he would have a son.

The Talmud[59] discusses the influence of the red planet Mars on a persons' life. "He who is born under the influence of Mars will be a spiller of blood." Rabbi Ashi, however, comments that is not totally fated. It is up to the individual person whether he will chose to be a murderous thief, a blood–letter (doctor), a ritual slaughter or a ritual circumciser.

"Man is capable of changing the world for the better if possible," Viktor Frankl explains, "and of changing himself for the better if necessary."[60] Psycho–physiological responses can be modified according to Dr. Howard Friedman; they are means to create a healing personality.[61]

"Man," Rabbi Soloveitchik says, "can be the architect of his own personality. He has the ability to fashion his own character and map out the path he will follow. Indeed, man is capable of determining in advance what his reactions will be to a given phenomena and events in the course of his life."[62]

In the next chapter we will learn how.

14

Character

Nearly all men can stand adversity, but if you want to test man's character give him power.

Abraham Lincoln

Character cannot be developed in ease and quiet.

Helen Keller

Character, not circumstances, makes a man.

Booker T. Washington

Parents can only give children advice; the final forming of a person's character lies in their own hands.

Anne Frank

Looking back, I can see clearly that my faith was a belief in perfecting myself. I tried to perfect mentally—I tried to perfect my will—I perfected myself physically. The beginning of it all was moral perfection; but that was soon replaced by perfection in general: by the desire to be better, not in my own eyes or those of God, but in the eyes of other people . . . Lying, robbery, adultery of all kinds, drunkenness, violence, murder—there was no crime I did not commit, and for all that people praised my conduct, and my contemporaries considered me to be a comparatively moral man.

So I lived for ten years . . . Life in Europe and my acquaintance with leading Europeans confirmed me yet more in the faith in which I believed, of striving for perfection. This I lived another six years till my marriage . . . My striving after self–perfection in general was now again replaced by my effort simply to secure the best possible conditions for myself and my family. So another fifteen years passed . . . Had a fairy come and offered to fulfill my desires I should not have known what to ask . . . I returned to what belonged to my earliest childhood. I returned to the belief that the chief and only aim of my life is to be better. I returned to a belief in God, in moral perfection.

Once again I turn to Tolstoy. Best known for *War and Peace* and *Anna Karenina*, at the height of his career, he underwent a profound spiritual awakening, as excerpted above from his 1872 work *A Confession and What I Believe*. These passages are but a brief chronological highlight of his of thoughts on the moral crisis his life faced.

Tolstoy epitomized what Carl Jung wrote: "we wholly overlook the essential fact that the achievements which society reward are won at the cost of a diminution of personality."[1] Like Tolstoy, I realized that to be better in character; better in moral perfection was what God had intended for mankind. Jewish sources confirmed that thought.

Maimonides was certainly one of the most influential Jewish scholars of the Middle Ages; the unsurpassed medieval philosopher, physician, and astronomer. His fourteen–volume opus, *Mishnah Torah*, is still considered a canonical authority as a codification of Talmudic law.

Maimonides' first volume began his oeuvre with the foundations of the Jewish faith. You might think naturally that the next tome to follow would perhaps deal with the laws of what a Jew can and cannot eat; maybe the laws of family purity; prayers or festivals; torts and damages; but no. Maimonides' second volume is titled the *Laws of Character Development*.

Pause for just a moment. The *Mishnah Torah* is a canonical ordering of Talmudic law. What has character development to do with Jewish law? The answer is provided by one of the foremost Talmudist, Kabbalist, and Jewish leaders of the past few centuries, Rabbi Elijah Kremer, affectionately known as the *Vilna Gaon*; the saintly genius from Vilna.

In his eighteenth century work entitled *Even Sheleimah* Rabbi Elijah Kremer wrote, "All God's service is dependent upon the improvement of one's character. Character traits are fundamental to the performance of all commandments and to Torah principles. Conversely, all sins stem from unimproved character traits. The prime purpose of man's life is to constantly strive to beak his bad habits. Otherwise, what is life for?"[2]

The prime purpose in life is to improve character traits—otherwise what is life for! Now we can appreciate why Maimonides listed the laws of character development second after the religious foundations. Lest you think this is only a Jewish idea, I assure you it is the universal goal of man.

Rick Warren is the founding pastor of the Saddleback Church, a 30,000–member congregation in California. Pastor Warren is also the author of best selling non–fiction hardback book in history, *The Purpose Driven Life: What on Earth Am I Here For?* In his book, Pastor Warren writes, "God's ultimate goal for your life on earth is not comfort, but character development.[3] Much confusion in Christian life comes from ignoring the simple truth that God is far more interested in building your character than anything else."[4]

The obvious question should be why is character development so crucial? Didn't God, after all, make man in His own image? If God is perfect then we shouldn't we be too? The 15th century rabbi, Joseph Albo, I think provides an answer.

Writing in his the classic work on the fundamentals of Judaism, *Sefer ha–Ikkarim*, Rabbi Albo tell us that the Bible says good at the end of each day of creation except after the day man was created. He explains there are two kinds of perfection: of nature and of man. Nature consists of its being, man in his becoming. Nature is always present; therefore judgment could be passed upon it. As it was created, so it was completed. Man, however, is goal–directed; he was, therefore, incomplete at creation. Man's evaluation had to be left in abeyance.[5]

"There is just one purpose for man and for the world: self–improvement towards perfection!" according to Rabbi Wolbe, "No man is born perfect. He must work to perfect himself."[6] Rabbi Dr. Twerski writes, "Man's mission is thus to develop himself into the being that God desired, and to transform the physical world into holiness."[7] Rabbi Yisroel Salanter said, "The purpose of man's existence is to purge every negative trait and character attribute from his heart."[8]

Maimonides explains with regard to all traits: a man has some from the beginning of his conception, in accordance with his bodily nature. Some are appropriate to a person's nature and will be acquired more easily than other traits. Some traits he does not have from birth. He may have learned them from others or turned to them on his own. This may have come as a result of his own thoughts or because he heard that this was a proper trait for him, which he ought to strive. He accustomed himself to it until it becomes a part of him.[9]

Although written in the 12th century, Maimonides' approach is comparatively modern. Each and every person possesses many character traits that are very different and distant from the others, Maimonides says. One type is wrathful; he is constantly angry. There is the calm individual who is never moved to anger, or, if at all, he will be slightly angry, during a period of several years.[10]

The *Mishnah* lists four types of temperaments: Easily angered and quick to forget—his gain is overridden by his loss; slow to anger and slow to forget—his loss is overridden by his gain; quick to grasp and slow to forget—this is a good portion; slow to grasp and quick to forget—this is a bad portion.[11]

Yet, the more I learned about the Jewish view of character traits, I realized anger and similar behaviors were anomalous to the secular understanding of personality traits, i.e. extraversion, intuition etc. After thinking about it for a long while, I began to put the pieces together.

Rabbi Moshe Luzzatto explains that man is veritably placed in the midst of a raging battle. For all the affairs of the world, whether for the good or for the bad are trials to a man: poverty on the one hand and wealth on the other; serenity on the one hand, suffering on the other; so that the battle rages against him on all fronts.[12]

Pastor Warren writes, "When you understand that life is a test, you realize that nothing is insignificant in your life. Every day is an important day, and every second is a growth opportunity to deepen your character, to demonstrate love or to depend on God.[13] Every problem is a character building opportunity and the more difficult it is, the greater the potential for building spiritual muscle and moral fiber."[14] *Good sailors are not made on calm seas!*

Character is not just an indication of a disease prone capability. It is mirrored reflection of who we are to ourselves, our loved ones, our family, our co–workers, and to humanity at large. The lesson Tolstoy and I learned was that we need not to change our characters only in order to live longer, but because primarily *that is our purpose—to be better humans*. It is not whether we are extraverted or Type XYZ which is crucial, rather whether we are prone to behaviors such as anger, etc as the *Mishnah* says in its four temperaments.

We can change our character traits, but we must do it for the right reasons. Rabbi Eliyahu Dessler, the renowned 20th century master of Mussar, provides an additional incentive for change, "One can appreciate the attributes of God only to the extent that we possess some of those attributes ourselves."[15]

Maimonides writes the development of character traits is nothing but the healing of the soul and its powers.[16] Rabbi Dr. Twerski adds, "Spirituality requires that one seek to improve oneself and to grow in character."[17] Rabbi Abraham Heschel says, "It is not by the rare act of greatness that character is determined, but by everyday actions."[18]

The *Zohar*, the main Kabbalistic work of mysticism in Judaism, explains God created man in this world and gave him the faculty to prefect himself in His service and to direct his ways so as to merit the enjoyment of that celestial light which God has hidden and reserved for the righteous.[19]

Rabbi Dessler writes that the personality one brings with him from this world is the personality he will have in the world to come.[20] Again this is universal; Pastor Warren agrees: "When you transfer into eternity, you will leave everything else behind. All you are taking with you is your character."[21]

The Jewish concept of hell, Rabbi Dessler clarifies, is to burn away the part of one's personality corrupted by sin, as a surgeon cauterizes a wound which has festered.[22] Doesn't it make sense to avoid the fires of hell? Isn't it better to spend the energy in this life to be a better person? And what if all people on earth understood this to be their life's work? Isn't that what John Lennon sang about—*Imagine*!

Man confronts a crucial test, Rabbi Luzzatto says. For if he allows himself to be allured by this world and drawn away from his Creator, he will debase himself and debase the world along with himself. But if he masters himself, cleaves to his Creator, and uses the world as an aid to serve Him, he will be elevated and the world itself will be elevated along with him.[23] In Hebrew this is called *Tikkun HaOlam*—a rectification of the world.

Though he held no official position, Rabbi Abraham Karelitz, known as the *Chazon Ish* after his *magnum opus*, was of the most widely recognized 20th century authorities of Jewish law and life. He writes in his classic work, *Faith and Trust*, an example that encompasses these ideas:

> What we see in life is a person like Reuben, who is a moral person, always speaking of trust in God, condemning excessive efforts in life, and expressing his abhorrence of constant pursuit of financial means. Indeed, he is a successful person; he lacks no customers in his store, and he does not need to expand his efforts in that direction.

And suddenly, we are surprised to see Reuben, that great truster in God, conferring secretly with his assistants and consultants as to how to stop a potential rival who plans to open a store just like his. Reuben is very upset by this threat. At the beginning he keeps his feelings to himself because he is embarrassed to reveal them to his acquaintances, fearing their derision. But with time he loses his sense of shame, and begins to act openly with the aim of preventing the rival from carrying out his plan. Gradually he gravitates towards the crooked path, and his sense of shame evaporates: he commits low and deplorable actions—in public.

Competition between him and his rival becomes widely known, and is the talk of the town—and still he feels no shame, but comes up with baseless and untrue reasons and explanations to justify his actions. Over time he becomes even more sophisticated and adds new explanations, claiming, that everything he is doing is for the sake of Heaven and is morally acceptable. He fools himself into believing this and fools others as well.[24]

How can Reuben, a man of devout living, truster in God, stoop so low in his behavior? The sages who expound *Mussar* say that within everyone is a sleeping tiger. When life goes well, the tiger rests quietly, but let us be embattled over money, issues of pride, threats to our personal hegemony, estranged from our spouse, then we see the tiger claw its way to the surface, mauling everyone in its sight, including ourselves. And after the tiger retreats to its lair, we stand in shock at the collateral damage done to our lives.

The story is told that during a 19th century convention of German university deans to discuss curricula, a professor said, "There is an area of knowledge that is studied in only one institution in the world, in a yeshiva in a Russian town named Kelm. That subject is *Mussar*—the correcting man's character traits."

Rabbi Lopian asks, what is *Mussar*?—Reflection. A man must simply learn to reflect upon his ways. He must supervise and guide his thoughts, his speech, and his deeds, not permitting them to run wild.[25]

Rabbi Karelitz teaches at the root of all character traits there is only one good trait and one bad trait. The bad trait is that of leaving natural life to its natural processes. If a person makes no effort to the contrary, he will become skilled in all the bad traits. The good trait is the absolute determination to put moral feeling above the desire, and from that starting point a person can fight against all bad traits together.[26]

The mere acquisition of knowledge does not help a person to conduct himself in an upright fashion, Rabbi Salanter writes. The principles he has learned must be inculcated within his heart—bound and joined to him so that they and he are united as one.[27] Rabbi Karelitz says the only way to correct the heart is to correct the deeds. Gradually he will become accustomed to doing what is good, and it will become an inherent tendency.[28]

Character change follows change in behavior. Since we are what we do, if we want to change who we are, we must begin by changing what we do undertaking a new mode of action.[29] Asks Maimonides, how one be can trained to follow good temperaments to the extent that they become a permanent part of him? He should perform—repeat—and perform a third time. He should do this constantly, until these acts are easy for him and do not present any difficulty. Then, these temperaments will become a fixed part of his character.[30]

During the time I worked in the Old City of Jerusalem, I was able to be a member of a *Mussar* group lead by Rabbi Lawrence Kelemen. Our purpose was to meet weekly in order to study one of the Jewish works dealing with character improvement. As Rabbi Karelitz advised, "To read a book on character traits written by a sage in his sagacity—that is the cure for the soul. When one studies it constantly—that is the correction of one's bad traits."[31]

Rabbi Yisroel Salanter explains, "In most cases, however, man does not have the innate strength to master his desires, which are based in the subconscious and are naturally very powerful. But just as in the realm of intellectual endeavor, each session of 'clarification learning' makes an impression on the subconscious. It is important to point out that the only way a learned skill can be made second nature is through initial conscious effort—for if this weren't true, it would be unnecessary to employ conscious study in order to generate 'reflex' knowledge in the subconscious."[32]

Up close and personal. After many months studying with Rabbi Kelemen, I asked for a private meeting. During our time I poured my heart out about the disharmony between my wife and myself, the dysfunctionalism that prevailed at home and its tragic effects on our sons, the pressures at work, and the uncertainties of my health.

Rabbi Kelemen took it all in and responded honestly, he had no initial response, but asked to give him a week; which I haltingly did. In a week's time we sat again. He explained that he took my situation to a sage greater than himself and was told simply to sit with me and learn a passage that had been written by Rabbi Wolbe in his work, *Aleh Shor.*

> The quality of suffering encompasses still more than what we have discussed thus far. We would be unable to grasp all its components were we to continue describing them in terms of practical application. So if we cannot delineate these points in practical terms, we can at least learn them in theory.
>
> Let us deepen our understanding by first quoting what our Sages have learned:[33] 'They who accept being shamed and do not shame others, they who listen to insult without responding in kind, they who serve out of love and who remain joyful even whilst being afflicted—of them the verse speaks, saying, 'And they who love Him are as the rising sun in its splendor.'

'The rising sun in its splendor' is the ultimate expression of the sun in its brilliance. To whom would we think to attribute such glory? Surely to those individuals whose multiple actions affect many others? But our Sages see it rather differently. They single out for praise the person of forbearance; the one who suffers affliction yet retains a joyful disposition. Such a person shows the greatest ultimate strength!'

'Others look upon a person with afflictions with pity. No greatness is attributed to such an individual. Nevertheless, such a person may be greater than the man of action. May God protect him from affliction, yet we must know that suffering affliction and carrying it with joy and without becoming broken in spirit causes that individual to be ranked among the greatest of the great. Lost in a seemingly hopeless situation, with no one to turn to, this individual may also find himself on a higher level than when he was previously a man of many activities.'[34]

That was it; no suggestions, no sagely advice, no compassionate counseling, we just sat down and learned the above passage. One of the basic tenets of Orthodox Judaism is having faith in our learned rabbis. Even when their advice seems counterintuitive, we trust that it contains truths steeped with the wisdom of our religion. I left with a Xerox copy of what we had studied during out brief meeting.

With resolve, I read the passage three times a day before each session of prayer. Days, weeks, months elapsed without anything falling from the heavens, yet I zealously read on. Then after about a year I began to notice subtle changes. It was a different me that now faced the challenges of my life. I no longer jousted with my wife in arguments. As a matter of fact, I realized I was holding my tongue quite a bit at work, dealing with my sons, and listened understandingly to my wife's shaming. Even my neighbor commented one day to me, "I still hear the arguments coming from your house, but now there is only one voice."

They who accept being shamed and do not shame others, they who listen to insult without responding in kind, they who serve out of love and who remain joyful even whilst being afflicted. By a miracle people no longer pushed my buttons. As a matter of fact, with an electricians' skill I began rewiring the buttons of my life. The *Mussar* approach to character development had worked. My thrice daily affirmation of Rabbi Wolbe's words made an impression on my subconscious.

Coincidentally, the focus of Rabbi Wolbe's weekly lecture I had recently attended at the time was focused on Nahmanides' letter he had written to his son in Spain after he immigrated to the Holy Land. In the letter Nahmanides, the 13th century Catalan rabbi, philosopher, physician, Kabbalist and biblical commentator, counseled his son to accustom himself always to speak all of his words softly to all people every person, at all times, and with this he will be rescued from anger, the bad trait that brings mankind to sin.

Rabbi Wolbe explained, "It is very hard to work on anger. How can a person work on his anger? He does not want to get angry and then something that really irritates him comes along, and he bursts out in fury. Rather, says Nahmanides, he should endeavor always to speak softly; with every person, in every situation, at every time."[35] There I had it; a way to control anger; I expanded my affirmations to include Nahmanides' letter.

Sometime later, in another lecture, Rabbi Wolbe taught that "acknowledgment of goodness that a person owes another person who did him a good is a great principle in building one's character traits and really enriches the core of a person, and all of a person's relations with others. A true wealth comes out of this character trait."[36]

Rabbi Dessler says the subconscious mind is amenable to training, like some animals. If one gives clear and repeatable commands, it will obey.[37] This is the major premise of *Mussar* thought; returning knowledge into the heart. Or to put another way: letting the knowledge of the conscious mind penetrate the subconscious, achieved by use of the imagination; vivid imagery combined with reflection can make a lasting impression.[38]

Imagery and imagination are fundamental in changing of character traits and therefore our behavior. I remember once Rabbi Wolbe advising young scholars to pause for a moment at their front door before entering. They should reflect on their day; of how well they had learned in the yeshiva, how good they felt about their accomplishments and anxiously waiting to share their day with their wife. Then, he counseled, they should reflect on the day of their wife: taking care of small children, cleaning the home, shopping for necessities, ironing the endless stream of white shirts, etc. In other words envision what he will find when he opens the door. One can only imagine the new behavior he opts for as he open the door.

The big question is what character traits we possess are good and which ones we want to change? I believe the answer can be found in a saying by King Solomon in the Book of Proverbs:[39] "*As water reflects a face back to a face, so is the heart of man reflected in the heart of another man.*" Remember Rabbi Lopian defined *Mussar* as reflection.

If you want to know what character traits you should change, look at other people's behavior. What you find distasteful in them are the very traits you also possess that need change. The traits that you admire most in others are the ones you need to acquire. It sounds counterintuitive, but I assure you it is not.

In time I realized that most of our negative traits are in fact just defense mechanisms we have nurtured since we were young. Rescripting, reframing and reparenting the inner child can and will help change out negative traits and therefore help us change our behavior. I have seen its success with people I have worked with; I have seen its success within myself.

One of the guided imageries I often used was to take a relaxed person to an old apothecary shop, somewhere in the past. I told them that the proprietor inside can help them trade in elements of their character for ones they do not have or would like more of. The session focused on a self-evaluation; "a face to face, heart to heart appraisal," and always it had a cathartic effect.

The disease prone personalities have a single common thread: unhealthy behaviors and practices. If you correct the basis of a distorted past, resolve earlier adversities, reframe the past, present and create a new future, then unhealthy behaviors resolve themselves. The all encompassing term is called growth. And growth is the only way to achieve self–sustainability.

Rabbi Karelitz says as long as a person is alive he is obligated to make every effort to grow.[40] The work of character growth is not a magic pill you take once and are cured. If you stop watering plants, they will halt their growth. Plants need constant nurturing to develop, the same with a person. Maimonides says a person who has perfected his character traits should always analyze his personal qualities, weight carefully his conduct and evaluate the inclination of his soul every day.[41] Please do not think I have perfected my character traits and all I do is a daily assessment. I am a work in progress, I can assure you.

Just how does a person know whether he has been effective in changing his personality, character, etc? Rabbi Wolbe says the main channeling of character qualities is in one's dealings with other people.[42] It is to the crucible of relationships we turn next.

15

Relationships

Each of us comes for a short visit not knowing why, yet sometimes seemingly for a divine purpose. However, there is one thing we do know: that we are here for the sake of others.

Albert Einstein

In a world in which God is believed to exist, the primary fact is relationships.

Rabbi Sir Jonathan Sacks[1]

Life's deepest meaning is not found in accomplishments, but in relationships.

Gary Chapman[2]

Our survival depends on the healing power of love, intimacy and relationships.

Dr. Dean Ornish[3]

This bronze. Yes, now's the moment; I'm looking at this thing on the mantelpiece, and I understand that I'm in hell. I tell you, everything's been thought out beforehand. They knew I'd stand at the fireplace stroking this thing of bronze, with all those eyes intent on me. Devouring me. What? Only two of you? I thought there were more; many more. So this is hell. I'd never have believed it.

You remember all we were told about the torture chambers, the fire and brimstone, the "burning marl." Old wives' tales! There's no need for red–hot pokers. L'enfer, c'est les autres, Hell is—other people!

Probably most Boomers have encountered *Huis Closis*—*No Exit*, the existentialist French play by Jean–Paul Sartre. In our time it was widely featured in college literature anthologies. The play was presented for the first time in May 1944 at the Theatre du Vieux–Colombier in Paris.

Three damned souls, Joseph Garcin, journalist, man of letters from Rio; an unmarried Inès Serrano; and the Parisian Estelle Rigault are brought to the same drawing room in Hell depicted in Second Empire style with a massive bronze ornament standing on the mantelpiece. Inès died by a gas stove; Estelle from pneumonia; Garcin by twelve bullets through his chest.

In the soliloquy quoted above Garcin concludes existentially that rather than torture devices or physical punishment, hell is other people—*L'enfer, c'est les autres*. But Sartre got it wrong. Other people are not hell. *Other people and our relationships with them are where a person can ascend to heaven.*

To most people the Bible represents many things. To some it is the literal word of God. To others it is an ethical code of morality by which man can achieve fulfillment of the good life. To a few it is the primordial book of cosmology. To the Jewish people, the Bible is the divine law that permeates our every thought, action or contemplation.

In reality, however, the Bible is simply a book of relationships. Between man and woman, husband and wife, parents to children, children to parents, sisters to sisters, brothers to brothers, kings to vassals, nations to nations, mankind to the earth, humanity to God, and God to His creations. All of the Ten Commandants are about relationships, between man and God and people to people. God even tells us, "It is not good for man to be alone."[4]

Relationships are what separate humans from other species. "We are not animals because we are self–conscious," Rabbi Sir Jonathan Sacks says, "but because we are aware of ourselves as individuals and we are capable of forming relationships of trust."[5]

In his commentary on Psalm 33:15: "*He, who fashions their hearts for one another,*" Rabbi S.R. Hirsch says, "Humanity that distinguishes from beast is present only when man has acquired the virtues of sympathy, altruism, preparedness to act on behalf of the welfare of others. Only then does man fulfill his purpose. It is for this living for one another that God has fashioned the hearts of men, and it is in the light of this criterion that He evaluates all their deeds."[6]

The *Zohar* says, "For it is this purpose that God creates souls in couplers and sends them down to the world, so that there may be companionship both on high and below. And the well spring of all may be blessed."[7]

In the *Mishnah*[8] Hillel sums up the predicament we all face in life with regard to relationships. "If I am not for myself, who will be for me? And if I am only for myself, what am I?" Hillel also advises, "Do not separate yourself from the community."[9]

The Talmud relates a story that shows just how important relationships really are. Rabbi Beroka one day was walking through the market with Elijah the prophet. "Is there anyone here that you think is destined for the world to come?" asked Rabbi Beroka. After walking a few paces the prophet pointed out two men. "What is it you do?" Rabbi Beroka asked the men. "We are comedians. We cheer up people who are depressed. As well, whenever we see two people involved in a quarrel, we make every effort to make peace between them."[10]

Our relationships with others also influence our relationship with God. Rabbi Dosa ben Harkinas said, "In one whom people delight, God delights. In one in who people do not delight, God does not delight."[11]

"Real relationships to God cannot be achieved on earth if real relationships to the world and to mankind are lacking," Martin Buber explains. "Both love of the Creator and love of that which He has created are finally one and the same."[12] An inner religious development of the highest significance corresponds to the tendency, the striving to bridge the gulf between the love of God and the love of man. This is shown by the interpretation of this command, Buber adds. It is not just written, *Love thy neighbor as thyself,*[13] as though the sentence ended there, but it goes on: *Love thy neighbor as thyself, I am the Lord.*[14]

Our bodies and minds are hard–wired for relationships. Connection between social pain and physical pain illustrates the links between our emotions and physiological processes of our body. Social pain just does not cause emotional pain; it affects our physical being.[15]

Could pain killers that reduce the brain's response to physical pain also subdue social pain? Researchers discovered that when given Tylenol® a group reported feeling less social pain than the placebo group. Taking Tylenol® had made the brain's pain network less sensitive to the pain of rejection.[16] Tylenol® really does reduce the neural response to social rejection.[17]

Being cared for promotes opioid–based pleasure processes in the brain. We reach for the Snickers bar because the dopaminergic signals tell our brains that if we eat the Snickers bar, we will feel loved. In simple terms, we gravitate toward things that the brain has learned to associate with dopaminergic release.[18]

As I mentioned in Chapter 7—Addictions, Rabbi Dr. Twerski says we may form a relationship with food to compensate for the absence of relationships with people. Relating to food is safe because food can never reject you.[19] Unlike people, the Snickers bar will always be there for you; when you bite into it, you can always count on that feeling of being cared for. There was a certain truth in the advertisement, "My old pal Ovaltine."

We do care what other think of us. When a person contemplates doing something a little out of the ordinary, the first thing we do is look around to see if anyone is looking. Even just the thought that someone might be watching us is enough to determine our actions and behaviors. "Seeing ourselves as others would see us is sufficient to engage our self–control to overcome our unsocialized impulses in order to fall in line with societies expectations."[20]

Research indicates that just imagining what others think of you is sufficient to activate rVLPFC region of the brain. Right VLPFC sub regions are consistently active during motor inhibition. Input from the environment is sufficient to drive cognition in a bottom up fashion resulting in the production of appropriate behavior.

rVLPFC have also been implicated as a key region in the mirror neuron system. Mirror neurons are cells that respond both to the execution of an action and to observing someone else performing the same action.[21] The most striking finding on panoptic self–control is that merely seeing yourself, with no one else around, can promote self–restraint as well.[22]

In an experiment when subjects could see themselves in the mirror, fewer than 10 percent took more than one piece of candy. Just seeing one's reflection is enough to bring out our self–control to overcome impulse to snag some extra candy.[23] Imagine wall to wall mirrors in our kitchens and dining rooms and a perpendicular mirror facing the fridge. I have watched how people eat. Believe me; putting a mirror in front of you as you eat would be an eye opener.

Among the many significant findings of the Harvard Grant study was it is not the bad things that happen to us that doom us; it is the good people who happen to us at any age that facilitate enjoyable old age. Healing relationships are facilitated by having the capacity for gratitude, for forgiveness, and for taking people inside.[24]

Remember Rabbi Wolbe's lesson about gratitude and building character? "Acknowledgment of goodness that a person owes another person who did him a good is a great principle in building one's character traits and really enriches the core of a person, *and all of a person's relations with others*."[25] The Harvard Grant study proved Rabbi Wolbe to be right.

How many friends do we have? A survey in 1985, 59 percent of people listed they had three friends. By 2004 only 37 percent had three friends. In 1985, 10 percent had no friends and by 2004 no friends had risen to 25 percent.[26]

The fewer social relationships a person has, the shorter his or her life expectancy, and the worse the impact of various infectious diseases. Relationships that are medically protective can take the form of marriage, contact with friends and extended family, church membership or other group affiliations.[27]

Mortality rates in the United States for all causes of death, and not just heart disease, are consistently higher for divorced, single, and widowed individuals of both sexes and all races.[28] The Harvard Grant study observed that the divorced die more often only from illnesses made worst by the very factors that may have lead to the divorce.[29]

Compared with participants who felt most connected to others, socially isolated participants demonstrated a two to threefold increased risk of death from heart disease and all other causes. Strikingly, these results were independent of other cardiac risk factors.[30] Lonely people take longer to get better and if the illness is a serious one, they are more likely to die from it.[31]

Being divorced and having a higher mortality rate for all causes of death seemed to me to be counterintuitive. After my divorce, I felt much less stressed and healthier than I did while married. In fact, a few years after my divorce I encountered the young rabbi who was my learning partner when I was studying for rabbinical ordination. He looked at me and said, "Gosh, you look different. You are thinner, smiling and even look healthier. Are you still married?"

"Enmeshed or fused relationships are generally unhealthy, closed, ridged, and tend to discourage the fulfillment of one another's needs and rights," says Dr. Charles Whitfield. "They tend not to support the mental, emotional and spiritual growth of each person. Healthy relationships are open, flexible, allow the fulfillment of one another's needs and rights, and support the mental, emotional and spiritual growth of each person."[32]

Dr. Dean Ornish confirms that your immune system is less effective when you are in conflict with your spouse or companion, even when you just got married or are otherwise happy. Instead of being a source of refuge, love and support, it is particularly distressing when your spouse is a source of conflict.[33]

I answered my conundrum after I read *A Cry Unheard: The Medical Consequences of Loneliness*. In it Dr. James Lynch explained that it is not marriage per se that is the health factor. Rather, it is the lack of a confident, the lack of friends or other sources of social support.[34]

The lack of a confident. Dr. Ornish makes it clear "anything that promotes a sense of isolation often leads to illness and suffering. Anything that promotes a sense of love and intimacy, connection and community is healing.[35] The key for healing is relationship. Being loved is about having a place safe enough to express yourself, to express your feelings."[36]

Having a place safe enough to express yourself, to express your feelings. Dr. Ornish further explains an important reason why early family relationships are so predictive of later illness is that these patterns of relating do not change very much over time. Whether or not it was safe for you to be open and intimate in your family while growing up may determine to a large degree how safe it feels to be in an intimate relationship now.[37]

"In the child's body," Ernst Becker says, "is mirrored the whole quality of his relationship to his parents, the whole atmosphere of their approach to the world and life. The long experiences of the first five years of life are a kind of heavy emotional memory of how the world is, and what one must do to conform to it."[38]

Dr. T. Berri Brazelton explains we can't experience emotions that we never had, and we can't experience the consistency and intimacy of ongoing love unless we've had that experience with someone in our lives.[39] Robert Firestone adds that many people spend their entire lives in futile pursuit of the love that never existed or that was withheld from them by their parents.[40]

Harvel Hendrix is an author and with his wife the creator of Imago Relationship Therapy. In his book *Getting The Love You Want* he explains most of us seeking a relationship end up in unconscious marriages:

> Our unconscious expectation that we bring into marriage is that the partner we have chosen will love us in away our parents never did.[41] After all, people don't get married to take care of their partner's needs—they get married to further their own psychological and emotional growth. Once a relationship seems secure, a psychological switch is triggered deep in the old brain that activates all the latent infantile wishes. It is as if the wounded child within takes over.[42]
>
> At some point in their marriage, most people discover that something about their partners that awakens strong memories of childhood pain.[43] We enter marriage with the expectation that our partners will magically restore this feeling of wholeness. Their failure to do so is one of the main reasons for our eventual unhappiness.[44]
>
> A conscious marriage is a marriage that fosters maximum psychological and spiritual growth; it's a marriage created by becoming conscious and cooperating with the fundamental drives of the unconscious mind: to be safe, to be healed, and to be whole.[45]

The late Judith Wallerstein was a psychologist and researcher who created a 25–year study on the effects of divorce on the children. In her seminal study on divorce she validates Hendrix. "Men and women alike spoke sorrowfully of a pervasive sense of being uncared for. The most frequently mentioned complaint was a sense of having important, pressing needs which were unacknowledged, as well as unmet by the marital partner. Interestingly, no one blamed the children."[46]

Dr. Dean Ornish says the people we choose to be within a relationship and how we relate to that person can either help overcome adverse childhood experiences or reinforces them.[47] Gary

Chapman, the author of *The 5 Love Languages*, explains our most basic emotional need is not to fall in love but to be genuinely loved by another, to know a love that grows out of reason and choice, not instinct. I need to be loved by someone who chooses to love me, who sees in me something worth loving.[48]

After my divorce I went online in hopes of finding a new wife. Boy was that ever an experience! After about a year I planned on writing a book about online dating and began doing research. I joined a popular site; one that was very infrequently visited by Orthodox Jewish women to preserve objectivity.

In the course of a few weeks, I analyzed hundreds and hundreds of dating profiles of men and women of all ages. Unexpectedly, the site permanently blocked me. Their computer was very cagey; no matter how I tried to enter, no success.

I pondered over the data I collected but realized that it fell short of what I needed for my proposed book. I joined another site, but soon realized that their profile format made combining data impossible. Besides, that was the time I changed directions and starting researching *Until 120*.

But I did manage to accumulate enough data for some eye–openers about Boomers' relationships. I will share with you only one question asked by the online dating site, "What I Learned From My Relationships."

The following are the results of 1000 Baby Boomer profiles of women and men from the cities of Atlanta, Chicago, Dallas, Los Angeles, and New York. I chose these cities because I felt they would give a view of the entire country. There were minor regional differences but nothing worth pointing out. Surprisingly, it seemed both men and women learned much the same lessons from their marriages and relationships. Pity we didn't know these things *while* we were in those relationships.

Total Woman and Men	Women	Men
1. Communication	1. Communication	1. Communication
2. Honesty	2. Honesty	2. Honesty
3. Mutual Respect	3.Mutual Respect	3.Trust
4. Trust	4.Can't Fix or Change	4. Mutual Respect
5. Can't Fix or Change	5.Trust	5.Can't Fix or Change
6.Mutual Goals & Values	6.Mutual Goals & Values	6. Emotional Availability
7. Emotional Availability	7. Emotional Availability	7. Listening
8. Compromise	8. Friendship	8. Takes Effort & Work
9. Friendship	9. Trust Intuition	9. Compromise
10. Listening	10. Compromise	10. Friendship

In answer to the question, "what did you learn from your past relationships?" communication, honesty, respect, and trust were the most important lessons. Younger women and men under the age of 35 answered the question "what are you looking for in a partner?" by listing chemistry, love, passion, romance and affection as the top choices. In what Boomers were looking for in a partner, those things were also listed but not near the top ten. *Experience is always the best teacher.*

Close to 50 percent of first marriages fail. Two thirds of second marriages fail, and almost three–quarters of third marriages fail. Practice doesn't help us, apparently. After thinking about it, there seems to be much confusion about love and marriage. In the next chapter, I'll share with you what I learned about those topics.

16

Divorce, Marriage, Love

A person who does not love is a person who is barely alive.

Dr. Peter Breggin[1]

Man or woman, our first marriage is often to someone with the personality of our mother.

Nancy Friday[2]

A lack of self–esteem is often the root of serious problems in marriage.

Rabbi Dr. Abraham Twerski[3]

The opposite of love is not hate; the opposite of love is indifference.

Elie Wiesel

Why do we divorce? What is marriage? And what is love? These were the three questions that intrigued me most after my divorce because obviously I realized I hadn't a clue how to answer them. I am a two–time looser as we say. But I am lucky. I have friends who have lost many more times.

Since my divorce, I almost tied the knot a few times. I didn't because after the internal work I have done on myself; living life now in tandem with my inner child, I constantly battle my unconscious desires with my conscious knowledge.

Among the many legacies Boomers will leave to posterity will certainly be divorce. Over 58 percent of unmarried Baby Boomers are single through divorce. Eighty–seven percent of Baby Boomers have married at least once by the time they reached age 46. Of those who had married, 45 percent had experienced at least one divorce. More than a third of us are still single. And at our age, gray divorces are initiated by women more than double by men.[4] Why?

You were there. It was the time of the sexual revolution. We burned bras, scorned old values, and were determined not to follow in our parent's footsteps in anyway. Carly Simon sang it for us: *"Their children hate them for the things they're not. They hate themselves for what they are."*[5]

Our courtships went as follows: We met, we talked for a while trying to eat at the same time, we went to the movies where we did not talk to each other, and then we had sex. What the hell did we know about each other? We only knew with that first kiss, we tasted the effects of a Snickers bar. We wanted more. After sex, we felt like we'd eaten a family size pizza with all the toppings. Yum!

Tina Turner warned us but did we listen? *"You must understand that the touch of your hand makes my pulse react, that it's only the thrill . . . It's physical, only logical. You must try to ignore it, that it means more than that. What's love got to do with it, what's love got to do with it?"*

Matt Ridley is a British journalist who has written several popular science books and also member of the House of Lords. Ridley says, "Blindly, automatically and untaught, we bond with whoever is standing nearest when the oxytocin receptors in the medial amygdala get tingled."[6]

What we understood in a prehistoric manner was the other person gave us a feeling we did not want to live without. And when the pizza started giving us heartburn, we looked for another person who made pizza with a different recipe. No one ever told us that we could take an antacid and perhaps save a relationship.

We were taught every day in college that man was only an animal, glorified at best. You need only alter but a few genes and you get a primate. "If man is judged to be nothing more than a kind of higher animal," Rabbi Eliezer Berkovits says, "then to love him would mean mainly to satisfy his biological needs and love between the sexes would require only that they service each other is the most efficient manner."[7] *Ditto!*

The Boomer generation was weaned on consumerism and the disposability of goods. Everything is cheap. A watch, toaster or a relationship stops working; it doesn't pay to fix it. As Rabbi Sir Jonathan Sacks says, "A consumer–driven, advertising–dominated culture militates daily against attachments. A society saturated by market values would be one in which relationships were temporary, loyalties provisional and commitments easily discarded. It would, in short, be one in which marriage made little sense—and that, by and large, is what has happened."[8]

After graduate school, I became a practicing Sabbath observing Jew with all the trimmings. One of the first things I learned in encountering the teachings of our rabbis was a counterrevolutionary approach to sex. Rabbi Berkovits explained it may therefore very well be that how a man deals with personalizing the impersonal in his sex life is the core of all human morality.[9]

Rabbi Joseph Soloveitchik offers the Jewish way of personalizing the impersonal. "Marriage is basically supposed to accomplish the redeeming of the sex life from the aesthetic and hedonic and its conversion to an ethical moral experience whose intensity is not weakened through repetition."[10]

Orthodox Jews have a practice that goes beyond not engaging in pre–marital sex. *We do not even touch!* But the first time I heard about this practice was not when I was learning about Orthodox Judaism. Actually, I initially heard it in a strange way in college.

A friend of mine was dating a girl attending a neighboring college. One weekend he invited me to go with him so I could keep his girlfriends' roommate occupied. I agreed. Well, Friday night being a healthy male primate, I thought I would score big with the roommate. She was very good looking and we seemed to hit it off over prime rib. But later at her apartment instead of making time, I got a lecture about not engaging in pre–marital touching because it could lead to sex out of wedlock. I was stunned. Bill Graham sat between us on her couch.

She'd transferred from a Bible college. Rhetorically she asked me why men only think with their penis. I am sure today she is very happily married more than 40 years and proudly shares her grandchildren's selfies on Facebook. I, on the other hand, oh well.

Love marriages, sex resulting in blind romance, are doomed almost always to fail. Boomer divorce rates bear this out. The *Mishnah*[11] says any love that depends on a specific cause, i.e. sex, when that cause is gone, the love is gone; but if it does not depend on a specific cause, the love will never cease. What sort of love is depended upon a specific cause? The love of Amnon for Tamar.

Amnon, the son of King David, was in love with his half–sister Tamar. So desirous of her, he feigned illness, asking David to have Tamar bring him some food, dumplings. When Tamar arrived, Amnon revealed his true intentions. Tamar begged he refrain "because deeds like that are not done in Israel." Where could she go bearing such shame?

But he refused to heed her words and violated her. After the act, he despised Tamar, ordering her to leave. She pleaded in vain to stay. Amnon called his servant and sent Tamar away locking the door behind her. Devastated, she received little compassion from her brother Absalom. When David heard he grew angry. Absalom never spoke to Amnon; Tamar dwelled alone in Absalom's house.[12]

Sex blinds love. Martin Buber says, "As long as love is blind—that is, as long as it does not see a whole being—it does not yet truly stand under the basic word of relation."[13] "Infatuation makes us blind," Victor Frankel says, "Real love enables us to see."[14]

Regina: You hate me that much.

Horace: No.

Regina: Oh, I think you do. Well, we haven't been very good together. Anyway, I don't hate you either. I have only contempt for you. I've always had.

Horace: From the very first?

Regina: I think so.

Horace: I was in love with you. But why did you marry me?

Regina: I was lonely when I was young.

Horace: You were lonely?

Regina: Not the way people usually mean. Lonely for all the things I wasn't going to get. Everything in this house was so busy and there was so little place for what I wanted. I wanted the world. Then, and then—Papa died and left the money to Ben and Oscar.

Horace: And you married me?

Regina: Yes, I thought—but I was wrong. You were a small town clerk then. You haven't changed.

Horace: And it wasn't what you wanted?

Regina: No. No, it wasn't what I wanted. It took me a little while to find out I had made a mistake. As for you—I don't know. It was almost as if I couldn't stand the kind of man you were—. I used to lie there at night, praying you wouldn't come near.

Horace: Really? It was as bad as that?[15]

Little Foxes, a play by Lillian Hellman, starred Tallulah Bankhead in the 1939 Broadway production and Bette Davis in the movie. Directed by William Wyler, *Little Foxes* was nominated for nine Academy Awards.

Regina Hubbard Giddens is a 1900's Southern aristocrat who cares more for wealth than people. She has only contempt for her husband as she impatiently waits his death to inherit. In the next scene Horace suffers a heart attack but Regina makes no effort to get him his medicine from upstairs. Horace tries to climb the stairs but collapses on the way up. "What is a man in a wheelchair doing on a staircase?"[16] Hellman portrays a difficult marriage in the extreme, but unfortunately to many it may not be so farfetched.

Wallerstein in her study of divorce[17] found that men and women alike spoke sorrowfully of a pervasive sense of being uncared for. The most frequently mentioned complaint was the sense of having important and pressing needs which were unacknowledged, as well as unmet by the marital partner.[18]

Remember, relationships are disease prone if there is the lack of a confident and only promote health if the relationship means having a place safe enough to express yourself and your feelings. "To be truly open to another person's signals," Daniel Siegel says in his book, *The Mindful Therapist: A Clinician's Guide to Mindsight and Neural Integration*, "we need to transcend our own prisons of memory and move toward an open state of presence. To attune freely, we need to be fully receptive."[19]

Wallerstein reported divorces occurred in families where martial unhappiness had not been a special source of concern to either partner. The response to external stress, in other words, ricocheted into the family. The psychological mechanisms that lead from such stress to divorce can be explained by the stressed person's need to take flight to ward off the depression that threatens to overwhelm him or her.[20]

We flee from marriages that lack a confident we can share our stressors with and we feel are not safe enough to express ourselves. Remember, the number one lesson Boomers learned from past relationships was that communication was paramount.

Up close and personal. At some time after my divorce, independently each of my sons asked, "why did you divorce Mommy?" I had assumed that having been witness to our struggles, they would have understood. I gave each of them some sort of canned reason, which

I can no longer remember. But the question brought before my eyes a passage in the Talmud that always struck me as odd, even though I understood it.

The Talmud says, "Even the Temples' altar sheds tears for whoever divorces his first wife." [21] Why specifically should the altar cry tears when a couple divorces? I can hear God sheds tears, the Patriarchs and Matriarchs, maybe Moses, buy why stones?

Not so long ago I heard a response that Rabbi Paysach Krohn gave that answers my question. "The altar cries," Rabbi Krohn says, "because it expects animals to be sacrificed—not children." Rabbi Krohn's interpretation sadly is correct as I now know. Whenever we divorce, we render our children up to the altar.

Interestingly, Wallerstein found no one blamed the children for the divorce. [22] Wallenstein's research found: only thirty–four percent of the children and adolescents appeared to be doing especially good at the five year mark; [23] over one third of the children were consciously and intensely unhappy and dissatisfied with the life in the post divorce family; [24] and thirty–seven percent of all children and adolescents were moderately to severely depressed. [25] She also found parents who treated their children poorly were more likely to treat their marital partners badly as well. [26]

Years later I finally realized why I asked my wife for a divorce. In retrospect, it was none of the reasons I thought at the time. When I read a comment in Dr. Dean Ornish's *Love and Survival* for the first time I understood my reason. "When a person begins to feel accountable for his or her own actions rather than blaming the other person in the relationship, then the relationship transforms. Either the relationship may grow and become more authentic and intimate, or one person or both may decide to end a destructive relationship and choose another who is more compatible or who has a greater capacity for intimacy at that time." [27] Enough said.

"Once upon a time," said Rabbi Bunam, "in a simple public house in Warsaw, I heard two Jewish porters at a neighboring table tell each other all kinds of things over their brandy. One of them asked: 'Have you learned the Scripture portion for this week?' 'Yes,' the other said. 'So have I,' said the first one, 'and I find one thing hard to understand. It says there concerning our Father Abraham and Abimelech, the king of the Philistines: 'They made, these two, a covenant.' I asked myself why it says: 'These two.' That seemed superfluous.' 'A good question,' cried the other. 'But how do you answer that question?' 'I think,' the other answered, 'they made a covenant, but they did not become one; they remained two.'"[28]

This excerpt from *For The Sake of Heaven*, Martin Buber's fictional chronicle of legendry Hasidic life, portrays best my ultimate understanding of marriage. I had always been told a marriage was like a corporation: a merger to maximize goods and services between two people. Once I even heard marriage referred as a Mr. and Mrs. Company. "Hey, I got an idea. Let's pool our resources and get married."

But Rabbi Soloveitchik says, "Marriage is not a utilitarian transaction, a partnership agreement, a casual relationship. It is an existential commitment, a uniting of two lonely, incomplete souls to share a common destiny with its joys and sorrows. It is not an association but an integration.[29] The main value of marriage is to be found not in its collective utility, but in its creating a personal experience that enriches and enhances the lives of two individuals who were drawn to each other.[30] Each one finds self–fulfillment and completeness redeeming him or her from the devastating experience of loneness."[31]

In the corporation model, husband and wife are both expecting immediate returns on their investment. In reality, investment in a marriage has a very long period of amortization. A good marriage is not for those who depend only on immediate gratification.

Rabbi Berkovits says formal marriage is not to be based on the present love that at this moment unites two human beings, but on the trust in the self–transcending power of that love, in its as yet unfathomed potential that through care, devotion, and practice of basic humanity and decency will carry two human beings to the richest bio–psychic fulfillment of which they are capable.[32]

Marriage is also a covenantal union, according to Rabbi Soloveitchik. Two strangers decide to unite their destinies, to share the same fate, to suffer and rejoice together, to travel together and pay the toll of the road jointly.[33]

A covenantal union. "Covenantal relationships," Rabbi Sir Jonathan Sacks says, "where we help others and they help us without calculations of advantage are where trust is born. Contracts, social or economic, mediate relationships between strangers. But if we were always and only strangers to one another, we would have no reason to trust one another."[34]

Covenant is a bond, Rabbi Sacks continues, not of interest or advantage, but of belonging. Covenants are made when two or more people come together to create a 'We'. They differ from contracts in that they tend to be open–ended and enduring. They involve a commitment of the person to another, or to several others. They involve a substantive notion of loyalty—of staying together even in difficult times. They may call, at times, for self–sacrifice. The simplest example of a covenant is a marriage.[35]

Matchmaker, Matchmaker,
Make me a match,
Find me a find, catch me a catch
Matchmaker, Matchmaker
Look through your book,
And make me a perfect match.

In the 1964 Broadway hit, *Fiddler on the Roof*, Hodel knew what every girl in the *shtetl* knew: "A girl from a poor family must take whatever husband Yenta, the matchmaker, brings." Among many Jewish Ultra–Orthodox today, arranged marriages are still the norm.

Arranged marriages usually take place in religious environments, with people of the same faith, and they each know that they're going to get married because they want to have children, they expect love to grow in the family context and they're often not overly fantasizing about what it's all supposed to look like. They're more practical and down to earth in some respect.

Many studies indicate that couples who participate regularly in religious activities (e.g. church attendance) report greater marital happiness and satisfaction and may be less likely to divorce compared to their less religious counterparts.[36] Jewish Hasidic communities have established a mentoring system in which new couples are partnered with established couples, meeting regularly to deal with the challenges marriage and home life.

Rabbi Eliyahu Dessler explains the simple truth is that when a man choose a wife for himself, he finds, once the first intoxication has worn off, that she is not at all as he thought and that he has made a great mistake.[37] "People know very well that no one can rely on their own judgment in these matters. So, they purposely arrange for other people to make the decision for them. In a matter which one cannot trust one's own judgment one has to seek the advice of others, and if he doesn't rely on them he will most certainly do the wrong thing."[38]

The *Aleinu Marital Satisfaction Survey*[39] targeted the Orthodox Jewish community and focused upon the many facets of marital satisfaction and dissatisfaction. Of those who responded, 72 percent of men and 74 percent of women rated their marriages as "Very Good" or better. In contrast, only a small minority—about 13 percent—responded that their marriages were "Fair" or "Poor. And 74 percent of their spouses would marry them all over again if they could.

This compares with the *National Marriage Project* survey of the same year polling the general population. Only 62.9% percent of men and 59.5% percent of women in the *National Marriage Project* survey rated their marriages as "very happy."[40]

A pioneer in the study of arranged marriages is Robert Epstein, former editor–in–chief of *Psychology Today* and a PhD in psychology from Harvard University. In India, roughly 90 percent of marriages are arranged yet it has one of the lowest divorce rates in the world, even though divorce is legal there.

Dr. Epstein says, "There's a very interesting study done in India comparing the love in 'love' marriages to the love in arranged marriages that found something quite spectacular. In the love marriages, there's a lot of love at first, but then it weakens over time. In arranged marriages, there's not that much love at first, but it tends to grow over time, and it surpasses the love in the love marriages about five years out. Ten years out it's twice as strong."[41]

"The biggest result or insight we got was that commitment is a factor that seems most responsible for the growth of love," Dr. Epstein says. "That has to mean real commitment, not the kind we so often make in our marriages here, almost as if we're keeping our fingers crossed behind our backs. Real commitment meaning, 'I'm really going to be with you through thick and thin, through sickness and in health.' This has led me to develop the Vulnerability Theory of Emotional Bonding. 'I am entirely vulnerable to you. No matter what is happening, I will be there for you.'"[42]

Vulnerability. Sound familiar? Remember Bené Brown saying vulnerability is the birthplace of love, belonging, joy, courage, empathy, and creativity; the source of hope, empathy, account–ability, and authenticity. If we want greater clarity in our purpose or deeper and more meaningful spiritual lives, vulnerability is the path.[43] Vulnerability is the core of all emotions and feelings. To feel is to be vulnerable.[44]

In a paper[45] presented at the 95th annual meeting of the Western Psychological Association, Dr. Epstein said support was found for a "vulnerability theory of emotional bonding" according to which the strength of various aspects of an emotional bond can be predicted by independent measures of the vulnerability that each of two persons shows with respect to one another, where vulnerability is defined by self–reported measures of states of need and empathy. As predicted, bonds were weakest between subjects in low need and empathy states.

Covenant, existential commitment, arrangement, and vulnerability; so, *what's love got to do with*? Martin Buber explains love does not invalidate the 'I'; on the contrary, it binds the 'I' more closely to the 'Thou.' It does not say: 'Thou art loved' but 'I love Thee.'[46] "Man becomes an 'I' through a 'You.'"[47] *Ich und Du!*

In my research, I came across many meaningful definitions of love from a variety of well–respected people:

Harry Stack Sullivan: When the satisfaction or security of another person becomes as significant to one as is one's own satisfaction or security, then the state of love exists.[48]

Rollo May: We define love as a delight in the presence of the other person and affirming of his value and development as much as one's own. Thus there are always two elements to love—that of worth and good of the other person, and that of one's own joy and happiness in the relation with him.[49]

M. Scott Peck: I define love thus: The will to extend one's self for the purpose of nurturing one's own or another's spiritual growth.[50]

Victor Frankel: Love is living the experience of another person in all its uniqueness and singularity.[51]

There is another aspect of true love many people overlook. According to Pastor Rick Warren, you can give without loving but you cannot love without giving.[52] Rabbi Eliyahu Dessler adds that love and giving always come together. Is the giving a consequence of the love, or is perhaps the reverse; is the love the result of giving?[53]

Finally, the Bible[54] simply tell us what true love is and when does it occur. Abraham sent his servant to find a wife for Isaac. When Abraham's servant returned, he told Isaac all he had done. Isaac brought Rebecca into Sara's tent, she became his wife, and he loved her. From all I have newly learned, this seems to be the proper sequence to achieve a long lasting healthy marriage.

Portia Nelson was a renaissance woman: author, singer, actress, composer, lyricist, painter and photographer. She appeared in such films as *The Sound of Music, Dr. Dolittle, The Trouble with Angels,* and *The Other;* on the television soap opera, *All My Children,* as Mrs. Gurney for many years, my mother's favorite soap; on Broadway in the award–winning musical *The Golden Apple.* As a singer, a soprano with a silvery tone, she recorded five show albums for Columbia Records, and was included in the Smithsonian collections: *Cole Porter Songs* and *The American Popular Singer.*

Ms. Nelson had two bouts with cancer: breast cancer and throat and tongue cancer which Nelson, who never smoked, blamed on her years of singing in smoky nightclubs.

Her book, *There's A Hole In My Sidewalk,* is a sought after classic and well known to anyone who has been a member of a recovery twelve–step group. Her poem from that work, *Autobiography in Five Short Chap*ters, has been reprinted numerous times. That poem reflects the new street hopefully I now walk down after much inner work, as so many people have done:

197

Autobiography in Five Short Chapters [55]

By Portia Nelson

I walk down the street.
There is a deep hole in the sidewalk.
I fall in.
I am lost…
I am helpless.
It is not my fault.
It takes forever to find my way out.

I walk down the same street.
There is a deep hole in the sidewalk.
I pretend I don't see it.
I fall in.
I can't believe I am in the same place.
But it isn't my fault.
It still takes a long time to get out.

I walk down the same street.
There is a deep hole in the sidewalk.
I see it there.
I still fall in . . . It's a habit . . . but
My eyes are open.
I know where I am.
It is my fault.
I get out immediately.

I walk down the same street.
There is a deep hole in the sidewalk.
I walk around it.

I walk down another street.

17

Doctored

God heals and the doctor takes the fee.

Benjamin Franklin

Never go to a doctor whose office plants have died.

Erma Bombeck

The art of medicine consists in amusing the patient while nature cures the disease.

Voltaire

One must not forget that recovery is brought about not by the physician, but by the sick man himself.

Dr. Georg Groddeck

I must confess that I am spoiled in my opinions of physicians. I grew up in rural Georgia being cared for by an iconoclastic country doctor. Dr. John Lewis was practicing medicine well before the Twentieth Century turned. As a child many were the times my mother would call Dr. Lewis, handing me the phone and after our few minute conversation, he would diagnose, tell my mother my temperature, and call in a prescription to the local pharmacy for my mother to pick up. Payment was never the critical factor. I am really not sure if my mother ever paid for those calls.

The Talmud[1] interesting enough tells an applicable story. Once in the study hall they were discussing who had received greetings from Heaven. Abaye received greetings every Friday before the Sabbath arrived; Rava annually at Yom Kippur, but Abba the physician would receive greetings from the Heavenly Academy every day; a fact which caused Abaye distress. Abaye's colleagues explained that Abba the physician preformed deeds he was unable to do. And what were deeds of Abba the physician? He had a private place in which patients would deposit the coins he took so whoever did not have payment would not be embarrassed. *Those were the days my friends…*

It wasn't always the case that sick people consulted doctors to cure an illness. When the Jewish Temple stood in Jerusalem, people turned to prophets for healing. The Talmud[2] tells us that in addition to the forty–eight prophets and seven prophetesses which are recorded in the Bible, there were well over a million prophets in Israel at the time. Only those prophets whose prophecies were needed for future generations were recorded.

Nahmanides, the 13th century Spanish Biblical commentator, explains that if the Israelites keep the commandments given at Sinai, then God promised, "I shall remove illness from your midst."[3] He makes clear that God promises "food and drink that will bless you to extent that no illnesses will befall your bodies."[4]

In his commentary, Nahmanides points out that if a righteous person lives by the commandants and God keeps illness at bay, it would be less than miraculous because the wicked at times also live healthy long lives. But if it happens to an entire people, the Israelites, then the world would recognize that this came from God and would appreciate His reverence to the Jewish people.

The underlying principle according to Nahmanides is when the nation of Israel is perfect in observing the commandments, then as a group nature does not guide their affairs. "For God blesses their bread and their water and He will remove illness from their midst and they will not need a doctor."[5] This is how the righteous lived during the age of prophecy. If illness did occur because of some sin, they would consult a prophet rather than a doctor. "What business," asks Nahmanides, "does a doctor have in the home of one who fulfills the will of God?"

As is usually the case in the Talmud,[6] a dispute ensues: whether or not it is proper to seek out doctors for a cure. One side says before going to a doctor, a person should say the following prayer, "May it be Your will, God, that this treatment cure me, for only You are the true healer and only Your cures are real. Alas, but we have accustomed ourselves to seek out doctors."

Yet, the other side argues that we should not pray accordingly at the doctor's office because it is God, Himself, who sends us to doctors. The Bible says, "And he shall provide for healing."[7] From here the Jewish sages learn that permission was given in Heaven for doctors to offer medical treatments.

We saw previously[8] that King Hezekiah crushed the copper serpent because the people no longer looked to God as the healer of all illness. As a matter of fact, the Talmud in several places tells us "Everything is in the hands of Heaven except for the fear of Heaven."[9] And in another reference the Talmud says "a person does not stub his toe down below, unless it has been decreed upon him from above."[10] If that is really true, then why did God give His blessing to doctors to heal?

To answer this question, we must turn to Rabbi Eliezer Papo, the 18th–19th century rabbi of Sarajevo who was a proponent of the rabbinic–Kabbalistic school of *Mussar*. In his best known work, *Pele Yoetz*, he poses our question:

> You may ask since God gives life and death, what is the point of a doctor? If it is determined that a person will die, then all the doctors in the world won't be able to save him. And if the Almighty wants him to live, then He can find ways to cure him without a doctor.
>
> The answer to this and many similar questions is that there are three types of Divine Providence. If a person merits living, he will live even if the doctor administers the wrong treatment. If the person has, Heaven forbid, been decreed to die, no doctor will be able to

save him. There is a third type of situation where a person has, because of his sins, been subjected to the rules of nature. If he takes care of himself, he will live; if not he will die. Every person should consider himself to be in the third category.[11]

And indeed, the Talmud[12] gives credence to Rabbi Papo's answer by finally stating that all is in the hands of heaven except for illnesses brought about as a result of cold and inflammation. We will revisit this Talmudic statement in a later chapter.

Even though doctors are seemingly sanctioned in Judaism and every Jewish mother dreams of her son becoming a doctor, does reverence for the profession necessarily follow? The Talmud[13] argues about appropriate trades for children to learn. One side says not to teach sons to be sailors, shepherds, storekeepers, donkey, camel, and wagon drivers.

An opposing view says that camel drivers are righteous and sailors are pious, but adds that "the best of physicians go to hell." *Boy, talk about not mincing words.* BTW, fewer than half of the doctors in the United States say they would choose the same career if they had it to do over.[14]

Many are the commentaries explaining this statement: at times physicians refuse to treat patients who lack payment, they do not exert themselves properly as a doctor should, when a physician does not know the cause of an illness and how to treat it but yet still claims expertise he causes the patient's death, physicians not acknowledging God as the true Healer, etc. In today's parlance, it would be appropriate to say that many physicians view MD to mean *medical deity*.

Baby Boomers in high school world history were taught about the Babylonian Code of Hammurabi which dates back to about 1754 BCE. However, most people do not realize it was also probably one of the first recorded efforts to regulate the medical profession:

If a physician: makes a large incision with a bronze lancet, and kills him, or opens a tumor with the operating knife, and cut out the eye, the physicians hands shall be cut off; makes a large incision in the slave of a freed man, and kill him, the physician shall replace the slave with another slave; opens a tumor with a bronze lancet, and puts out his eye, the physician shall pay half his value; heals the broken bone or diseased soft part of a man, the patient shall pay the physician five shekels in money; operates on a man for a severe wound with a bronze lancet and saves the man's life; or if he opens an abscess of a man with a bronze lancet and save that man's eye, he shall receive ten shekels of silver.

During the past millennium the medical profession has to some extent been regulated in all cultures with just cause. For all medicine, the first principle is *primum non nocere*—first do no harm. Yet, throughout the ages this was unfortunately the exception not the rule. Doctor's cures invariably killed more patients that they saved.

In Talmudic times the theory of diseases was highly influenced by ideas of an imbalance of the basic "four humors;" a theory known as dyscrasia for which the main treatment was bloodletting which remained the norm for centuries and was considered modern medicine. The barber and the physician often shared the same identity. George Washington was literally bled to death by his physicians.

Let me ask a question. What are the three leading causes of death in the United States today? Almost everyone will place cancer and/or heart disease in the number one and two slots. Number three is a little more problematic. Is it chronic lower respiratory diseases; cerebrovascular diseases; Alzheimer's disease; diabetes mellitus; influenza and pneumonia?

The U.S. Department of Health and Human Services annually publishes the leading causes of death in the United States. Their methodology is based on information from all death certificates filed in the 50 states and the District of Columbia. Cause–of–death statistics are based upon the International Classification of Diseases and are ranked according to the number of deaths assigned to rankable causes of death.

But the third leading cause of death is *not* included in the International Classification of Diseases and most often *does not* appear on death certificates. The number three cause of death in the United States is iatrogenic illness: unnecessary surgery, medication errors in hospitals, nosocomial infections in hospitals, other errors in hospitals, and nonerror—adverse effects of medications.[15]

Iatrogenic illness is derived from the Greek *iatro* meaning doctor and *genic* meaning caused by. Therefore, iatrogenic illness refers to doctor created illnesses. Iatrogenesis is basically the inadvertent or unintended adverse effects or complications caused by medical treatments or medical advice.

Gary Null in an article in *Journal of Orthomolecular Medicine*[16] explained iatrogenic morbidity, mortality, and financial loss in outpatient clinics, transitional care, long–term, rehabilitative and home care, practitioner's offices, and hospitals, are also due to:

1. X–ray exposures of mammography, fluoroscopy, CT scans.
2. Overuse of antibiotics in all conditions
3. Carcinogenic drugs
4. Immunosuppressive drugs, prescription drugs
5. Cancer chemotherapy
6. Surgery and surgical procedures.
7. Unnecessary surgery
8. Medical procedures and therapies
9. Discredited, unnecessary, and unproven medical procedures
10. Doctors themselves
11. Missed diagnoses

Dr. Barbara Starfield, in an article published in the *New England Journal of Medicine*[17] proposed a relationship between iatrogenic effects and type of care received. The results of international surveys document the high availability of technology in the United States. The United States is second only to Japan in the availability of magnetic resonance imaging units and computed tomography scanners per million population. Japan, however, ranks among the highest on health; the United States ranks among the lowest.

It is possible that the high use of technology in Japan is limited to diagnostic technology not matched by high rates of treatment, whereas in the United States, high use of diagnostic technology may be linked to the cascade effect and to more treatment. [Emphasis added]

This is exactly the point. Dr. Starfield's comparison between the US and Japan exemplifies the difference between Oriental Medicine and Western Medicine. Where Western biomedicine seeks a pathological mechanism behind the veil of symptoms, Chinese medicine rarely looks further than the patient.[18]

Recently, *Bloomberg*[19] ranked countries efficiency of their health–care systems. Countries with populations of at least five million, GDP per capita of at least $5,000 and life expectancy of at least 70 years were ranked by life expectancy, relative per capita cost of health care; and absolute per capita cost of health care:

1. Singapore
2. Hong Kong
3. Italy
4. Japan
5. South Korea
6. Australia
7. Israel
8. France
9. United Arab Emirates
10. United Kingdom

The United States was ranked #44 ahead of Bulgaria, Iran, Columbia, Azerbaijan, Algeria, Brazil and Russia. The top ten is very diverse globally so regional influences seem not to play a role. Nor is the amount of money spent on health a factor. The US spends $8,895 per capita on health care, the largest of any country, which is 72.7% more than #1 Singapore and 74.2% more than #7 Israel where I live. It is interesting also to note that four of the top five countries are historically based on Oriental medicine.

Dr. Bradley Bale, co–author of *Beat the Heart Attack Gene: The Revolutionary Plan to Prevent Heart Disease, Stroke, and Diabetes*, points out, "Most doctors are not disease detectives. They're trained to look for symptoms of active disorders and treat them; they're forced to rely on medical guidelines that are designed for the general population. Consequently, patients are screened and treated according to the average results from large studies, receiving one–size–fits–all care instead of tests and therapies tailored to their individual needs."[20]

And this is one of the major opportunities for iatrogenic illness to occur. A doctor sees twenty patients in a day with the same symptoms of runny nose, cough, sore throat, etc. Diagnosis: a virus. The next patient that comes in with the same symptoms gets the same diagnosis, "A virus; it's going around."

But in that next person it is not viral, but an undiagnosed bacterial infection with a world of difference in complications. Instead of discomfort for a few days, she ends up in an ICU ward fighting for her life. Etc, etc, etc! In one study physicians who diagnosed their patients as having pneumonia reported an 88 percent confidence but proved correct only 20 percent of the time.[21]

In a study published in the *Journal of General Internal Medicine*[22] twenty–six acute care nonfederal hospitals throughout the U.S. were studied for voluntary electronic reporting of medical errors and adverse events. The most commonly reported events within medication and infusions were wrong dose, omitted drug, wrong drug, drug reaction–allergy, wrong time–frequency, wrong form–infusion rate, wrong patient.

Of the reported medical errors and adverse events, 67% caused no harm, 32% temporary harm, 0.8% life threatening or permanent harm, and 0.4% contributed to patient deaths. Among 80% of reports that identified level of impact, 53% were events that reached a patient, 13% were near misses that did not reach the patient, and 14% were hospital environment problems.

Though the proportion of very serious adverse events was small, it was not negligible: slightly more than 1 per 1,000 admissions. The authors concluded that if this rate was applied to the entire population of 33.7 million inpatients in nonfederal acute care hospitals in the U.S. during the year of the study, an estimated 34,000 patients per year could be permanently injured or die during hospitalization because of an adverse medication event.

Of all adverse reports in the study, registered nurses reported 47%, pharmacists and pharmacy technicians 16%, laboratory technicians 10%, unit clerks/secretarial staff 10%, licensed practical nurses and nursing assistants 3%, and physicians 1.4%. Physicians contributed less than 2% of all reports. The authors said that physicians operate within a belief system of self–blame and personal responsibility, rather than viewing such events as the end process of a series of systematic deficiencies. Additionally, physicians may not report because of "professional courtesy," concern for implicating colleagues, or fear of repercussions.

I believe that a major underlying cause of iatrogenic illness is that doctors in their zeal to ride the wave of technologic advancements they have over looked the most important item: the patient.

Dr. William Osler, a Canadian physician who died in 1919, is frequently described as the "Father of Modern Medicine." One of the four founders of Johns Hopkins Hospital, he created residency as a program for specialty training and was the first to bring medical students to the patient's bedside for clinical training. Dr. Osler said,

"The good physician treats the disease; the great physician threats the person who has the disease."

The iconoclastic country doctor is to me the forgotten model of health care which we lack today. I was curious what Dr. John Lewis was taught in his 19th century medical training that made him so special to so many? I partially found my answer looking back through medical texts of the time

One book I read published in 1909 was *Preventable Diseases* by Dr. Woods Hutchinson. Dr. Hutchinson was a Professor of Anatomy, University of Iowa; Professor of Comparative Pathology and Methods of Science Teaching, University of Buffalo; Lecturer, London Medical Graduates' College and University of London; State Health Officer of Oregon, and also the author of A *Handbook of Health*, *Conquest of Consumption*, and *Instinct and Health*.

A century ago, Dr. Hutchinson advised doctors, "Don't rush for some remedy with which to club into insensibility every symptom of disease as soon as it puts in an appearance. Give nature a little chance to show what she intends to do before attempting to stop her by dosing yourself with some pain–reliever or colic cure."[23]

Hippocrates, the Father of Medicine, twenty four centuries ago told his disciples in Greece that disease is not only suffering, *pathos*, but also toil, *ponos*, which is the fight of the body to restore itself. There is *vis medicatrix naturae*—a healing force of Nature which cures from within.[24] Maimonides concurs by quoting a passage in Aristotle's *Perception and the Perceptible*: "Most of those who die, die from the treatment because of the ignorance of most physicians about Nature."[25]

But of all Dr. Hutchinson's advice, I think the following accents the root cause of iatrogenic illness. "Small wonder that the shrewd advice of a veteran physician to the medical student should be: The first step in the examination is to look at your patient; the second is to look again, and the third to take another look at him; and keep on looking all through the examination."[26]

Dr. Hutchinson is not the only 19th century physician I think has a lot to teach modern medical doctors. Another is Sir Joseph Bell. Bell was a professor at the University of Edinburgh Medical School. A pioneer in forensic pathology, he was the author of many texts including the *Manual of the Operations of Surgery*.

Whenever Queen Victoria visited Scotland, Dr. Bell was her personal surgeon and physician. Bell also achieved notoriety as Sir Arthur Conan Doyle's model for his legendary sleuth, Sherlock Holmes. Doyle was a medical student in Edinburgh who studied under Professor Bell.

In his TED TALK,[27] Dr. Abraham Varghese tells of an exchange between Bell and his medical students that Conan Doyle chronicled. Doyle describes a conversation between Bell and a woman with a child:

> The woman says, "Good Morning." Bell says, "What sort of crossing did you have on the ferry from Burnt Island?" She says, "It was good." And he says, "What did you do with the other child?" She says, "I left him with my sister at Leith." And he says, "And did you take the shortcut down Inverleith Row to get here to the infirmary?" She says, "I did." And he says, "Would you still be working at the linoleum factory?" And she says, "I am."
>
> And Bell then goes on to explain to the students. He says, "You see, when she said, 'Good morning,' I picked up her Fife accent. And the nearest ferry crossing from Fife is from Burnt Island. And so she must have taken the ferry over. You notice that the coat she's carrying is too small for the child who is with her, and therefore, she started out the journey with two children, but dropped one off along the way.
>
> You notice the clay on the soles of her feet. Such red clay is not found within a hundred miles of Edinburgh, except in the botanical gardens. And therefore, she took a short cut down Inverleith Row to arrive here. And finally, she has dermatitis on the fingers of her right hand, a dermatitis that is unique to the linoleum factory workers in Burnt Island."

Dr. Varghese adds, "And when Bell actually strips the patient, begins to examine the patient, you can only imagine how much more he would discern. And as a teacher of medicine, as a student myself, I was so inspired by that story."

In a popular contemporary textbook of cardiovascular medicine the authors wrote the following:

> There is a temptation to carry out expensive and occasionally uncomfortable or even hazardous procedures to establish a diagnosis when a detailed, thoughtful history and through physical examination are sufficient. The overreliance on laboratory tests has increased as physicians attempt to use their time more efficiently by delegating responsibility for taking the history to an assistant or nurse or by even limiting the history to a questionnaire.
>
> First, it must be appreciated that the history remains the richest source of information concerning the patient's illness and any practice that might diminish the quality or quantity of information is likely ultimately to impair the quality of care. Second, the physician's attentive and thoughtful taking of a history establishes a bond with the patient. [28]

Talking about patient histories, recently I was telling my doctor about my history of having had two polyps at an early age; that my mother died from colon cancer; and three years ago my colonoscopy found one small polyp. The conversation lasted about twenty minutes. I then said there was another issue I wanted to discuss. He said, "Next time." I looked at him and said, "Next time?" He responded "next time" and rose signaling the visit's end. Doctor's visits in our time have become more like *speed dating*!

I made an appointment a few days later with my doctor to discuss the other problem which I knew was not serious. God forgive me for having violated the sacrosanct 12 minute patient encounter during the previous visit. But I asked myself, what if I had been a normal patient. By normal, I mean the typical person who does not proactively self–advocate his medical treatment and shows up for an office visit armed with studies from the likes of the *New England Journal of Medicine*, the *British Medical Journal, American Journal of Clinical Nutrition, Journal of General Internal Medicine*, etc like I do. What if someone's other problem was excruciating chest pains, rectal bleeding, a nondescript lump or some other such unknown? *What the hell has happened to the medical profession of Dr. John Lewis?*

According to one study,[29] the corporatization of American medicine has extended into all parts of the health care system. Wall Street and the interests of shareholders have replaced Main Street in shaping the organization of health care, the market, and even clinical decisions. About two–thirds of HMOs are for–profit corporate organizations. Almost half of the nation's Blue Cross–Blue Shield plans are now for–profit. For–profits are typically driven by the market with a strong focus on managing costs rather than care.

The study says that for–profit versus not–for–profit makes a big difference as was shown by a recent finding. The two largest health insurers in California are Kaiser Permanente (not–for–profit) and Blue Cross (for–profit); Kaiser spent 96% of every premium dollar on medical care, whereas Blue Cross spent just 76% on medical care. *For investor–owned health care corporations, money is the mission, not the public interest.* [Emphasis added]

Medicine is slowly changing. The rise of complementary–alternative medicine (CAM) therapies is forcing the change. Given patients' demands and utilization of complementary–alternative medicine therapies, despite the lack of evidence, family physicians are faced with questions related to the integration of CAM in their patient management and an increasing need to address how CAM therapies can be integrated into conventional medical systems.[30] As Dr. Bernie Siegel says, "When you are told what day you are going to die and all hope is taken away, why not seek alternative therapies?"[31]

A century ago there was much over lap even in medical school training. The Carnegie Foundation commissioned Abraham Flexner in 1910 to survey and report on the quality of medical schools in the United States and Canada. The Flexner report effectively drew the line between allopathic medicine and other dogmas. Doctors would no longer be trained in complementary and alternative medicine, just allopathic medicine. For more than a century, allopathic (drug medicine) and homeopathic (natural medicine) have slugged it out. The American Medical Association, the AMA, was originally founded to protect the financial interests of allopathic medicine.

The AMA spent the ensuing years since Flexner discrediting and eliminating all but allopathic medicine. I won't go through the AMA's unscrupulous history of destroying competition except for one example. In 1974 five chiropractors sued the American Medical Association for violation of the Sherman Anti–Trust Act known as the Wilk suit. In 1987 the court found the AMA was guilty of conspiring to "contain and eliminate the chiropractic profession."

Dr. Elisabeth Kubler–Ross in her seminal work *On Death and Dying* asked a series of rhetorical questions which I think it are worth quoting:

> What happens in a changing field of medicine, where we have to ask ourselves whether medicine is to remain a humanitarian and respected profession or a new but depersonalized science in the service of prolonging life rather than diminishing human suffering? Where the medical students have a choice of a dozen lectures on RNA and DNA but less experience in the simple doctor–patient relationship that used to be the alphabet of every successful family physician? In a professional society where the young medical student is admired for his research and laboratory work during his first years of medical school while he is at a loss for words when a patient asks him a simple question?[32]

Doctors have become so specialized that the traditional role of a caregiver who focuses on healing and wellness has disappeared. Some doctors and patients are unsatisfied with a focus on using pharmaceuticals to treat or suppress a specific disease rather than on helping a patient to become healthy. Recognition of the harmful effects of health care interventions, and the likely possibility that they account for a substantial proportion of the excess deaths in the United States compared with other comparably industrialized nations have created a new medical revolution, one albeit with an old approach.

Integrative medicine is a combination of complementary and alternative medicine with evidence–based medicine which treats the "whole person," focuses on wellness and health rather than on treating disease, and emphasizes the patient–physician relationship. Critics unjustly claim that integrative medicine compromises main stream medicine by using ineffective complementary remedies.

In integrative medicine patients and physicians are partners in the healing process. The whole person including all aspects of lifestyle—embracing mind, body and spirit that influence health, wellness, and disease—are utilized. And where possible, interventions that are less invasive and natural are used.

In 2011, a survey[33] was commissioned to determine how integrative medicine was currently being practiced across the United States. The study found strong affiliations to hospitals, healthcare systems, and medical and nursing schools as well as the centers' collaborative work with, and growing referrals from their own health systems reveal that integrative medicine is now an established part of healthcare in the United States.

From a list of 20 clinical conditions, respondents chose the top 5 for which they perceive integrative medicine to be most successful at their centers. These are: chronic pain, gastrointestinal conditions, depression, stress and cancer. The interventions prescribed most frequently across all conditions are: food, nutrition, supplements, yoga, meditation, traditional Chinese Medicine, acupuncture, massage and pharmaceuticals.

The Consortium of Academic Health Centers for Integrative Medicine, which encourages the spread of CAM education, was founded in 2000 after an initiative by eight academic medical centers and now boasts 46 medical school members.

A clinical study[34] on integrative medicine in China makes clear an important point:

> The coexistence of Western medicine and traditional Chinese medicine began to appear when Western medicine was introduced to China from the middle of 16th century. Integrative medicine is not only an innovative China model in clinical practice, but also the bridge for traditional Chinese medicine toward the world. The history of man's science development showed that the crossing and blending of two kinds of knowledge systems will be able to set up a new knowledge system. Integrative medicine, an unprecedented task in present world, is a new pattern of medicine.

Martin Jacques in his book, *When China Rules the World*, points out the value of Chinese medicine and its efficacy:

> Chinese medicine, rather like the world's cuisines, is a product of thousands of years of trial and error, of everyday experience and resourcefulness of hundreds of millions of people and their interaction with their plant environment. Western medicine is a rigorous product of the scientific method and the invention and refining of chemicals. There is a widespread and growing acceptance in the West that medicinal palliatives and cures derived from civilizational experience are a valid and important part of medicine, even if we do not understand how the great majority of them actually work.[35]

To me, a striking example of "the coexistence of Western medicine and traditional Chinese medicine" is the fact that in China open heart and brain surgery are routinely performed while the patient is fully awake, utilizing acupuncture instead of modern anesthesia!

Still more is needed in the medical revolution. Dr. Siddhartha Mukherjee in his Pulitzer Prize winning book, *Emperor of All Maladies: A Biography of Cancer*, made the following observation. "We now know there is a link between nutrition and the risk of particular forms of cancer, but this field remains in its infancy. Low fiber, red meat rich diets increase the risks of colon cancer, and obesity is linked to breast cancer."

I ask you then, how is it possible that studies conducted by the Centers for Disease Control and Prevention and others consistently show that less than 30% of physicians give advice on diet and lifestyle changes to cancer survivors; only one in four give exercise recommendations and less than half ever ask about smoking habits?

Dr. Mukherjee's quote highlights a major problem of medicine today: nutrition education. A survey published in the *American Journal of Clinical Nutrition* showed that the majority of medical schools are not providing adequate nutrition instruction.[36] A study in *Academic Medicine* found that only 27 percent of medical schools currently meet the minimum target, set by the National Academy of Sciences, of 25 hours for class time about nutrition. Twenty–five hours? Just guess how many hours medical students are in class during their training.

Although nutrition as a science, an article in the *British Medical Journal* explained, has always been part of conventional medicine, doctors are not taught, and therefore do not practice, much in the way of nutritional therapeutics. Nutritional interventions generally fall outside the mainstream.[37] Eight hundred years ago Maimonides admonished all medical practitioners not to employ medication if they can manage the sick by regulating nourishment alone.[38]

A report by the World Health Organization:

> Nutrition is coming to the fore as a major modifiable determinant of chronic disease, with scientific evidence increasingly supporting the view that alterations in diet have strong effects, both positive and negative, on health throughout life. Most importantly, dietary adjustments may not only influence present health, but may determine whether or not an individual will develop such diseases as cancer, cardiovascular disease and diabetes much later in life. [39]

The World Health Organization Study Group called for a shift in the conceptual framework for developing strategies for action, placing nutrition—together with the other principal risk factors for chronic disease, namely, tobacco use and alcohol consumption—at the forefront of public health policies and programs.

The eminent inventor Thomas Alva Edison believed, "The doctor of the future will give no medicine, but will interest his patients in the care of the human frame, in diet, and in the cause and prevention of disease." The future is now!

There are nationally known doctors such as Neal Barnard, Caldwell Esselstyn, Joel Furman, Michael Greger, Mark Hyman, Michael Klaper, John MacDougall, Dean Ornish, Andrew Weil and others like Colin Campbell, author of *The China Study,* who today are living proof of Edison's prophecy.

If you have never heard these names I encourage you to enter them in Google and YouTube. They can provide you with a wealth of information on lifestyle changes that as aging Baby Boomers you should think about making now before it is too late.

Welcome back, Dr. Lewis!

18

Big Parma

It is difficult to get a man to understand something when his salary depends upon his not understanding.

Upton Sinclair

This American system of ours, call it Americanism, call it capitalism, call it what you will, gives every one of us a great opportunity if we only seize it with both hands and make the most of it.

Al Capone

What you put at the end of your fork is a more powerful medicine than anything you will find at the bottom of a pill bottle.

Dr. Mark Hyman

The Jupiter study was a great breakthrough in the battle to find things to prescribe to people who don't need them.

Stephen T. Colbert, D.F.A

Baby Boomers grew up with television police shows: Robert Stack as Elliot Ness in *The Untouchables*, Broderick Crawford in *Highway Patrol*, Telly Savalas as *Kojak*, Peter Falk as *Colombo*, Jack Lord in *Hawaii Five–O*, etc until the genre changing *Hill Street Blues*. But by far, the best cop in the naked city was Sergeant Joe Friday portrayed by Jack Webb in *Dragnet*. The popular series ran from 1951–1959. Webb brought the show back in 1967 and in color with Harry Morgan of *M*A*S*H* fame as his partner. *Dragnet* always began by the announcer saying, "Ladies and gentlemen, the story you are about to see is true. The names have been changed to protect the innocent."

This chapter deals with the pharmaceutical industry and as you will see is one of the main reasons I chose to become proactive and self–advocating in my health. But unlike the *Dragnet* announcer, I can only say that the story you are about to read is true, but the names *have not* been changed to protect the innocent. Unfortunately, there are no innocents in the pharmaceutical industry.

Sergeant Joe Friday's most remembered line was, "Just the facts, ma–am." This chapter contains only *some* of the facts about the pharmaceutical industry. There is much, much more to the story. "*We were working the day watch . . .*"

A criminal enterprise is defined by the FBI as a group of individuals with an identified hierarchy, or comparable structure, engaged in significant criminal activity. These organizations often engage in multiple criminal activities and have extensive supporting networks.

Title 18 of the United States Code, Section 1961(4), the Racketeer Influenced and Corrupt Organizations (RICO) statute, defines an enterprise as "any individual, partnership, corporation, association, or other legal entity, and any union or group of individuals associated in fact although not a legal entity."

The FBI defines organized crime as any group having some manner of a formalized structure and whose primary objective is to obtain money through illegal activities. These organizations often engage in multiple criminal activities and have extensive supporting networks. Such groups maintain their position through the use of actual or threatened violence, corrupt public officials, graft, or extortion, and generally have a significant impact on the people in their locales, region, or the country as a whole. For all practical purposes the terms Criminal Enterprise and Organized Crime are similar and often used synonymously in the practice of law.

Big Parma

A study[1] in *Journal of the American Medical Association*:

Participants were a sample of the adult admissions in two tertiary care hospitals over a six month period. The adjusted rates per 100 admissions were 6.5% for adverse drug effects and 5.5% for potential adverse drug effects.

Conclusion: Adverse drug effects are a major cause of iatrogenic injury that many are preventable, and for every preventable adverse drug effect there are almost three potential adverse drug effects. Of the adverse drug effects in the study: 1% fatal (non–preventable), 12% life–threatening, 30% serious and 57% significant. Of the total 28% were deemed preventable, *but among the life–threatening and serious adverse drug effects, 42% were preventable.* [Emphasis added]

A study[2] in the *New England Journal of Medicine*:

Of the adverse drug events, 13% were serious, 28% were ameliorable, and 11% were preventable. Of the ameliorable events, 63% were attributed to the physician's failure to respond to medication–related symptoms and 37% to the patient's failure to inform the physician of the symptoms.

Conclusion: Adverse drug events are common in outpatient care, that they have important consequences, and *that more than one third of such events are preventable or ameliorable.* [Emphasis added]

A study[3] in the *Journal of General Internal Medicine*:

Of the 400 patients, 45 developed an Adverse Drug Events (ADE) following hospital discharge. Of these, 27% were preventable and 33% were ameliorable. Injuries were significant in 32 patients, serious in six, and life threatening in seven. Patients were less likely to experience an ADE if they recalled having side effects of prescribed medications explained. *Risk increased with prescription number.* [Emphasis added]

A study[4] in the journal *Current Aging*:

> The Centers for Disease Control indicated that 70–80% of
> humans diagnosed with one or another form of senile dementia,
> including Alzheimer's disease, are not basically sick *but are suffering
> from huge overdoses of legally prescribed medicines.* [Emphasis added]

Drugs can either be a panacea or purgatory whether inside a
hospital or outpatient use at home. They are dangerous in the hands
of the untrained. They are dangerous in the hands of the trained.
Another of Dr. William Osler's cogent comments a century ago
was, "The person who takes medicine must recover twice, once
from the disease and once from the medicine." However, today this
is only half true. It is becoming increasingly more and more difficult
to recover from the medicine.

We routinely take medications without a thought to the small
print warnings about side effects because we have trust in our
medical professionals. "If it would be harmful they would know and
they would warn us."

But the medical profession also relies on the trust of those in the
"top down" to give them accurate and reliable information about
the pharmaceuticals they prescribe. Doctors prescribe medication in
good faith based on the information they receive from the tier
above them. And those at the top, the government regulatory
agencies such as the Food and Drug Administration, upon whom
do they rely?

Academic medicine, the universities that conduct the research,
run the clinical trials, sign off on the trustworthiness and reliability
of the results, etc are the pivotal cog in the wheel of our system of
checks and balances that the patient, the physician, and the
regulating agencies rely. They all have Pollyanna confidence that the
pharmaceutical industry, the top of the pyramid, is honest and
above reproach.

Big Parma

In an article[5] in the *New England Journal of Medicine* appropriately titled 'Is Academic Medicine for Sale?' Marcia Angell, editor in chief of the *Journal* at the time, thought it reasonable to disclose to its readers that the ties between the pharmaceutical industry and academic medicine "were becoming fairly common." She cited one study[6] with a drug for the treatment of chronic depression appearing in the issue as an example:

> No one could have foreseen at the time just how ubiquitous and manifold such financial associations would become. The authors' ties with companies that make antidepressant drugs were so extensive that it would have used too much space to disclose them fully in the Journal. We decided merely to summarize them and to provide the details on our Web site.

Angell further wrote "finding an editorialist to write about the article presented another problem. Our conflict–of–interest policy for editorialists established in 1990 is stricter than that for authors of original research papers." The problem Angell explained that at the time the *Journal* required editorialists "have no important financial ties to companies that make products related to the issues they discuss."

The *Journal's* policy was analogous to the requirement that judges recuse themselves from hearing cases if they have financial ties to a litigant. Just as a judge's disclosure would not be sufficiently reassuring to the other side in a court case, "so we believe that a policy of *caveat emptor* is not enough for readers who depend on the opinion of editorialists."

"But as we spoke with research psychiatrists about writing an editorial on the treatment of depression," Angell continued, "we found very few who did not have financial ties to drug companies that make antidepressants."

I am sure you have already realized the inherent problem: conflict of interest. The article went on to explain the problem in detail:

Researchers might undertake studies on the basis of whether they can get industry funding, not whether the studies are scientifically important. That would mean more research on drugs and devices and less designed to gain insights into the causes and mechanisms of disease.

It would also skew research toward finding trivial differences between drugs, because those differences can be exploited for marketing. Of even greater concern is the possibility that financial ties may influence the outcome of research studies.

There is now considerable evidence that researchers with ties to drug companies are indeed more likely to report results that are favorable to the products of those companies than researchers without such ties.

When the boundaries between industry and academic medicine become as blurred as they now are, the business goals of industry influence the mission of the medical schools in multiple ways.

A few years later, Marcia Angell put it all in a bestselling book, *The Truth About the Drug Companies*. Allow me to quote an excerpt from *The New York Review of Books*[7] summary she wrote:

The pharmaceutical industry is not especially innovative. As hard as it is to believe, only a handful of truly important drugs have been brought to market in recent years, and they were based on taxpayer–funded research at academic institutions, small biotechnology companies, or the National Institutes of Health (NIH).

The great majority of "new" drugs are not new at all but merely variations of older drugs, called "me–too" drugs, already on the market. "If I'm a manufacturer and I can change one molecule and get another twenty years of patent rights, and convince physicians to prescribe and consumers to demand the next form of [an existing drug] just as my patent expires, then why would I be spending money on a lot less certain endeavor, which is looking for brand–new drugs?"

In a comparative study[8] on the relationships between physicians and the drug and device industry published in the *American Journal of Law and Medicine* the author categorically states:

> Patients are not well served by current systems for marketing of drugs and devices, the goal of which seems to be the distortion, indeed the corruption, of medical judgment through financial inducements.
>
> Drug and device companies should be prohibited from giving any gifts to professionals who have the authority to prescribe or order their products, to the families or employees of such professionals, or to undergraduate or graduate professionals in training.
>
> Drug and device companies should be absolutely prohibited from funding medical education, including continuing medical education, directly or indirectly.
>
> Physician–industry relationships present conflicts of interest because the physician's primary commitment to patients in clinical practice, students in education, and science (and patients) in research comes into conflict with a secondary commitment to a drug or device company that offers the physician an opportunity for financial gain.

Conflict of interest is not the only problem with the current system of drug testing. The pharmaceutical industry spends millions on the development of drugs. Years are spent isolating molecules, lab testing, animal testing, and human clinical trials. Each new drug is under market pressure to be approved so the pharmaceutical company can begin to recover its capital expenditure. *Time is money!*

Everyone would agree that pharmaceutical companies should make a profit; that is free market capitalism. Yet, in 2001 during a time of recession, the top 10 U.S. drug companies increased their profits by 33%, whereas the overall profits of Fortune 500 companies declined by 53%.[9]

Ridged controls, however, are placed upon drug trials for good reason. Before drugs are peddled to the public, the consumer has the inherent right to know that they are effective, they are safe, and that they perform as advertised. Drugs involve life and death matters. The pharmaceutical industry capitalizes on that fact in not necessarily ethical ways. "People are waiting to be cured by our drugs! Let's not waste valuable time getting the drugs into the market."

As a result often drug trials are stopped after only interim results are determined and do not wait the long term trials to end. Is this wise? An article published in the *British Medical Journal*[10] said "most of the recent clinical trials that were stopped early were used in support of an application at the European Medicines Agency or the US Food and Drug Administration."

The article goes on to say if you are going to stop a trial claiming superiority for a new treatment you need proof beyond a shadow of a doubt. That is not usually the case. Reporting requirements are voluntary not mandatory. The pharmaceutical company decides if it publishes testing results or not and what kind of information it reveals. The FDA is not allowed to reveal the results it has because the industry claims they are "proprietary" information.

The article cited a study[11] in the *Journal of the American Medical Association* whose conclusion was that "randomized controlled trials stopped early for benefit are becoming more common; often fail to adequately report relevant information about the decision to stop early, and show implausibly large treatment effects, particularly when the number of events is small. These findings suggest clinicians should view the results of such trials with skepticism."

The trials studied were typically industry funded evaluated drugs in cardiology, cancer, and HIV. In 94% of the trials identified, the papers failed to report at least one of the following pieces of information: the planned sample size, the interim analysis after the drug trial was stopped, whether the predetermined stopping rule was adhered to, or if there had been an adjusted analysis that accounted for interim monitoring and truncation of the trial.

Another wide spread problem is that the authors of the research are many times not the ones who write the final reports. There are several large medical writing firms that regularly produce reports for the pharmaceutical industry.

Ghostwriting is the practice whereby a pharmaceutical company will typically ask an external medical writing company to draft papers that are favorable to the company's product. In a large industry study on depression which resulted in approximately 124 papers, at least 45 were acknowledged to have been written by a single author who was also a science fiction author.[12]

Then they will invite outside prominent researchers or key opinion leaders to list themselves as the authors, in an attempt to increase the credibility of the paper. As economist Jeffery D. Sachs says in his book,[13] *The Price of Civilization: Reawakening American Virtue and Prosperity*, "Industry has shown time and time again that it is possible to find people with a PhD in their title to sign off on just about any fraudulent scientific claim, if the fee is right."

Sometimes the pharmaceutical industry crosses the legal line by off–label marketing to physicians. It is common for pharmaceutical companies to promote drugs for conditions that the drug doesn't have a license for.

A significant proportion of drug company financial penalties relate to off–label marketing and some of the largest corporate fines indeed include penalties for off–label promotion. Although it is not legally permitted, off–label marketing generates colossal additional revenue for the pharmaceutical industry. Sometimes they do get caught with their hands in the cookie jar.

Dr. Peter C. Gøtzsche who heads the Nordic Cochrane Centre in Copenhagen decided in 2012[14] to do a random Google search combining the names of the ten largest drug companies with the term "fraud" selecting *only* the most prominent case described in the ten hits on the first Google page. The most common criminal offences were illegal marketing, recommending drugs for non–

approved (off–label) uses, misrepresentation of research results, hiding data on harms, and Medicaid and Medicare fraud.

The ten cases Dr. Gøtzsche cited were from 2007 to 2012 and all related to the United States:

Pfizer pleaded guilty to misbranding drugs "with the intent to defraud or mislead," and was found to have illegally promoted four drugs for uses which had not been approved by the drug regulators.

Novartis unlawfully marketed Trileptal® and five other drugs causing false claims to be submitted to government health care programs. The company paid kickbacks to health care professionals to induce them to prescribe Trileptal® and five other drugs.

Sanofi–Aventis deliberately misquoted the prices, underpaying rebates to Medicaid and overcharging some public health agencies for the medications.

GlaxoSmithKline pleaded guilty to having marketed a number of drugs illegally for off–label use, paid kickbacks to doctors, and failed to include certain safety data in reports to the FDA.

AstraZeneca illegally marketed one of its best–selling drug antipsychotic drugs to children, the elderly, veterans and inmates for uses not approved by the FDA and targeted its illegal marketing towards doctors who do not typically treat psychotic patients and paid kickbacks to some of them.

Roche convinced US and European governments to spend billions on the purchase of Tamiflu® in preparation for the mild 2009 influenza epidemic based on unpublished trials despite the fact there is no convincing evidence either that Tamiflu® prevents influenza complications or reduces the spread of influenza to other people. *Roche* had omitted publishing most of their clinical trial data and refused to share them with independent Cochrane researchers. *Roche* also used ghost writers.

Johnson & Johnson and its subsidiary *Janssen* had lied about the potentially life–threatening side effects and hidden risks associated with the antipsychotic drug Risperdal®.

Merck had failed to pay the appropriate rebates to Medicaid and other government health care programs, and had also paid kickbacks to doctors and hospitals to induce them to prescribe various drugs.

Eli Lilly successfully marketed off–label use for its top–selling antipsychotic drug, Zyprexa® including Alzheimer's, depression and dementia, particularly in children and the elderly, although the harms of the drug are substantial, inducing heart failure, pneumonia, considerable weight gain and diabetes.

Abbott promoted the sale of the epilepsy Depakote® for uses that were not approved by the FDA as safe and effective; made false and misleading statements about the safety, efficacy, dosing and cost–effectiveness of the drug for some unapproved uses; improperly marketed the product in nursing homes; and paid kickbacks to induce doctors and others to prescribe or promote the drug.

Dr. Gøtzsche concluded, "The drug industry is clearly playing hardball, running calculated risks and corrupting people on a large scale, which lead to the unnecessary loss of thousands of lives every year and great costs for our national economies. I therefore believe that what we are seeing has similarities to organized crime. *Many crimes would be impossible to carry out, if doctors weren't willing to participate in them.*" [Emphasis added]

And then there was Vioxx. Vioxx® was a non–steroidal anti–inflammatory drug (NSAID) approved by the U.S. Food and Drug Administration (FDA) for the treatment of arthritis and menstrual pain. After it went on the market, Vioxx® was found to have an increased cardiovascular risk.

Instead of pulling the drug from the shelves, *Merck* agreed to allow a label change to reflect the heart risks but continued to publicly deny any problems. Finally *Merck* was forced to initiate a worldwide recall of Vioxx®. But by the time of the recall, 25 million Americans had taken Vioxx® with millions more having taken the drug worldwide. *Up to 38,000 people died from heart attacks or strokes after taking Vioxx® with a total of about 160,000 patients injured.*

Merck set up a $4.85 billion settlement fund and paid nearly 35,000 complaints. *Merck* agreed to pay $950 million and plead guilty to a federal misdemeanor related to its marketing practices.

"*Merck* was accused of misleading doctors and patients about the drug's safety, fabricating study results to suit the company's needs, continually thwarting an FDA scientist from revealing the drug's problems and skirting federal drug regulations."

The clinical results for Vioxx® were published in the *New England Journal of Medicine*, but no one knew that it was missing some information. *Merck* scientists left out key data on heart patients to make the drug seem safer. Eventually it was concluded that high doses of Vioxx® increased the risk of heart disease 3.7 times.

Dr. William Castelli, the former director of the Framingham Heart Study, said in an interview[15] "We have these patients, you know, they want the golden bullet. Doctor, give me that magic bullet so I can go out and eat anything I want. Well, we don't have a therapy like that. It's much better if you can get people on a diet."

I want for the rest of this chapter to talk about one of the most popular golden bullets today: statins. I choose satins because it was a drug I took for a number of years and because in researching this book I kept coming across a plethora of studies concerning statins.

After my angioplasty, I was given the golden bullet: a 10 mg simvastatin. Additionally, I was also very cautious about what I ate. I had given up red meat and chicken, but still ate fish, low fat cheese, whole grains and beans, plenty of "heart healthy" olive oil, etc and tried to limit processed foods to only those with low fat content: the typical Mediterranean Diet. Even with successfully balancing my blood lipids for a number of years, my doctor wanted me to increase the dosage of my statin to 20 mg.

During those intervening years, I read prolifically about heart disease and at every junction I ran into the same panacea: a plant–

based no fat diet. I also read online about one of the side effects of statins I was experiencing: memory problems. At times, I could not remember simple things like did I turn the stove off, did I take my pills, a sentence I had just uttered in a conversation, etc. In fact, I was reading a lot about other statin side effects that worried me.

A seminal paper[16] by Dr. Geoffrey Rose, 'Sick Individuals and Sick Populations' published in the *International Journal of Epidemiology* was an eye opener for me. Dr. Rose began his paper by stating it is an integral part of good doctoring to ask not only, what is the diagnosis and what is the treatment? But why did this patient get this disease at this time and could it have been prevented?

In the paper Rose advocated that to find the determinants of prevalence and incidence rates, we study characteristics of population not characteristics of individuals. Drug studies are base on population samples and not on the results of the individual in the trial.

When a doctor prescribes a drug, he is not telling you that this golden bullet will cure your disease, ailment or problem. What he is really saying is "that from the information I know, that if X number of people take this pill, then Y number will be helped." For example: rosuvastatin, a statin medication. To prevent a single cardiovascular event, 95 people would be required to take the statin treatment for two years.[17]

Rose admitted that the population strategy had drawbacks; the most prominent being the prevention paradox. "A preventative measure which brings much benefits to the population offers little to each participating individual." *Few will benefit but all have to take part.*

So what was the eye opener I saw in Dr. Rose's paper? "If a doctor accepts that he is responsible for an individual who is sick today," Rose said, "then it is a short step to accept responsibility for the individual who may well be sick tomorrow."

My doctor would never take responsibility for my being sick in the future; *only I could!* The old adage hit me square between the eyes: *an ounce of prevention is worth a pound of cure.* I asked myself if taking the increase in the satin medication my doctor was advocating was going to prevent *my* recurrence of coronary artery disease since my blood lipids were in the normal range.

We agreed that I would increase the dosage of my statin to 20 mg and after three months take another blood test to see its efficacy. However, I took the prescription for the statin increase but did not fill it; continuing only with the 10 mg simvastatin. After much thought I finally decided to completely change my diet and give it a try.

For next three months I would eat *only* a 100% a plant–based, no fat diet without any processed foods, olive oil, added sugar, not even fish, just whole grains, beans, veggies, fruits, and fungus in the form of mushrooms. *It was time to either sink or swim!*

Following a Mediterranean Diet and taking a 10 mg statin, my blood cholesterol level the week before I met with my doctor was 210 mg/dl. Before my angioplasty, diet change and statins, my cholesterol hovered around 250–280 mg/dl. *Drum roll* . . . after three months of a 100% a plant–based diet, the follow up blood test reported my blood cholesterol level was 131.2 mg/dl.

My doctor was elated. I, on the other hand, immediately stopped taking the 10 mg simvastatin and after six more months and another blood test two important facts emerged. First, my blood cholesterol level stayed at the same low level despite not *taking any statin.* Second, my memory problems began clearing up and within a year vanished. It was then I admitted to my doctor that I never increased the statin dosage, quit taking any statins and that my dramatic cholesterol drop was due solely to diet change without any golden bullets.

We then discussed the memory side affect. She admitted knowing about the memory problem and explained that as a physician, she had to weigh the risks against the benefits. Realize before you take any golden bullet, there is always a calculated risk involved. I am not faulting my doctor at the time for not mentioning the memory problem; she happens to be one of the best physicians I know.

If I had the opportunity to change one thing about the medical profession, I think it would be to increase the 12–minute patient encounter by adding a couple of more minutes. During those few extra minutes I would have your doctor read to you the side effect warnings that accompany the medication he or she suggests you take; discuss them with you and together *both of you* weigh the calculated risks involved.

When I moved to Eilat, my new doctor in our first meeting read about my angioplasty, my single vessel coronary artery disease and without a blink of an eye said I should be taking a statin. But before he wrote the prescription, he wanted to discuss side effects. I was in shock! A doctor was going to discuss side effects of medication? My shock quickly dissipated when he asked if I ate pink grapefruits. Pink grapefruits?

He explained that of the two statins he was considering, one had efficacy complications when combined with pink grapefruits. He finally decided on rosuvastatin, writing me a prescription for Crestor® manufactured by *AstraZeneca*.

That first meeting drew the lines of our new patient–doctor relationship. I told him I refused to take a statin under any circumstances and explained my memory problems. He answered back that the memory side effect was never substantiated. I told him it was and besides the fact that after six months of taking no statins, my problem started clearing up and has not returned since was all the proof I needed.

Then he justified my taking a statin because my HDL–cholesterol was low, 32 mg/dl, when it should be greater than 40 mg/dl. I countered by quoting a letter Dr. Dean Ornish had written to the *New England Journal of Medicine*:[18] "A low HDL in a person consuming a diet low in fat, cholesterol, and animal protein may have differing prognostic implications from a low HDL in a person consuming a typical American diet." We parried!

Why am I so adamant about not taking a statin? Let's look in depth at statin medication using Crestor® as an example. Obviously we take medicines for the prevention of an illness, disorder or disease when other ameliorative means are not successful. Basically, prevention has two aspects: primary and secondary.

Primary prevention means taking medication before an illness has occurred. A person can be at low–risk, moderate risk or high risk depending on the established criteria. Assessing risk determines the level of treatment warranted.

Secondary prevention means an illness has already manifested itself, i.e. you had a heart attack. Then medication is prescribed to prevent a recurrence, to mitigate the effects of the illness, or keep the illness developing into a greater disease occurrence.

Crestor® began its life with the JUPITER (Justification for Use of Statins in Prevention: Intervention Trial Evaluating Rosuvastatin) study.[19] The lead author for the JUPITER trial was Dr. Paul M. Ridker. Although planned as a 5–year study, the trial was stopped after *only 1.9 years.*

The study population was not diagnosed with either coronary heart disease or diabetes and had normal LDL levels but high levels of c–reactive protein (CRP), a nonspecific indicator of inflammation which reflects general health and is a stronger predictor of cardiovascular events than LDL levels. The JUPITER population, however, was not totally healthy with 41% having metabolic syndrome, 16% smoked and 12% had a family history of heart disease.

When the study results were published, JUPITER took headline health by storm. *AstraZeneca*'s press release stated that the trial had reduced nonfatal heart attacks by 54% and nonfatal strokes by 47%. Approval was given by the FDA on August 12, 2003. Controversy immediately followed. The first of which were the author's conflict of interest:[20]

Dr. Paul M Ridker received grant support from *AstraZeneca*, Novartis, Merck, Abbott, Roche, and Sanofi–Aventis; consulting fees or lecture fees or both from *AstraZeneca*, Novartis, Merck, Merck–Schering–Plough, Sanofi–Aventis, Isis, Dade Behring, and Vascular Biogenics; and is listed as a co–inventor on patents held by Brigham and Women's Hospital that relate to the use of inflammatory biomarkers in cardiovascular disease, including the use of high–sensitivity C–reactive protein in the evaluation of patients' risk of cardiovascular disease. These patents have been licensed to Dade Behring and *AstraZeneca*.

Dr. Francisco Fonseca received research grants, lecture fees, and consulting fees from *AstraZeneca*, Pfizer, Schering–Plough, Sanofi–Aventis, and Merck.

Dr. Jacques Genest received lecture fees from *AstraZeneca*, Schering–Plough, Merck–Schering–Plough, Pfizer, Novartis, and Sanofi–Aventis and consulting fees from *AstraZeneca*, Merck, Merck Frosst, Schering–Plough, Pfizer, Novartis, Resverlogix, and Sanofi–Aventis.

Dr. Antonio M. Gotto received consulting fees from Dupont, Novartis, Aegerion, Arisaph, Kowa, Merck, Merck–Schering–Plough, Pfizer, Genentech, Martek, and Reliant; serving as an expert witness; and receiving publication royalties.

Dr. John Kastelein received grant support from *AstraZeneca*, Pfizer, Roche, Novartis, Merck, Merck–Schering–Plough, Isis, Genzyme, and Sanofi–Aventis; lecture fees from *AstraZeneca*, GlaxoSmithKline, Pfizer, Novartis, Merck–Schering–Plough, Roche, Isis, and Boehringer Ingelheim; and consulting fees from *AstraZeneca*, Abbott, Pfizer, Isis, Genzyme, Roche, Novartis, Merck, Merck–Schering–Plough, and Sanofi–Aventis.

Dr. Wolfgang Koenig received grant support from *AstraZeneca*, Roche, Anthera, Dade Behring and GlaxoSmithKline; lecture fees from *AstraZeneca*, Pfizer, Novartis, GlaxoSmithKline, DiaDexus,

Roche, and Boehringer Ingelheim; and consulting fees from GlaxoSmithKline, Medlogix, Anthera, and Roche.

Dr. Peter Libby received lecture fees from Pfizer and consulting fees from *AstraZeneca*, Bristol–Myers Squibb, GlaxoSmithKline, Merck, Pfizer, Sanofi–Aventis, VIA Pharmaceuticals, Interleukin Genetics, Kowa Research Institute, Novartis, and Merck–Schering–Plough.

Dr. Alberto J. Lorenzatti received grant support, lecture fees, and consulting fees from *AstraZeneca*, Takeda, and Novartis.

Dr. Borge G. Nordestgaard received lecture fees from *AstraZeneca*, Sanofi–Aventis, Pfizer, Boehringer Ingelheim, and Merck and consulting fees from *AstraZeneca* and BG Medicine.

Dr. James Shepherd received lecture fees from *AstraZeneca*, Pfizer, and Merck and consulting fees from *AstraZeneca*, Merck, Roche, GlaxoSmithKline, Pfizer, Nicox, and Oxford Biosciences.

Dr. Robert J. Glynn received grant support from *AstraZeneca* and Bristol–Myers Squibb. [Emphasis added]

The study concluded "no other potential conflict of interest relevant to this article was reported." Nine authors were specifically linked *AstraZeneca* and eleven of the fourteen listed authors by their own disclosure had deep ties with the pharmaceutical industry.

Crestor® is the most prescribed brand name drug in the US, with 22.3 million prescriptions filled and $5.8 billion in sales. A few months ago I too was curious about how *AstraZeneca* was doing with the law. So, like Dr. Gøtzsche, I did a Google search with "*AstraZeneca*," "fraud" and the date.[21]

I straight away got two hits: both from the Department of Justice Office of Public Affairs:

FOR IMMEDIATE RELEASE
Monday, July 6, 2015 AstraZeneca and Cephalon to Pay $46.5 Million and $7.5 Million, Respectively, for Allegedly Underpaying Rebates Owed Under Medicaid Drug Rebate Program. AstraZeneca LP has agreed to pay the United States and participating states a total

of $46.5 million, plus interest, to resolve allegations that it knowingly underpaid rebates owed under the Medicaid Drug Rebate Program, the Justice Department announced today.

FOR IMMEDIATE RELEASE

Wednesday, February 11, 2015 AstraZeneca to Pay $7.9 Million to Resolve Kickback Allegations. AstraZeneca LP, a pharmaceutical manufacturer based in Delaware, has agreed to pay the government $7.9 million to settle allegations it engaged in a kickback scheme in violation of the False Claims Act, the Justice Department announced today.

Next on my list is the *truth* about the real reduction in heart attacks in the JUPITER trial. *AstraZeneca* reported a 54% reduction in heart attacks. But this was only *relative risk* not the *absolute risk* reduction. Technically this is correct but is extremely misleading because absolute reduction is the most important measure. Allow me to explain.

In the placebo group, 0.76% of the people suffered a heart attack; the statin group was 0.36%. So, if you do the math, 0.76% minus 0.36% equals a difference of only 0.41%. *The absolute reduction in heart attacks was only* 0.41% not 54%. So where did the 54% reduction come from? Do the math again: multiply 0.76% by 54% and you get 0.41%. 54% is a relative not actual risk reduction. *AstraZeneca's* press release[22] stated that the risk of heart attack was cut by more than half: 54%. It neither reported whether the reduction risk as relative or absolute.

An article in *Drug Design, Development and Therapy*[23] pointed out that 25 people needed to take Crestor® for five years in order to prevent the first heart attack, an absolute risk reduction of only about 4%. The study noted that in primary prevention this baseline risk and event rate is low. In fact, aspirin alone could potentially have prevented 72 of the 99 heart attacks that occurred during the JUPITER trial.[24]

Additionally, a meta–analysis did not find evidence for benefit of statin therapy on all cause mortality in high risk primary prevention set up.[25] The results of the [JUPITER] trial do not support the use of statin treatment for primary prevention of cardiovascular diseases and raise troubling questions concerning the role of commercial sponsors.[26]

The claimed mortality benefit of statins for primary prevention is more a measure of bias than a real effect. The reduction in major coronary heart disease serious events with statins as compared to placebo is not reflected in a reduction in total serious adverse events.[27]

Translating JUPITER's findings without first carefully considering their implications would not be prudent. For any one individual, even with no hyperlipidemia, but elevated hs c–reactive protein, JUPITER's findings offer only a small chance of benefit.[28]

Side effects are another concern of mine. There was reported a 27% increase in diabetes in rosuvastatin–treated patients compared to placebo–treated patients. Memory problems I already highlighted.

For several years I suffered with osteoarthritis in my knees. Sometimes the pain was so debilitating that I had to lie down; on the ground, in bed, on the floor etc, just to get relief. But miraculously, after I discontinued the statins, the osteoarthritis disappeared and never returned. To me it was clear that I never in fact had osteoarthritis; it was joint pain caused by taking the statin; a well known side effect. Etc, etc, etc!

However, of all the side effects listed in the Crestor® patient package insert: constipation, nausea, headache, sick feeling, dizziness, abdominal pain, debilitation, weakness, muscle pain, urine protein, diabetes, skin rash, itching, hives, severe allergic reaction–including swelling in the face, lips, tongue, difficulty swallowing or breathing, jaundice, hepatitis, blood urine, joint pain, memory loss, breast enlargement in men, confusion, interstitial lung disease, diarrhea, edema, insomnia, sexual problems, depression, respiratory problems, and constant muscle weakness, the one that most concerned me *is a side effect that is not even listed.*

Every cell in the human body is a self–contained molecular factory whose purpose is to support our life. The power plants that keep our cells going are called mitochondria, tiny organelles inside our cells that generate our energy in the form of APT (adenosine diphosphate). Mitochondria enable us to use oxygen.[29]

In mammals, mitochondria produce energy from the breakdown of food. As mitochondria burn up food using oxygen, smog in the form of free–radical sparks escape damaging adjacent structures in the cell nucleus occasionally causing irreversible DNA mutation; enduring alterations in gene sequence.[30]

Plants, unlike mammals, convert sunlight and CO_2 into sugars for mitochondria to produce energy. One byproduct of photosynthesis is also the release of too many free oxygen radicals. An example is coral bleaching in the ocean. Crank up the photosynthesis which is the case with global warming and you crank up free radicals. Free radicals harm the coral; the algae are ejected and the white carbonate skeleton becomes visible through the translucent tissue layer.[31]

Human free radical damage to the DNA causes a mitochondrial dysfunction implicated in: diabetes, Huntington's disease, cancer, nogenesis, Alzheimer's disease, Parkinson's disease, bipolar disorder, schizophrenia, anxiety disorders, cardiovascular disease including atherosclerosis, sarcopenia, chronic fatigue syndrome, fibromyalgia,[32] and multiple sclerosis.[33]

Mitochondria are also directly connected to cellular apoptosis, programmed cell death. Free radical damage can stop cellular apoptosis resulting in the uncontrollable growth of cancer cells. And according to the Free Radical Theory of Aging, the rate of accumulations of spontaneous mutations in our mitochondrial DNA is the principle determinate of the rate of aging.[34]

A reduction of mitochondria DNA (mtDNA) content leads to more aggressive forms of breast cancer; mtDNA may serve as a biomarker for how to identify and treat cancers that more quickly metastasize.[35] Mitochondrial function is deregulated in cancer. Different tumor types may be more or less sensitive to mitochondrial function depending on which oncogenic lesions drive the tumor.[36]

The alteration of the mitochondrial and glycolytic proteomes is a hallmark feature of breast cancer further providing relevant markers to aid in the prognosis of breast cancer patients.[37] The mechanisms that promote the repression of mitochondrial activity in tumors will contribute to transform cancer into a chronic disease.[38]

Studies identify mitochondria as the target and the origin of major pathogenic pathways leading to the progression of myocardial dysfunction. Mitochondrial defects lead to metabolic remodeling, deficit in cardiac energetics and increased oxidative stress.[39]

The extraordinary dependence of neurons on mitochondrial oxidative metabolism energy is directly linked to neurodegenerative conditions. The central role of mitochondria in neurodegeneration has become apparent over the last decade.[40]

The body's defense against free radicals is intracellular antioxidants which safely remove free radicals before they can damage the cells. Coenzyme Q_{10} (CoQ_{10}) is a natural antioxidant synthesized by the body which protects cells from free radical damage and additionally helps to produce energy your body needs for cell growth and maintenance.

However, the richest sources of antioxidants come from richly colored vegetables and fruits. Antioxidants from fruits and vegetables make it easier for the mitochondria to neutralize the free radicals.[41]

CoQ_{10} is beneficial for heart health in maintaining the normal oxidative state of LDL cholesterol, helps assure circulatory health, and supports optimal functioning of the heart muscle and may also help support the health of vessel walls. It is not rocket science: *the more CoQ$_{10}$ the greater number of healthier mitochondria.*

So, what has this got to do with statins? A LOT! Medications have now emerged as a major cause of mitochondrial damage, explaining many adverse effects.[42] All classes of cholesterol medications such as statins have been documented to damage mitochondria, as well as psychotropic drugs, cancer (chemotherapy) medications, analgesics such as acetaminophen and many others. Medications damage mitochondria directly by inhibiting mtDNA transcription, the synthesis of an RNA copy of DNA, or indirectly by inhibiting enzymes like CoQ$_{10}$ required for energy production.

Yes, you understood correctly. All statins and most of the medications we take create a mitochondrial dysfunction. *If that's not shooting yourself in the foot I don't know what is.* Statins like Crestor® totally block the body's production and reduce circulating levels of CoQ$_{10}$. Mitochondrial function may be impaired by statin therapy.[43]

Let me go through the logic again: Mitochondria are vital to our life. CoQ$_{10}$ is a natural antioxidant which the body produces to protect us from free radical damage and aids in cellular energy production. Free radicals cause mitochondrial dysfunction which in turn is responsible for a cornucopia of diseases and illness. The older we Baby Boomers get, the less CoQ$_{10}$ our bodies naturally produce. Statins and other medications inhibit the body's ability to produce CoQ$_{10}$ and cause direct mitochondrial damage. *Why the hell would anybody want to take a statin more less another medication if there was another way you keep from getting sick?*

I am not over stating the importance of CoQ$_{10}$:

Those who benefit most from CoQ$_{10}$ supplementation are the elderly, athletes, those receiving statins or HMA Co–A reductase inhibitors, given the high risk of mitochondrial dysfunction from CoQ$_{10}$ deficiencies in this group.[44] The Shanghai Women's Health Study, with relatively larger sample size and longer follow–up time, suggests an inverse association for plasma CoQ_{10} levels with breast cancer risk in Chinese women.[45]

Supplementing 100 mg CoQ_{10}, 10 mg riboflavin and 50 mg niacin to breast cancer patients along with tamoxifen reduces the serum tumor marker level and thereby reduce the risk of cancer recurrence and metastases.[46] Analysis of our findings suggests that baseline plasma CoQ_{10} levels are a powerful and independent prognostic factor that can be used to estimate the risk for melanoma progression.[47]

Current studies support a role for CoQ_{10} supplementation in patients with endothelial dysfunction.[48] The study revealed up–regulation of lipid peroxidation, oxidative DNA damage and deficiency of CoQ_{10} in coronary artery disease showing CoQ_{10} supplementation may have cardio–protective effects in coronary artery disease.[49] A higher level of plasma CoQ_{10} was significantly associated with reducing the risk of coronary artery disease.[50]

CoQ_{10} can be considered as an evidence–based approach to the treatment of hypertension.[51] CoQ_{10} may be a promising therapeutic strategy for ameliorating glutamate excitotoxicity and oxidative stress in glaucomatous neurodegeneration.[52] CoQ_{10} supplementation at a dosage of 150 mg appears to decrease the inflammatory marker interleukin–6 (IL–6) in patients with coronary artery disease.[53]

CoQ_{10} levels were statistically significantly lower in post–cardiac arrest patients than in healthy controls; lower in human subjects with return of spontaneous circulation (ROSC) after cardiac arrest; and lower in those who died, and a poor neurologic outcome.[54] CoQ_{10} may provide a promising therapeutic potential for ameliorating oxidative stress–mediated mitochondrial dysfunction in ischemic retinal injury.[55]

Oral administration of CoQ_{10} increases both brain and brain mitochondrial concentrations; providing evidence that CoQ_{10}

can exert neuroprotective effects that might be useful in the treatment of neurodegenerative diseases.[56] Extensive pre–clinical studies have strongly supported CoQ_{10} as a potential agent in providing neuro–protection and slowing disease progression in neurodegenerative diseases.[57]

I truly believe in the importance of CoQ_{10} and put my money where my mouth is. Even though I eat only a plant–based diet, the richest source of antioxidants that neutralize the effects of free radicals, I take a 200 mg gel cap of CoQ_{10} ubiquinone every day. *It ain't cheap!*

But the real kicker for me is in the patient insert *AstraZeneca* includes: "Crestor® is *indicated* to lower high levels of cholesterol and triglycerides in the blood *when changes in diet and exercise have failed to do so.*" [Emphasis added] Duh! Changes in diet and exercise have been proven to lower high levels of cholesterol and triglycerides in the blood and *never* fail to do so.

What this means is that no one needs ever take a statin if they are willing to change their lifestyles; but we don't. An article in the *British Medical Journal*[58] concedes "not with any realistic hope of changing population lifestyle, our study suggests that both nutritional and pharmaceutical population approaches have the potential to have a significant effect on population mortality."

Dr. William Castelli additionally said,[59] "Now if I would put everyone on a vegetarian diet and drive their numbers down by diet, we would get rid of all the atherosclerosis in America. As I have said, there are a billion people out there somewhere around the world where they're on that kind of diet and they don't get this disease."

Adopting a Mediterranean diet after a heart attack is almost three times more powerful in reducing mortality than taking a statin. Pharmacology can assuage the symptoms but can't alter the pathology.[60] Weight loss, especially in with exercise and dietary changes, are powerful techniques to lower cardiac risk and c–reactive protein levels, and in fact would be preferred to statins.[61]

Current dietary recommendations, diets low in saturated fats expanded to include food high in viscous fibers (oats and barley) and vegetable protein foods (soy) and nuts, appear to reduce LDL levels similarly to statins.[62]

Focusing on optimizing therapies known to reduce mortality in patients with heart failure rather than adding a statin in an attempt to alter the atherosclerotic process appears to be a better approach.[63] Statins are not the only means of reducing risk of cardiovascular disease. People at high cardiovascular risk can reduce their risk by making lifestyle changes.[64]

And the previously mentioned study in *Drug Design, Development and Therapy*[65] that said 25 people needed to take Crestor® for *an absolute risk reduction of only about 4%* also pointed out "it is instructive to compare the improvement in absolute risks achieved using the Mediterranean Diet as an intervention, *which may exceed 5% in some situations.*" [Emphasis added]

Finally, Boomer women should also be aware that a study[66] of women 55–74 years of age who took statins 10 years or longer showed that these women had a 1.83–fold increased risk of invasive ductal carcinoma (IDC) and a 1.97–fold increased risk of invasive lobular carcinoma (ILC); nearly double compared to never users of statins. Among women also diagnosed with hypercholesterolemia, users of statins for 10 years or longer had more than double the risk of both IDC and ILC breast cancers compared to never users.

The French playwright Jean–Baptiste Poquelin, known by his stage name Molière (1622–1673) said it best, "My lord Jupiter knows how to sugarcoat the pill."

19

Fat Lies

We've never had a heart attack in the Framingham Heart Study in 35 years in anyone who had cholesterol under 150.

William Castelli, M.D.

Learning to eat as Mother Nature intended her children to eat does not mean giving up something. It means gaining health, youthful energy and appearance, increased mental capacity, a joy in living you never dreamed was possible.[1]

Dick Gregory

In my own laboratory we have shown in experimental animals that cancer growth can be turned on and off by nutrition, despite very strong genetic predispositions.[2]

Colin Campbell, PhD

I can say with confidence that my rapid transformation from middle–aged couch potato to *Ultraman*—to, in fact, everything I've accomplished as an endurance athlete—begins and end with my Plant Power Diet.[3]

Rich Roll

Those who would deny global warming contend, without convincing evidence, that the rise in global temperature is in fact the result of long term climate cycles, or a consequence of changing solar activity operating on a time line invisible to our science because we have not been looking long enough. But the minority view is totally debunked by the deep time record of past CO_2 and past climate changes. However, it does not seem like a minority view if you tune in to politically conservative radios and telecasts.[4]

What Peter Ward wrote in his book, *The Flooded Earth: Our Future in a World Without Ice Caps,* about global warming accents a ubiquitous phenomenon about our life in general: cognitive dissonance. Leon Festinger developed his Theory of Cognitive Dissonance[5] to explain the uncomfortable feeling we have when we begin to understand that something we believe to be true is contradicted by evidence.

When contrary facts arise that threaten our cardinal beliefs, we reverently cling to our beliefs despite incontrovertible proof of their falsehood. Festinger says we spend our lives paying attention only to information which supports our beliefs and constantly avoid information which does not.

Deniers are people who refuse to admit the truth of a concept or proposition that is supported by the majority of scientific or historical evidence. The most famous of which in modern times have been those who deny the Holocaust ever happened. In their excellent exposé, *Merchants of Doubt: How a Handful of Scientists Obscured the Truth on Issues from Tobacco Smoke to Global Warming,* Naomi Oreskes and Eric Conway document serious consequences to society denier's force upon us.

Inherently deniers know that their positions are false and without basis. But their goal is not to refute opposing evidence, rather to merely cast doubt. Orchestrated doubts are enough to feed and reinforce our cognitive dissonance. The tobacco industry knew long ago that smoking was hazardous to health and that nicotine was very addictive. Yet, they injected doubt for decades until finally a federal judge decisively said that the tobacco industry had lied, willfully deceiving the public.

In 2002, Gary Taubes wrote an article in the *New York Times*[6] entitled, *What If It's All Been a Big Fat Lie?* Taube challenged more than thirty years medical science that eating fat was unhealthy. The American medical establishment, Taubes contended, ridiculed the late Dr. Robert Atkins dietary recommendations only to discover "the unrepentant Atkins was right all along." If you want to lose weight, Atkins advised, "eat truly luxurious foods without limit, lobster with butter sauce, steak with béarnaise sauce and bacon cheeseburgers."

Yes, you will lose weight, but the short term benefits of weight loss are outweighed by the long term cardiovascular harms. As a study published in *Preventive Cardiology* pointed out, those following a high–fat diets may have lost weight, *but at the price of increased cardiovascular risk factors, not only increase the risk of heart disease, but also the risk of strokes, peripheral vascular disease, and blood clots.*[7][Emphasis added]

So began the war of information challenging the public to live in a state of perpetual cognitive dissonance. Taubes and many others filled the shelves with contra–evidence supporting the view that fat, particularly the saturated fat of meat and dairy products, *was not* "the primary evil in the American diet."

As far as our eating habits are concerned, we are told that we have changed little from Paleolithic man. "Eat like a caveman" has become the modern mantra. The only problem with this idea is that the pristine portrait of the hunter–gather is wrong. Today we are encouraged to have a *Flintstones'* image of Paleolithic man. Fred and Barney come home from the quarry; stoke the coals with some Mesquite chips soaked in Scotch, smoke up a couple of Brontosaurs steaks while Wilma and Betty cool the beer.

The fact is that Paleolithic man more often survived primarily by what his gatherer wife foraged. Gathering can be just as critical as hunting because men sometimes return with nothing, in which case the family must rely entirely on gathered foods.[8]

Besides, *Homo Erectus* had small jaws and small teeth that were poorly adapted for eating the tough meat of game animals.[9] Cereals (wild wheat and barley) and small–grained grasses made up the largest component of the Stone Age diet, not meat.[10]

245

Today starchy foods make up more than half, 63 percent on average, of the diets of tropical hunter–gathers and may well have been eaten in a similar quantity by our human and pre–human ancestors in the African savannas.[11] Evidence for plant food processing, the grinding and pounding of wild food plants, from the recovery of flour residues on coarse tools were found across Europe up to 30,000 years ago.[12]

As an article in *Scientific American*[13] lucidly points out:

> We are not biologically identical to our Paleolithic predecessors, nor do we have access to the foods they ate. And deducing dietary guidelines from modern foraging societies is difficult because they vary so much by geography, season and opportunity. The Paleo diet not only misunderstands how our own species, the organisms inside our bodies and the animals and plants we eat have evolved over the last 10,000 years, it also ignores much of the evidence about our ancestors' health during their—often brief—individual life spans.

A recent study published in *International Journal of Exercise Science* found that after ten weeks on the modern unrestricted Paleolithic diet, LDL ("bad") cholesterol increased by 12.5 mg/dL and total cholesterol by 10.1 mg/dL. Triglycerides also increased slightly. *The worst outcomes were seen among the subgroup that had been the healthiest before starting the diet.*[14][Emphasis added]

Trying to understand the relationships between dietary patterns, fat and cholesterol with disease is much like answering the rhetorical question: which came first the chicken or the egg? But in this case it was neither the chicken nor the egg. Actually, it was the rabbit.

In 1908, the preliminary work of A.I. Ignatowski suggested that rabbits might develop atherosclerosis after eating non–vegetarian food, including meat and eggs. But it was Nikolai N. Anichkov who first demonstrated the role of cholesterol in the development of atherosclerosis. His classic experiments in 1913 paved the way to our current understanding of cholesterol's role in cardiovascular disease. Anichkov's research is often cited among the greatest discoveries of the 20th century.[15]

However, the Father of the diet–lipid–heart disease hypothesis was Ancel Keys. Keys, whose uncle was the silent movie star Lon Chaney, received his PhD in oceanography and biology from UC Berkeley, but it was his life work in nutrition that made him one of the greats in the field.

Little known is his moniker as the creator of K–Rations which continues to feed millions of soldiers worldwide; K stands for Keys. The story goes that while working for the Army Quartermaster Corps, he secured $10,000 from William Wrigley, Jr., water–tight boxes from the Cracker Jack Company and hard biscuits, dry sausage, hard candy, and chocolate from a local Minneapolis grocery store. K–Rations were thus born becoming a major staple of military nutrition.

After observing in southern Italy the highest concentration of centenarians in the world, Keys hypothesized that a Mediterranean–style diet low in animal fat protected *against* heart disease and that a diet high in animal fats *led* to heart disease. Keys launched the *Seven Countries Study* in 1958 after his research on the relationship between dietary pattern and the prevalence of coronary heart disease in Greece, Italy, Spain, South Africa, Japan, and Finland. His conclusion was that saturated fats as found in milk and meat have adverse effects opposite to the beneficial effects of the unsaturated fats found in vegetable oils.

Pragmatically, Keys never advocated the easy solution to the problem of fat by becoming a vegetarian as impractical. "A diet without meat," Keys said, "is extremely dull for most people."[16] "Civilized living is an intelligent search for durable satisfaction, a nice compromise between the pleasures of the moment and those of the future," Keys wrote. "So it is with eating; a balance should be struck between first impulse and appreciation of the consequences of such indulgence."[17] *Bravo!*

Today the diet–lipid–heart disease hypothesis is constantly under attack. In February 2015 the US Dietary Guidelines Committee (DGAC) reported that dietary cholesterol was no longer a "nutrient of concern," by citing available evidence that there was no relationship between consumption of dietary cholesterol and serum cholesterol. Gary Taube's vindication of Atkins seemed to be creditable. It became open season to eat meat, eggs, sausage and other high cholesterol foods.

But a hostile reaction immediately emerged within the medical community. Dr. Neal Barnard is the president of the Physicians Committee for Responsible Medicine; a Washington, D.C. based nonprofit public health organization advocating preventive medicine through proper nutrition which represents more than 10,000 physicians and 100,000 other healthcare professionals. Dr. Barnard in a response submitted to the *British Medical Journal Blog*[18] asks a definitive question: So how did the Dietary Guidelines Advisory Committee arrive at its not–guilty verdict that dietary cholesterol was no longer a "nutrient of concern"?

Dr. Barnard explained that the committee wrote that their finding was consistent with the 2014 report of the American Heart Association and the American College of Cardiology. The problem he explained was that "the AHA/ACC report did not actually reach this conclusion." They summarized evidence published since 1985, called for more research, "but did not suggest that there was no relationship between dietary cholesterol and serum cholesterol."

The question staring me in the face when I first read the BMJ/Blog was how could the Dietary Guidelines Advisory Committee possibly subvert the AHA/ACC report? I found a partial answer in Mexico. November 11–14, 2008, the global World Dairy Summit was held in Mexico City. The International Dairy Federation at the summit decided their main priority was to neutralize the negative impact of milk fat by regulators and medical professionals "using science to reposition milk fat and differentiate it from saturated fats."

The dairy industry set up a major, well–funded campaign to provide proof that saturated fat does not cause heart disease, assembled scientists who were sympathetic to the dairy industry, provided them with funding, encouraged them to put out statements on milk fat and heart disease, and arranged to have them speak at scientific meetings. Deniers were casting doubt again; shades of the tobacco industry. Studies began to blossom exonerating saturated fat from disease.

In a noteworthy interview, Dr. Martijn Katan, an emeritus professor of nutrition at the Vrije Universiteit Amsterdam and a world–renowned expert on diet and cardiovascular disease, explains why these new studies did not reach the same conclusions as the decades of research showing the culpability of saturated fat of meat and dairy products with disease:

> Not finding something can have two causes: either it's not there or the people who were searching didn't use the right method to search. The question is whether the observational studies that we're talking about are able to answer the question. If you look in detail at how these studies are done, everything works in favor of not finding an effect. The fact that saturated fat raises cholesterol, especially the bad LDL cholesterol, is beyond doubt. That has been shown in hundreds of trials that fed people different fats.[19]

The journal *Annals of Internal Medicine*[20] published a paper suggesting there is no evidence supporting the longstanding recommendation to limit saturated fat consumption. Dr. Walter Willett, Chair of the Department of Nutrition at Harvard School of Public Health, warned in response that the paper's conclusions are seriously misleading. Dr. Willett emphasized that because the meta–analysis contains multiple serious errors and omissions, conclusions of the study should be disregarded.[21]

Déjà vu. Why do I keep uncovering the same consistent underlying problem with the dietary guidelines as I have shown in previous chapters: conflict of interest? In a well documented article in the *Food and Drug Law Journal*[22] appropriately named 'Saving U.S. Dietary Advice from Conflicts of Interest,' Jeff Herman wrote:

> Recall that the Guidelines must be based on the preponderance of current scientific and medical knowledge. Congress clearly wanted the Guidelines to reflect the best science available, for good reason. With incomplete or inaccurate information, the government is unable to appropriately shape nutritional programs and people are deprived of the opportunity to make fully informed choices regarding their health.[23]
>
> Relationships with the food and drug industries are commonplace on the Advisory Committee: three out of 11 members on the 1995 Committee had past or present industry ties); seven out of 11 members on the 2000 Committee; 11 out of 13 members on the 2005 Committee; and on the 2010 Committee currently nine out of 13. These relationships are substantial.[24]
>
> For example, on just the 2000 Committee, members had past or present ties to: two meat associations; four dairy associations and five dairy companies; one egg association; one sugar association; one grain association; five other food companies; six other industry–sponsored associations; two pharmaceutical associations; and twenty–eight pharmaceutical companies.[25]
>
> Scientists with ties to the drug industry may feel pressure to not give advice that could have the effect of reducing reliance on these very profitable drugs. They may also not believe that diet or lifestyle is important or even necessary to control risk factors for chronic disease, when people can just take a pill.[26]

After uncovering documents under the Freedom of Information Act that revealed a money trail from the American Egg Board to universities where 2015 Dietary Guidelines Advisory Committee (DGAC) members were employed and persistent industry pressure to get limits on cholesterol removed, the Physicians Committee for Responsible Medicine filed a lawsuit alleging several DGAC members came from institutions that were funded by the egg industry and relied on egg–industry–funded research findings when they removed limits on dietary cholesterol. In allowing this to happen, the USDA and DHHS violated the Federal Advisory Committee Act, which mandates that the advisory committee "will not be inappropriately influenced by the appointing authority or any special interest."

Jeff Herman wrapped up the article in the *Food and Drug Law Journal* with a section asking how well the guidelines actually prevent chronic disease. His conclusion:

> The Dietary Guidelines for Americans, however, significantly underperform when it comes to preventing chronic diseases, though other diets—principally the Mediterranean diet and also Harvard's Alternate Index—perform much better, likely because they are more consistent with current scientific and medical knowledge.[27]

The Mediterranean diet, as advocated by Keys, emphasizes eating primarily plant–based foods, such as fruits and vegetables, whole grains, legumes and nuts; replacing butter with healthy fats, such as olive oil; using herbs and spices instead of salt to flavor foods; limiting red meat and chicken to no more than a few times a month; eating fish at least twice a week; and optionally drinking red wine in moderation.

We think it is only current scientific and medical knowledge that shows eating meat is unhealthy. The Bible, interestingly, I believe is the first historical record. In the beginning man was not permitted to eat meat. God said, "Behold, I have given you every herb bearing seed, which is upon the face of all the earth, and every tree, on which is the fruit yielding seed, to you it shall be food."[28]

251

"Man was confined, "Rabbi Joseph Soloveitchik explains, "to yield the soil. Only cereal food was assigned to him. He was not allowed to kill any living creature . . . this injunction against a carnivorous life includes a natural aversion to flesh and an ethical norm. At this crossroads' animal and man part. The former remains arrested within the biological automatism, the latter experiences it on a higher plane—an ethical opportunity."[29]

Rabbi Yaakov Culi, the 18th century Biblical commentator, in his celebrated anthology, *MeAm Lo'ez* explains:

It is often asked why people [in the Bible] lived so long in those times. We see that most of these individuals lived close to a thousand years. Rabbi Moshe Maimonides explains that one reason for the extreme longevity of these individuals was that they were very careful of their diet. They did not eat meat or animal products, nor did they ever drink wine or other intoxicating beverages. Their entire diet consisted of only natural, purely vegetarian products, and their only beverage was pure water. They also ate very carefully measured amounts, exactly the optimum portion. They never ate too much, since doing so has a tendency to weaken man's constitution.[30]

Check out the early Biblical longevity of humans: Seth lived to be 912, Enosh 905, Kenan 910, Mahalalel 895, Jared 962, Methuselah 965, etc. Obviously, many things changed after the flood including what we were allowed to eat. God recanted, "Every moving thing that lives shall be food for you, just as the green herbs I have given you." So, what happened to human longevity after we started eating meat? Eber lived till 464, Arpachshad 438, Shelah to 433, Peleg 239, Reu 239, Serug 230, Nahor 148, etc.

Believe or not the Talmud[31] talks about saturated fats in a fashion. Eating a dip called *kutach*, made from bread crumbs, salt and sour milk, was very popular in Babylonia. Yet, the Talmud cautions that eating *kutach* clogs the heart. And in other places, the Talmud[32] discusses things that will return a person's illness and make his sickness more severe: meat of an ox, fatty meat, roasted meat, poultry, roasted eggs, milk or cheese.

Probably the first recorded study into the benefits of a plant–based diet appears in the Book of the Prophet Daniel.[33] After the Babylonian King Nebuchadnezzar conquered Jerusalem, he instructed his chief eunuch to take Jewish youths skilled in wisdom, discerning in knowledge, and perceptive in understanding and prepare them for royal service in the king's court. They were to be given a daily provision of the king's food and wine.

Now Daniel and his three friends not wanting to eat the king's non–kosher food, struck a deal with the steward in charge to give them only vegetables and water to drink for ten days and then judge their appearances. At the end of the ten days on only a plant–based diet, Daniel and his friends appeared "fairer and fatter" than all the other youths who ate the king's food. The steward then decided to give everyone a plant–based diet.

Finally a *Midrash*[34] acquaints us with a story of two men who entered a shop to eat. "One ate course bread and vegetables while the other ate refined bread, fat meat, drank old wine and partook of an oily sauce and came out feeling ill. The man who had fine food suffered harm, while the one who had course food escaped harm." Classic Jewish sources are replete with such advice and tales.

Books and books have already been written discussing meat, saturated fats, dairy etc and their relationships to chronic illness and disease. When I first drafted an outline for this book, I considered including such chapters more or less as a *Readers Digest* approach dealing with topics of cancer, heart disease, diabetes, etc. Yet, as my research progressed, I came to a more holistic understanding of disease causes which I will soon share. But before I do that, I want to offer several quotes for you to consider:

Dr. Neal Barnard: It may be that the number of mitochondria you have depends on what you eat. Eating fatty food turned off/ disabled the genes that produce mitochondria.[35]

Colin Campbell PhD: Cow's milk protein should be considered a carcinogen: consuming it leads to cancer and cancer halts or goes into remission once milk protein consumption is stopped.[36] Plant proteins did not promote cancer growth at even high levels of intake.[37]

Dr. Gary Fraser: Vegetarian Seventh–day Adventists men and women had a greater longevity, ages at death, 81.2 men and 83.9 women, differences 9.5 men and 6.2 women years as compared with non–Adventists.[38]

Dr. Sir Richard Doll: The truth seems to be that there is quite good evidence that cancer is largely an avoidable disease. The ways in which diet influence the development of cancer are legion.[39]

A concluding quote. Everyone these days understands the problem with pesticides on the fruits and vegetables and is encouraged to buy organic. Rachel Carson in her groundbreaking book, *Silent Spring*, created an awareness of the unrestricted use of pesticides and the adverse health effects, spawning the environmental movement.

But we forget that more than half a century ago, Carson also warned us about another concern most people aren't aware of— pesticide contamination in meat:

In the diet of the average home, meats and any products derived from animal fats contain the heaviest residues of chlorinated hydrocarbons. This is because these chemicals are soluble in fat. Residues on fruits and vegetables tend to be somewhat less. Cooking does not destroy residues.[40]

I mentioned previously that the article, 'Sick Individuals and Sick Populations', by Dr. Geoffrey Rose opened my eyes to many new ways of looking at disease and illness. Rose also wrote, "Case centered epidemiology identifies individually susceptibility, but it may fail to identify the underlying cause of the incident; if cause can be removed, susceptibility ceases to matter.[41] Causes and susceptibility placed a new angle on my research: what make us susceptible to illness; what are the causes of susceptibility. Rose's key question was how to remove the cause of susceptibility.

Strangely enough, I found the answer reading the Book of Job. If I asked you to name the archetype of evil, I am sure you would name Satan. In the story of Job, God and Satan are more or less having a wager on Job's righteousness. Now imagine if Satan wanted to harm a person, surely he would do it in the worst way possible. The Book of Job tells us, "Satan departed from the presence of God and inflicted a sever inflammation on Job from the soles of his feet to his crown."[42]

Previously, I quoted the Talmud[43] that all is in the hands of heaven except for illnesses brought about as a result of cold and inflammation. We are, according to the Talmud, responsible for the inflammation in our bodies; nothing divinely devised. *Inflammation is both the cause and susceptibility of almost all disease and illness.*

An article[44] in the *Journal of Manipulative and Physiolological Therapeutics* confirmed that chronic pain and other degenerative conditions encountered in clinical practice have similar biochemical etiologies, such as a diet–induced pro–inflammatory state:

> The typical American diet is deficient in fruits and vegetables and contains excessive amounts of meat, refined grain products, and dessert foods. Such a diet can have numerous adverse biochemical effects, all of which create a proinflammatory state and predispose the body to degenerative diseases. It appears that an inadequate intake of fruits and vegetables can result in a suboptimal intake of antioxidants and phytochemicals and an imbalanced intake of

essential fatty acids. Through different mechanisms, each nutritional alteration can promote inflammation and disease.

We can no longer view different diseases as distinct biochemical entities. Nearly all degenerative diseases have the same underlying biochemical etiology, that is, a diet–induced proinflammatory state. Although specific diseases may require specific treatments, such as adjustments for hypomobile joints, beta–blockers for hypertension, and chemotherapy for cancer, *the treatment program must also include nutritional protocols to reduce the proinflammatory state.* [Emphasis added]

Odds of living to one hundred have risen from approximately 1 in 20 million to 1 in 50 for women in low–mortality nations due to interventions that reduced infectious diseases in the first part of the 20th century *and from less lifetime inflammation.*[45] [Emphasis added]

Inflammatory diseases usually end with the suffix—itis: appendicitis, arthritis, bronchitis, bursitis, colitis, dermatitis, gastritis, gingivitis, hepatitis, myocarditis, osteoarthritis, otitis media, peridontitis, phlebitis, rheumatoid arthritis, rhinitis, tendinitis, tendonitis, tonsillitis, etc. More importantly, inflammation plays a pivotal role in heart disease, cancer and Alzheimer's disease.

In heart disease, chronic inflammation is a source of cellular damage.[46] Tissue damage is a hallmark of chronic inflammation, which has a variety of harmful effects on the endothelium: the lining of the blood vessels.[47] Inflammation is fundamental reason for cholesterol being deposited in the arteries in the first place.[48]

Inflammation is the key player in destabilizing plaque, explaining why some people with relatively little buildup have heart attacks and strokes, while others with substantial plaque deposits never suffer these events.

Feelings of hostility—along with mild to moderate depression— in healthy men have also been shown to raise levels of a protein, IL–6, a marker of inflammation that may be involved in the process that causes arterial thickening.[49] A study published in *Israel Medical Association Journal*[50] corroborated this connection.

Immigrating to another country is a very stressful and at times a depressing experience even if the move is a wanted voluntary one. Believe me, I know from firsthand experience. The late Dr. David Servan–Schreiber says, "We know that the feeling of helplessness weakens the immune system and causes inflammation, which encourages the growth of tumors as well a host of other problems, including heart conditions, hypertension, diabetes, and arthritis."[51]

Recent immigrants from the former Soviet Union to Israel were studied to determine the causes for their high heart attack rates. "The worse profile and prognosis observed among patients who recently emigrated from the Soviet Union cannot be explained by traditional risk factors for coronary artery disease such as smoking, diabetes, hypertension, and lipid disorders."[52] *I am convinced chronic low–grade inflammation is the culprit!*

People who take low–dose aspirin for heart attack prevention also have a lower risk of several types of cancer, including of the breast, colon, and esophagus.

Infection is certainly a cause of bodily inflammation. More often, however, inflammation results from the foods we choose to eat. Pro–inflammatory foods are meat and dairy, omega 6 fatty acids, i.e. corn oil, cottonseed oil, peanut oil, sesame seed oil, saturated fat, processed foods and generally any product with a long shelf life or ingredients you cannot pronounce.

Some pro–inflammatory foods listed on several sites on the internet in alphabetical order are:

> bagels, breads, rolls, baked goods, candy, cake, cookies, cereals (except old fashioned oatmeal), cornstarch, corn bread, corn muffins, corn syrup, crackers, croissants, doughnuts, egg rolls, fast food, French fries, fruit juice, fried foods, flour, frozen yogurt, granola, hard cheese (except for feta and grating cheeses, such as Romano and Parmesan), honey, hot dogs, ice cream, Italian ices, jams, jellies and preserves, margarine, molasses, muffins, noodles, pancakes, pastry, pie, pita bread, pizza, pasta, popcorn, potatoes, pudding,

relish, rice (white), sherbet, shortening, snack foods, including: potato chips, pretzels, corn chips, rice and corn cakes, soda, sugar, tacos, tortillas and waffles.

The anti–inflammatory diet closely follows the Mediterranean diet! That is why the Mediterranean diet is good for the prevention of heart disease, cancer, obesity, diabetes, cataracts, macular degeneration, Alzheimer's, cognitive dysfunction, multiple sclerosis, osteoporosis, etc.

However, the diet I religiously follow is the one developed by Dr. Caldwell B. Esselstyn, Jr. in his book, *Prevent and Reverse Hearth Disease*.[53] Esselstyn's diet goes one step beyond the Mediterranean diet. "A giant leap for mankind" in my opinion! At first blush, Esselstyn's diet seems extreme. But is eating only fruits and vegetables more extreme than chemotherapy or by–pass surgery?

- You may not eat anything with a mother or a face (no eggs, meat, poultry, or fish).
- You cannot eat dairy products.
- You must not consume oil of any kind—not a drop.
- Generally, you cannot eat nuts or avocados.
- All vegetables except avocado. Leafy green vegetables; root vegetables; veggies that are red, green, purple, orange, yellow and everything in between.
- All legumes—beans, peas, and lentils of all varieties.
- All whole grains and products, such as bread and pasta made from them as long as they do not contain added fats.
- All fruits.

Confession: There is one item in Dr. Esselstyn's diet that I am an apostate. I eat nuts and seeds; specifically almonds, walnuts, Brazil nuts, pumpkin seeds, and brown sesame seeds. I started off without nuts but my research kept turning up study after study that convinced me to add nuts. For example:

Studies in the *American Journal of Clinical Nutrition*:

> Our meta–analysis indicates that nut intake is inversely associated with ischemic heart disease, overall cardiovascular disease, and all–cause mortality.[54]
>
> Nut consumption is associated with lower risk of all–cause, cardiovascular disease, and cancer mortality.[55]

A study in the journal *Nutrients:*

> There are consistent evidences from epidemiologic and clinical studies of the beneficial effects of nut consumption on risk of coronary heart disease, including sudden cardiac death, as well as on diabetes in women, and on major and emerging cardiovascular risk factors.[56]

A study in the *International Journal of Epidemiology*:

> Total nut intake was related to lower overall and cause–specific mortality (cancer, diabetes, cardiovascular, neurodegenerative diseases, respiratory, and other causes) in men and women.[57]

My new doctor was aghast when I told him the last cardiologist I saw was the one who preformed my angioplasty in 1999 and sent me straight to a cardiologist. In our first meeting the cardiologist, the head of angioplasty at largest hospital in Tel Aviv, reviewed my file while I explained my vigilant adherence to the Esselstyn diet.

When I finished, the cardiologist turned to me and said, "You know I have a seminar I give for my cardiology patients and during our sessions I tell them to do exactly what you are doing. I bring in chefs from top hotels to show my patients that vegan food can be appealing, tasty, appetizing, delectable, palatable, and delicious. And I have seen with my own eyes patients who I told nothing else could be done adopt a vegan diet and now are alive and healthier than they ever were."

Healthy eating may be best achieved with a plant–based diet. Physicians should consider recommending a plant–based diet to all their patients, especially those with high blood pressure, diabetes, cardiovascular disease, or obesity.[58] Of all diets, the vegan diet was the healthiest one; had the lowest total energy intake, better fat intake profile, lowest protein and highest dietary fiber intake; typical aspects: high fruit and vegetable intake, low sodium intake, and low intake of saturated fat.[59]

Experts agree on the optimal diet to prevent not only heart disease but also cancer and other chronic disease such as type 2 diabetes mellitus consists of a lot of fruit and vegetables, fish, less salt and sugar, more unrefined cereals, beans and nuts.[60]

So, who should you believe? One of the preeminent classic Jewish commentaries on Biblical commandants is 16th century work, *Sefer ha Hinnuch*, attributed to Rabbi Aaron haLevi of Barcelona Spain. Rabbi haLevi tells a parable which I consider is most appropriate:

> There was a man whom thousands upon thousands of people adjured not to drink the water of a certain stream, as they saw that the water killed those who drank it. They tested this matter a thousand times at various periods, and with persons from different countries. Yet one wise person, an expert physician, told this man, "Do not believe them all: for I tell you from the vantage point of wisdom that this water is not lethal, because it is pure and swift running, and the earth over which it passes is good. Drink to your heart's desire."
>
> Would it be good for that man to forget the widely–known testimony of all and do as this wise person said? Of course it would not be good; an intelligent person would not listen to him nor do as he advised.[61]

The overwhelming evidence is in favor of a whole–food, plant–based diet!

260

Earlier I wrote about what I considered my information theory of health and that to achieve wellness you need to correct the MIS–information in your life. For the remainder of this chapter I want to share some of the conclusions from a number of the studies on inflammation and its effect on disease and illness I read. *This kind of information is what convinced me to change my lifestyle.* Hopefully the following information might convince you as well.

Anti–Inflammation Diet

Inflammation is linked with cancer and dietary agents, derived from fruits, vegetables, spices, nutraceuticals, can suppress chronic inflammation and thus help prevent and treat cancer. Chronic diseases require chronic, not acute, treatment.[62] Developing a healthier diet with the addition of specific supplements designed to reduce oxidative stress and inflammation should be an important part of an overall palliative care plan. The majority of nutrients should be obtained via a wholesome diet.[63]

Variety in fruit and vegetable intake is associated with lower serum c–reactive protein.[64] The results indicate that one potential mechanism underlying the relation between fruit and vegetable intake and coronary heart disease may involve influencing the process of systemic inflammation.[65] It is clear that a role of oxidative stress is of some importance to these inflammatory conditions. The only near certainty is that a diet rich in fruit and vegetables is beneficial and resources are better spent on that than on expensive supplements.[66]

Higher intakes of fruit and vegetables were associated with a lower risk of the metabolic syndrome; a high intake of fruit and vegetables is associated with reduced plasma concentrations of inflammatory markers.[67] Flavonoids comprise an array of active compounds ubiquitous in plants whose therapeutic potential is fairly obvious. The areas that hold most promise are chronic inflammatory, allergic, coronary artery diseases and breast cancer.[68]

Energy restricted low–fat and very–low–carbohydrate diets both significantly decreased several biomarkers of inflammation. These data suggest weight loss is primarily the driving force underlying the reductions in most of the inflammatory biomarkers.[69]

Cancer

Why does chronic inflammation cause cancer in some individuals but not in others? The answer might lie in the relative ability of the individual to repair accumulated DNA damage caused by cytokines, free radicals, prostaglandins, and growth factors.[70] Inflammation has been demonstrated to play a major role in the initiation, progression, and prognosis of cancer.[71]

The use of anti–inflammatory agents decreases the incidence and recurrence of various cancers, and can improve the prognosis for patients. Overall this review provides evidence for a strong link between chronic inflammation and cancer. The lack of toxicity associated with natural anti–inflammatory agents combined with their cost provides additional advantages.[72]

We propose a unifying hypothesis that all lifestyle factors that cause cancer and all agents that prevent cancer are linked through chronic inflammation.[73] Inflammation is a key component of the tumor microenvironment. Recent efforts have shed new light on molecular and cellular pathways linking inflammation and cancer.[74]

Inflammatory cells have powerful effects on tumor development. Early in the neoplastic process, these cells are powerful tumor promoters, producing an attractive environment for tumor growth, facilitating genomic instability and promoting angiogenesis.[75]

Deregulation of inflammation associated miRNAs (small non–coding RNA molecules whose function is to regulate genes involved in differentiation, apoptosis, and inflammation) has the capacity to influence prostate cancer initiation and progression.[76]

Chronic and persistent inflammation contributes to cancer development and even predisposes to carcinogenesis; anti–inflammatory agents should be explored for both prevention and treatment of cancer.[77]

Inflammation can affect every aspect of tumor development and progression as well as the response to therapy. One of the major lessons learned from investigating the relationships between inflammation and cancer is that most cancers are preventable.[78] It is becoming increasingly apparent that activation of multiple inflammatory signaling pathways provides a critical link between obesity and cancer.[79]

Drugs that target cancer related inflammation have the potential to re–educate a tumor promoting inflammatory infiltrate, prevent such cells from migrating to the tumor site, or induce tumor inhibiting microenvironment, leading to suppression of cancer.[80]

Src, a transforming protein, might serve as a critical mechanistic link between inflammation and cancer, mediating and propagating a cycle between immune and tissue cells that can ultimately lead to the development and progression of cancer.[81]

In a setting of chronic inflammation, the persistent tissue damage and cell proliferation as well as the enrichment of reactive oxygen and nitrogen species contribute to a cancer–prone microenvironment.[82]

Macrophages are key orchestrators of chronic inflammation. These results highlight a direct connection between early, causative and sufficient oncogene rearrangement and activation of a pro–inflammatory program in human tumor.[83]

Long–standing inflammation secondary to chronic infection or irritation predisposes to cancer. Many inflammatory mediators, cytokines, chemokines, and eicanosoids, are capable of stimulating tumor cell proliferation.[84] The links between obesity and inflammation and between chronic inflammation and cancer suggest that inflammation might be important in the obesity–cancer link.[85] Inflammation enhanced ROS production induces DNA damage, inhibition of apoptosis, and activation of protooncogenes by initiating signal transduction pathways; thus increasing oxidative damage and promoting mechanisms of carcinogenesis.[86]

Breast cancer patients with the most elevated levels of blood proteins indicating chronic, low–grade inflammation were 2 to 3 times more likely to die regardless of tumor stage, age, race, cardiovascular disease or body mass index.[87]

Heart Disease

The results show that there is a strong association between chronic inflammation in the coronary arteries and reduction of the coronary lumen. Neither age nor cholesterol rich deposits had significant explanatory power.[88]

Low–grade inflammation and oxidative stress, that predicts an increased risk for chronic disease in adults and adolescence, are already present by early adolescence. Mechanisms as dietary antioxidants may inhibit the development of atherosclerosis.[89] Inflammation of the vessel wall plays an essential role in the initiation and progression of atherosclerosis, its final stages: plaque erosion or fissure and eventually plaque rupture.[90]

In the elderly inflammatory markers are non–specific measures of health and predict both disability and mortality even in the absence of clinical cardiovascular disease.[91]

Inflammation plays a major role in atherothrombosis, and measurement of inflammatory markers such as High–Sensitivity C–Reactive Protein (hsCRP) may provide a novel method for detecting individuals at high risk of plaque rupture.[92]

Alzheimer's disease

Oxidative damage, caused by free radical activity resulting in tissue inflammation, to brain cells may be a principle indicator of Alzheimer's disease activity.[93] This is the first study to link neuroinflammation independently to early death in Alzheimer's disease and, hence, a rapidly progressing disease. Our results suggest that inflammation is an independent underlying mechanism in the malignancy of Alzheimer's disease.[94]

Most neurological diseases are the result of a combination of multiple factors, but the systemic inflammatory response and the production of autoantibodies are common components and determinants in the onset, evolution, and outcome of these diseases.[95]

Although mechanisms underlying Alzheimer disease remain unclear, neuroinflammation seems to be a common feature to neurodegenerative diseases with an important contribution to the pathology, affecting among others, physiological processes with a repairing function such as the adult neurogenesis process.[96]

Inflammation is known to occur in the brains of both Alzheimer's disease and Down syndrome patients in response to the presence of neuritic plaques and neurofibrillary tangles.[97] Atherosclerosis and Alzheimer disease share a common infectious inflammatory pathoetiology; have similar age–dependence, vascular pathology, genetic underpinnings and association with infection.[98]

20

Timeless Aging

By the time you're eighty years old you've learned everything. You only have to remember it.

George Burns

I do not wish to achieve immortality through my works. I wish to achieve immortality by not dying.

Woody Allen

There shall be no more an infant who lives a few days nor an old man who has not filled his days; for the youngest shall die a hundred years old.

Isaiah 65:20–22

Those who think they have no time for bodily exercise will sooner or later have to find time for illness.

Dr. Edward Stanley

Dr. Robert Coleman Atkins died on April 8, 2003, at the age of 72. Nine days prior to his death, Dr. Atkins fell and hit his head on an icy New York pavement. Atkins official death certificate states the cause of death as "blunt impact injury of head with epidural hematoma."

A medical report issued by the New York medical examiner's office a year after his death showed that Atkins had a history of heart attack, congestive heart failure and hypertension. Atkins had suffered cardiac arrest in April 2002. It also noted that he weighed 258 pounds (117 kilograms) at death.

Seventeen months later, Ancel Keys died on November 20, 2004, two months before his 101st birthday in the Cilento region located on the southwest coast of Italy. Is it only anecdotal evidence that Key's lifelong adherence the Mediterranean–style diet helped him achieve centenarian status?

Perhaps it was spending the last 28 years of his life actually living in the Mediterranean region he studied so prolifically. Does it help to know his wife, Margaret Haney Keys, died two years later at the age of 97? Maybe Ancel and Margaret Keys discovered the elusive Fountain of Youth in their beloved Italian village Pioppi?

According to Wikipedia, the Fountain of Youth is a spring that supposedly restores the youth of anyone who drinks or bathes in its waters. Tales of such a fountain have been recounted across the world for thousands of years, appearing in writings by Herodotus in the 5th century BCE, the Alexander romance in the 3rd century CE and the stories of Prester John during the early Crusades.

Stories of similar waters were also evidently prominent among the peoples of the Caribbean during the Age of Exploration in the early 16th century who spoke of the restorative powers of the water in the mythical land of Bimini. The legend became particularly prominent by the Spanish explorer Juan Ponce de León, first Governor of Puerto Rico. Ponce de León was searching for the Fountain of Youth when he traveled to what is now Florida in 1513.

I know it sounds boastful, but during my research I discovered the true Fountain of Youth. Funny thing is that people were always looking in the wrong place. In actuality, the Fountain of Youth is not something you drink but what you eat and how much of it!

Blue Zones is a concept used to identify a demographic and/or geographic area of the world where people live measurably longer lives. John Robbins is an author who popularized the links among nutrition, environmentalism, and animal rights. In his book,[1] *Healthy at 100: The Scientifically Proven Secrets of the World's Healthiest and*

Longest–Lived Peoples, he discusses three areas: Hunza region of Pakistan, the valley of Vicabamba in Ecuador, and the Abkhasia portions of the Caucasus Mountains in the Soviet Union.

Dan Buettner is a *National Geographic* Fellow and *New York Times* bestselling author. In his book[2] *The Blue Zones: Lessons for Living Longer from the People Who've Lived the Longest* Buettner identifies the Seventh–day Adventists of Loma Linda, California; Okinawa, Japan; Sardinia, Italy; Nicoya Peninsula, Costa Rica; and Icaria, Greece.

What all Blue Zones have in common is a population that is statistically older, healthier and happier than the rest of us. Buettner lists nine lessons he learned from the centenarians:

> Moderate, regular physical activity.
> Life purpose.
> Stress reduction.
> Moderate calorie intake.
> Plant–based diet.
> Moderate alcohol intake, especially wine.
> Engagement in spirituality or religion.
> Engagement in family life.
> Engagement in social life.

Obviously, the nine are interrelated and form a synergistic pattern that explains why there are so many centenarians living in the Blue Zones. However, I want to discuss only three: plant–based diet, moderate caloric intake and moderate, regular physical activity. Diet and exercise are two of the most prominent reasons for longevity.

A study in *Arquivos de Neuro–Psiquiatria*:

> The biological clock cannot be stopped, but lifestyle changes, such as stress management, healthy eating habits and adoption of physical activity, can slow down the aging process; evidence of the impact of exercises on our cells' health is incontestable. [3]

A study in *Asian Pacific Journal of Clinical Nutrition*:

A nutritious diet, adequate physical exercise, and a harmonious family environment may be the key lifestyle factors for their longevity of centenarians in Chongqing, China. [4]

A study in *Aging Cell*:

A sensible balanced diet and regular exercise, combined with high quality health care, is still likely to provide the best current route to maintaining quality of life throughout the human lifespan and of decreasing risks of morbidity and early mortality. [5]

A study in *Archives of Internal Medicine*:

Well informed choices improve life expectancy. Choices regarding diet, exercise, hormone replacement therapy, body weight, and cigarette smoking, in combination, appear to change life expectancy by many years.[6]

A study in the *Journal of Nutrition Health and Aging*:

A dietary pattern including plenty of fruit while limiting meat and fried foods may improve the likelihood of ageing successfully. [7]

John Robbins explains the diets of two zones he cited:

Vicabamba diet is almost entirely vegetarian, made up primarily of whole grains such as corn, quinoa, wheat, and barley, tubers including potatoes, yucca, sweet potatoes, vegetables, fruits, seeds, beans and nuts, eat almost no meat and never any butter.[8]

Abkhasian formula: a great amount of exercise built into their daily routines, begin breakfast with a salad of green vegetables freshly picked from the garden, which are eaten raw, the people eat their "beloved abista," a cornmeal porridge, fresh cooked and served warm, eat very little meat, no fatty dishes, no sugar, little salt and almost no butter.[9]

Each of the Blue Zones has their characteristic qualities of diet and lifestyle. I would like to discuss the Blue Zone of Okinawa because although I adhere to Dr. Caldwell Esselstyn's heart disease prevention diet, I lean more to an Okinawan version rather than a Mediterranean one. Allow me to explain why. Studies on Okinawa show that:

> The high centenarian prevalence found for Okinawa can be largely explained by the very low mortality risk from cardiovascular disease and certain cancers.[10]

> The Okinawa way is associated with impressive health benefits; lower risk for obesity, diabetes, and numerous age–associated diseases such, i.e. cardiovascular disease and certain cancers.[11]

While the Mediterranean and Japanese diets are both known to be healthy, there is one major exception. The Mediterranean diet is characterized by a high consumption of cereals (wheat) think pasta, vegetables, fruit, fish, and olive oil. The Japanese also consume large amounts of cereal (rice) think sushi, vegetables, fruit and fish, but there is a much lower intake of oils and fats. Despite what headline health says about olive oil being "heart healthy," olive oil intake at high levels is not healthy.[12]

The traditional Okinawan diet deviates from the traditional Japanese diet. It contains 30% green and yellow vegetables, a tiny amount of fish usually less than half a serving per day, less rice than the average Japanese diet, more soy [tofu] as a principal protein and other legumes.

Okinawans eat an average of three ounces of soy products per day. Tofu may play a role in reducing the risk of heart disease.[13] Meat in the form of pork is usually only eaten during monthly festivals. However, the purple–fleshed Okinawan sweet potato is primarily its main staple counting for the majority of the diets' calories.

In fact, although the Okinawans consume the same total grams of fiber, their diet consists of: 25% less wheat, barley, and other grains, 38% less sugars, 24% less fish, 27% less meat and 30% more legumes than the traditional Japanese diet.[14]

Notable in the Okinawan diet is the intake of the antioxidant vitamins at rates higher than the recommended levels: vitamin C– 289%, vitamin E–190%, vitamin B6–221% as well as folate– 295%.[15] A study in the *Israel Medical Association Journal*[16] showed that strong nutritional support, providing supplements such as antioxidants as well as general macro– and micro– nutrient requirements, will sustain appropriate immune responses in a large fraction of older people.

We do not die of old age. Dr. Hans Selye, a pioneering endocrinologist on the response of an organism to stressors, said:

> Among all my autopsies I have never seen a person who died of old age. In fact I don't think anyone has ever died of old age yet. To die of old age would mean that all the organs of the body had worn out proportionally, merely having been used too long. This is never the case.[17]

The Oxford bio–gerontologist Aubrey deGrey says, "Aging is not an extension of development, but decay. Aging doesn't kill us; it only makes us steadily more killable.[18] The decline of the immune system is one of the most deadly effects of aging."[19]

A study in *Clinical Interventions in Aging*[20] appropriately named 'The aging process and potential interventions to extend life expectancy' highlights another important aspect of the Okinawan diet: life expectancy might be due to diet based on vegetables, grains, soy, fruits, fish and seaweed. *It is noteworthy that this diet is very similar to the*

caloric restriction interventions designed for experiments in animal models.
[Emphasis added]

Calorie or caloric restriction is a dietary regimen that reduces calorie intake without incurring malnutrition or a reduction in essential nutrients defined relative to a person's previous intake before intentionally restricting calories.

Okinawans do consciously practice calorie restriction; they have developed cultural habits that led to prudent food choices that maximize nutritional properties while minimizing caloric density.[21] Indeed, they appear to be one of the few populations in the world that may have experienced mild long–term caloric restriction without significant malnutrition, and this may help explain their exceptionally healthy survival.[22]

The beneficial effects of calorie restriction on longevity are partly mediated by improved mitochondrial function.[23] Calorie restriction lowers the generation of mitochondrial free radicals, toughens cell membranes against free radical assault and reduces the age–related accumulation of mitochondrial DNA mutations.[24] Calorie restricted mice have a lower metabolic rate proportional to their increase in lifespan, in line with the rate of living theory.[25]

Caloric restriction protects against the decline in cardiovascular function that occurs with increasing age, prevents diseases of the cardiovascular system and cancer, and may have a major beneficial effect on health span, life span, and quality of life in humans.[26]

It also attenuates the age–associated changes in the heart and major vessels which cannot be explained by the effect of lower body weight but are attributable to more intimate cellular mechanisms of calorie restriction itself.[27] Diet–induced obesity regimens result in an increase in colon tumor development, while calorie restriction decreases colon tumor development.[28]

We all can agree that we eat far too much. So, how are we supposed to restrict our caloric intake? Don't worry, be happy! Big Pharma is working diligently for a "golden bullet" for you to take to achieve calorie restriction benefits while still eating what you want. *You just can't make huge profits on fruits and vegetables like you can a pill.*

But as one study cautions, "we are on the verge of understanding calorie restriction which may allow the development of new drugs to provide some of the health benefits of this dietary regimen; however, *drugs will not create carte blanche for irresponsible living.*"[29] [Emphasis added]

To paraphrase author and social activist Naomi Klein's comment on geoengineering and climate change, caloric restriction pills similar to statins "are the very antithesis of good medicine, whose goal is to achieve a state of health and equilibrium that requires no further intervention." [30] By leaving ourselves at the mercy of Big Pharma "we effectively give up the prospect of ever being healthy again."

Moderate, regular physical activity is another component of the Blue Zone Fountain of Youth. Maimonides says "as long as one exercises, exerts himself greatly, does not eat to the point of satiation . . . he will not suffer sickness and he will grow in strength even if he eats harmful foods. Whoever is idle and does not exercise will be full of pain for all his days and his strength will fade away."[31] "What is termed exercise," Maimonides states, "is powerful or rapid motion or a combination of both, that is, vigorous motion with which the respiration alters."[32]

Today we define two kinds of exercise. Either aerobic exercise of low to high intensity like long distance running, jogging, swimming, cycling, and walking or anaerobic exercise that works muscles at a rate faster than that at which your body can supply them with oxygen to promote strength, speed and power as used by body builders to build muscle mass. Dr. Esther Sternberg an expert on neural–immune science in her book *Healing Spaces: The Science of Place and Well–Being* says that low grade exercise like walking produces results after just thirty minutes[33] and moderate exercise shows the greater response to boost the immune system.[34]

Another study found that older men who walked two miles a day had only half the rate of dementia found among men who walked less than a quarter–mile a day.[35] Henry David Thoreau said, "I have met with but one or two persons in the course of my life who understood the art of Walking." How true today!

Low calorie intake coupled with high physical activity levels appear to have contributed to a caloric restriction phenotype in older Okinawans.[36] People who exercised three hours per week are biologically nine years younger than those who exercised less than fifteen minutes a week.[37] Physical exercise acts directly on cytokines responsible for inflammation by lowering their level in the blood.[38]

The first Swanson brand TV dinner was introduced in 1953. Baby Boomers were nurtured and nourished by the tantalizing tastes of Salisbury Steak, Turkey and Dressing, Fried Chicken, pure white mashed potatoes with a square drop of margarine, tater tots, and the infamous perfectly round green peas while glued to the tube.

Blue Zones are not inhabited by Couch Potatoes who spend their free times in front of a TV eating. In fact, watching TV gives you higher odds of having metabolic syndrome: greater than twofold for women and by 82% for men who watch TV 3 hours per day vs. 0–1 hours per day. BMI also mediates the association between TV viewing and cardiovascular disease outcomes. There is even a lower metabolic expenditure for TV viewing than sitting doing office work.[39]

The strongest predictor of being obese among children, ages 10–12 years in eight European countries was TV watching at two meals. Promotion of family meals may be a way of avoiding eating in front of the television. The odds ratio of being overweight was lower for children who reported to never watch TV at meals.[40] *So much for TV trays!*

In fact, reduced TV viewing and prevention of infrequent activity have greatest beneficial associations for glucose metabolism among the obese and with benefits for other biomarkers across obese and non—obese groups.[41] FYI, I have not personally owned a TV since 1976.

More than a decade ago, I bought a treadmill because I realized my walking was intermittent at best due to the weather. Just like Goldilocks, some days were just too hot, others just too cold and some just too soggy to walk outside. Now I walk indoors which forces away my excuses not to walk. You can easily buy a used treadmill. Several of your neighbors I am sure have treadmills upstairs in their bedrooms that they are using to hang dry cleaning and laundry.

The treadmill takes care of my aerobic exercise. For anaerobic exercise, I work out with weights. When I played high school football, I could dead lift more than my total body weight with ease. Now I am content just to bench press sixty pounds (27 kilograms). Both walking and weightlifting together provide all the exercise I need and helps keep my body trim. It all paid off a few years ago when a woman I was dating complemented me by saying, "You know you have two qualities few men your age have—blue eyes and a flat stomach."

When I hear the word '*Bama* instantly I think of the legendary head coach of the University of Alabama football team Paul "Bear" Bryant. During his 25—year tenure as the *Crimson Tide's* head coach, he amassed six national championships and thirteen Southeastern Conference championships. Upon his retirement in 1982, Bryant held the record for most wins as head coach in collegiate football history with 323 wins.

More recently, I have come to associate the name Bama with a Blue Zone most people have never heard of. The road to Bama county China in southern Guangx region is lined with thick stands of bamboo, graceful eucalyptus, glossy chestnut trees and winds along a jade colored pristine river. Bama and its villages are in a remote mountainous area with few factories or pollution.

In recent years, Bama has gained notoriety as the home of villages with roughly five times more centenarians than China's average proportion to population. Today Bama is the center of attraction for thousands of tourists who come in hopes of learning the secrets of longevity.

Bama centenarians eat an anti–inflammation, alkalizing plant–based diet high on vegetables including pumpkins, tomatoes, amaranth leaves, sweet potatoes, pak choi, mushrooms, bamboo shoots and peppers; eat fruits such as bananas, guavas, grapes, and pears daily; consume hemp, corn, brown rice, millet, soy beans, tofu, lima beans, and mung beans regularly. Seldom do they eat meat. Their average consumption is only about 1500 calories daily and they moderately drink corn wine.

Although most of their food is steamed, not fried, they rely on hemp oil, nature's most perfectly balanced oil because of its 3:1 ratio of omega–6 to omega–3 essential fatty acids. I recently saw a Chinese documentary on Bama and hemp plants in the film were ubiquitous.

The Chinese emperor Shen–nung reportedly taught his people to grow hemp for fiber in the twenty–eighth century BCE. A text from the period 1500–1200 BCE documents knowledge of the plant in China—but not for use as fiber. In 200 CE the physician, Hoa–tho described the use of cannabis as an analgesic.[42] Dr. Hoa–tho also advocated exercise reminding his patients, "The door hinge will rust if it is not used."

I would not be a true Baby Boomer if I passed up an opportunity to talk about hemp. Hemp whether it is called cannabis, cannabis indicia, cannabis americanus, Indian hemp, or marijuana all refer to the same plant—pot.

Pot was just something everyone did during university days. Times have changed. Who would have thought then we would see not only cannabis legal for medical use worldwide, but also even totally legal in some states. (A disclaimer—the last time I smoked pot was in 1974 before I entered graduate school.)

A joint position statement (pardon the pun) by the Cancer Council of Australia and the Clinical Oncology Society of Australia on the medical use of cannabis reflects the current worldwide medical opinion:

> There is no current evidence that cannabis or cannabinoids are effective at inhibiting tumor growth or to treat or cure cancer in humans.

Marijuana should be brought back to clinical use because the therapeutic potential of Cannabinoid CB1 receptor agonists is huge, do not penetrate the blood–brain barrier, do not cause psycho–activity, but have various therapeutic effects.[43] The improvement in cancer related symptoms should push the use of cannabis in the practice of oncology palliative treatment.[44]

Among Israeli cancer patients, cannabis use is perceived as highly effective by some patients with advanced cancer.[45] In stark contrast to opioids and other pain medications, cannabis is relatively non–addicting and has the best record of any pain medication—no deaths attributed to overdose or direct effects of medication.[46]

Despite the worldview as expressed by the Cancer Council of Australia that there is no current evidence that cannabis or cannabinoids are effective at inhibiting tumor growth or to treat or cure cancer in humans, in my research I found plenty of evidence to the contrary.

The California Men's Health Study concluded: "Cannabis use only was associated with a 45% reduction in bladder cancer incidence. Although a cause and effect relationship has not been established, cannabis use may be inversely associated with bladder cancer risk in this population."[47] To me 45% is pretty big!

A study in *British Journal of Pharmacology*:

> Cannabinoids exert a number of effects depending on cell types, route of drug administration, timing of drug delivery and, last but not least, responsivity of tumor and normal cells. [48]

A study in *Oncology Reports*:

> Emerging research in (endo)cannabinoids show that these compounds have the ability of modulating cancer progression.[49]

A study in the *International Journal of Oncology*:

> Data reported in this review seem to confirm the ability of cannabinoids to induce cell death in different tumor models. [50]

I just wonder if the Bama tradition preserves something Dr. Hoa–tho knew about tetrahydrocannabinol (THC) in Chinese medicine we do not. George Washington in his *Farwell Address* advised, "Don't make entangling alliances." However, how many people know he also said, "Make the most of the Indian hemp seed and sow it everywhere!"

One last Blue Zone I want to mention is my apartment which I consider to be a candidate for a future Blue Zone. If you truly want to be a centenarian then you need to live like a centenarian. You do not have to move to the Mediterranean as Ancel Keys did, or I have done, nor travel to the orient. You can start today making your home wherever you live into a Blue Zone. Like Nike says: *Just Do It!*

Roll, 'Bama, Roll!

21

Inner Calm

Look deeply into nature and then you will understand everything better.

Albert Einstein

One psychological effect of serious meditation is to comprehend a new way of perceiving and relating to the world.

Larry LeShan[1]

Mindfulness is the final common pathway of what makes us human; our capacity for awareness and for self–knowledge.

Jon Kabat–Zinn[2]

As we keep or break the Sabbath day, we nobly save or meanly lose the last best hope by which man rises.

Abraham Lincoln.

Instead of being humble, I made the mistake of believing I had found the magic formula that would allow me to stay healthy and to give myself over completely to the projects I cared about. I told myself I was protected simply because I was still taking a number of precautions. I was careful about my diet. I meditated and did some yoga. I believed that this gave me license to ignore the fundamental needs of my body—such as sleep, rest, and a regular routine. In retrospect there are some lessons to be learned here. We must not exhaust and over exert ourselves. One of our best defenses against cancer is finding a place of inner calm . . . Personally, I never managed to find that calm, and today I regret it. I didn't manage to remain close to nature to its and my, natural rhythms. I am absolutely convinced that spending time in a forest, on a mountain, or by a river bank brings us something that is wonderfully revitalizing . . . to find balance and healing within ourselves.[3]

Dr. David Servan–Schreiber was a Clinical Professor of Psychiatry at the University of Pittsburg School of Medicine and cofounder of its Center for Integrative Medicine. Dr. Servan–Schreiber was also the author of the international bestseller, *Anticancer: A New Way of Life,*[4] in which he reveals his own personal confrontation with a diagnosis of a glioblastoma brain tumor and the lessons he learned that extended his life nineteen years after his initial diagnosis. Of all books, his was the one I chose to give my best friend recently when he was diagnosed with cancer.

Following a yearlong battle with a relapse of brain cancer, Dr. Servan–Schreiber died in July 2011. Yet, during that year he chose to painstakingly share his many personal questions he had about how we choose to live and how we prepare for death in a powerful, honest and truly inspiring book, *Not The Last Goodbye: On Life, Death, Healing and Cancer*, posthumously published. The excerpt at the beginning of this chapter was taken from that work.

"In the public perception of *Anticancer* the nutritional guidelines, such as eating raspberries and drinking green tea, tended to overshadow other recommendations," he said, "it's easier to eat fish and berries than it is to change your work habits or your relationship with your spouse.[5] In light of my own ordeal, I am tempted to emphasize the absolute necessity of finding and maintaining inner peace."[6]

Reading *Not The Last Goodbye* was a very emotional experience for me. It conjured up many past feelings going as far back as the day John Lennon died. On my way to the synagogue early that morning the car radio brought the news that Lennon had been shot. I was stunned beyond belief and passed the synagogues' entrance in a trance. The thought that the Beatles would never sing again was really the first time a feeling of mortality faced me. The beauty of a flower disappears forever with the winter snow despite the fresh blooms of the spring.

An epiphany came to me when I first finished the book—I too lacked an inner calm. I had believed in my own indestructibility and lived daily under the clouds of immortality—*I was Veggieman.* I rivaled anyone I knew in being healthy, but secretly I knew inside it wasn't enough. Servan–Schreiber said, "I am simply convinced that being at peace with yourself, and accepting your mortality, means you can direct all your energy toward the healing process."[7]

During the last few years I can honestly say that I have begun the process of inner calm; making peace with myself. And with it I have gained a feeling of equanimity, an evenness of the mind, I never knew before. So profound an experience that on an online dating site I was using, I listed equanimity as my occupation because it was occupying all of my waking moments. Boy did that have great effects; similar to walking in the park with a cute puppy, I got a dozen emails from women who asked me to explain what it meant.

A major part of my inner calm comes from my belief in God and the rest from mindfulness training, learning a form of breathing meditation, communing with nature, and continuing to strictly observe the Sabbath as restricted by Jewish law and custom.

My personal belief in God could fill volumes, but for now I will only speak to one aspect I found in the 16th Psalm,[8] *Shviti Hashem l'negdi tamid*—"I have set the Lord always before me." This excerpt is frequently inscribed above the ark where Torah scrolls are kept in a synagogue.

Rabbi Israel Baal Shem Tov, the founder of the 18th century Chassidic movement, explains that the word *shviti* is an expression of *hishtavut*–equanimity and is related to the Hebrew root–word *shaveh*–equal, to remove all unevenness.

The notion of equanimity is a fundamental principle in the pursuit of religiosity and piety. The Baal Shem Tov writes, "no matter what happens, whether people praise or shame you, and so, too, with anything else, it is all the same to you. This applies likewise to any food; it is all the same to you whether you eat delicacies or other things." [9] This is what Rabbi Wolbe meant by quoting the Talmudic passage: *They who accept being shamed and do not shame others, they who listen to insult without responding in kind, they who serve out of love and who remain joyful even whilst being afflicted.*

Rabbi S. R. Hirsch, the 19th century Biblical commentator and educator of the German Orthodox community, explains the 16th Psalm as follows:

> There are those who labor under the delusion that God must be conceived as Someone Who towers far above the earthly affairs and Who thinks all things terrestrial are far below Him. "But as for me," King David says, "my conception of Him is very different. I have perceived His presence on the level of my own earthly existence; I no longer seek Him in heights but I have set Him before my eyes in everything I do on earth. Nothing here below is so small or insignificant that God would be indifferent to it. Whatever I am, whatever I wish to accomplish, lies clearly before His eyes. I shall hold fast to this conviction, forever, and shall never again allow myself to succumb to even a moment of weakness."[10]

Yea, though I walk through the valley of the shadow of death, I will fear no evil; for Thou art with me; Thy rod and Thy staff they comfort me.[11] Knowing that there exists a personal God Who is always close at hand, there for you at every moment, brings a tremendous feeling of inner calm, unsurpassed by anything else. This feeling levels–*shaveh*–all the ups and downs life has to offer; an evenness of the mind called equanimity—*manuchas hanefesh*.

Mindfulness today is only associated with Buddhist practices, but nothing could be further than the truth. The Jewish sages have always spoken to being mindful as a true goal of living. The 18th century philosopher and Kabbalist, Moshe Chaim Luzzatto, wrote in his classic work, *The Path of the Just*, "Anyone who is not mindful, it is forbidden to pity him."[12]

Rabbi Luzzatto based his comment on a passage in the Talmud[13] meaning that God has endowed mankind with the capacity for understanding greater than any other creation. As such, man is under an obligation to use his mind to think and understand things creatively anew rather than act like other creatures that seemingly live a repetitive existence.

Ellen Langer, Professor of Psychology at Harvard, in her book, *Mindfulness*, writes we become mindless by forming a mindset when we first encounter something and then cling to it when we re–encounter that same thing.[14] When we learn something mindlessly, it does not occur to us to think about it later, irrespective of whether such thoughts would be acceptable to us.[15] The way we take in information, mindfully or mindlessly determines how we use it later[16] which can potentially create MIS–information.

Mindlessness limits our control by preventing us from making intelligent choices.[17] When our minds are set on one thing or on one way of doing things, mindlessly determined in the past, we blot out intuition and miss much of a present world around us.[18]

In contrast, mindfulness, according to Daniel J. Siegel, Clinical Professor of Psychiatry, UCLA School of Medicine, in his book, *The Mindful Therapist: A Clinician's Guide to Mindsight and Neural Integration*, is being conscientious and intentional in what we do, being open and creative with possibilities, or being aware of the present moment without grasping onto judgments—being mindful is a state of awareness that enables us to be flexible and receptive and to have presence.[19] *Mindfulness is the cure for cognitive dissonance!*

With mindfulness practice, Siegel writes, we may become more nonjudgmental, develop equanimity, be more aware of what is going on as it is happening, and develop the capacity to label and describe with words our internal world.[20]

Langer says that the ability to transcend context is the essence of mindfulness.[21] Changing contexts generates imagination and creativity as well as new energy. When applied to problem solving, it is often called reframing.[22]

I acquired mindfulness when I started reframing the past, present and future in all contexts of my encounters as I have previously explained. We can cultivate mindfulness simply by paying attention, which may seem easy enough to accomplish, but I assure it is not. The art of paying attention is developed and refined through a practice known as mindfulness mediation.

Rabbi Aryeh Kaplan was a 20th century scholar lauded as an original thinker and prolific writer and is most well known for his intimate knowledge of physics and Kabbala. Meditation, according to Rabbi Kaplan, consists of thinking in a controlled manner,[23] a focused awareness. Our mind in part is under control of our will which we call consciousness and in part *not* under the control of our will which we call our unconscious or subconscious.

One of the goals of meditation, Rabbi Kaplan explains, is to gain control of the subconscious part of our mind.[24] And in gaining control, we cultivate our ability to mindfully pay attention. Indeed, one of the most powerful benefits of meditation is control over the unconscious mind.[25]

Rabbi Kaplan states that most people learn to think as very young children, and throughout their adult lives, they do not think any differently than they did as children. Through meditation, you can control the thought process and learn to think in new ways, thus gaining new and richer mind experiences. Mindful meditation, learning to control your mind and thoughts, gives us the ability to transcend the ways of thinking we learned as children.[26]

The word used in Hebrew for meditation is *hitbonenut*. It is the reflexive of the root–word *bin* meaning to understand and literally means "making oneself understand" that is contemplating something so deeply and completely that one makes himself understand it in all aspects. I believe this is the understanding the Talmud referred to.

Rabbi Luzzatto says a person should constantly—at all times and during periods—set aside time for meditation.[27] Rabbi Chaim Vital, the 16th–17th Kabbalist often speaks of mental seclusion, "one must seclude–*hitboded*–himself in his thoughts to the ultimate degree."[28] Early generations of Jewish sages would spend hours in meditation before attempting to pray.

Most people think in order to meditate you must do something. Really, the opposite is the case: you meditate by *not* doing. Meditation is simply quieting down all parts of you mind and *not* concentrating on you immediate experience or what is happening around you. Success at mindful meditation is achieved by calming your heart and your mind and finding an inner balance with which to weather the storms of life.

For many years a neighbor of mine had lived in an ashram in upstate New York when he was younger where he taught busy executives and professionals how to survive the day. After my angioplasty he tried teaching me yoga. Well, I was the proverbial bull in the china shop. But my real triumph came when I started a meditation which entailed simply breathing.

Dr. Servan–Schreiber writes:

> Mindfulness means centering on yourself and your breathing . . . The object is to attain the highest level of physical self–awareness by focusing on the act of breathing. In so doing, we gradually rid ourselves of thoughts until we have as few as possible. The result is an extremely restful state in which we are in fact momentarily released from the tyranny of our egos. This state could be described as the physical sensation of being yourself at peace.[29]

Counting breaths is often called the mindfulness of breathing and specifically concerns inhalation and exhalation as part of mindfully paying attention to one's body in quietude. Our mind is a system of decoherence always absorbing unlimited sensory, auditory and visual inputs at a quantum level. The mind functions much like traffic police during rush hour traffic. If the cop wasn't there, we face grid lock. Dreams also help us like a cop which is one of the main reasons without proper sleep we literally cannot function. Think of dreams acting like the defragmentation of Windows® system tools.

I also believe that the meditation of counting breaths has a deep mystical connection. The Bible says,[30] "And the Lord God formed man of the dust of the ground and breathed into his nostrils the breath of life." The Book of Job[31] says, ". . . and the breath of the Almighty gives them understanding."

Jewish commentators explain that at this moment man received his soul from God. I think at this point man also acquired his ability to be mindful much like the intention of the passage in the Talmud. So, when I count breaths I also focus on my soul, mindfulness, and my animation as a being created in the image of God in addition to counting my breath.

So let's go! Sit in a quiet place, phones off, all distractions put aside. Close your eyes and fully inhale then slowly exhale. And with each exhalation count in ascending order:

Inhale—exhale—one
Inhale—exhale—two
Inhale—exhale—three
Inhale—exhale—four
Inhale—exhale—five

When you reach five repeat the sequence again and again for three minutes. Set a timer for three minutes or have someone with you who keeps the time. It may sound simple but I assure it is not. Concentrate just on breathing, counting and nothing else. Oh, I almost forgot when you realize that you have counted past five and are counting six or seven, just start over again with one . . . two etc. And when you become aware that you have stopped counting and are paying attention to your zillion wandering thoughts just start once again with one . . . two etc.

It took me weeks before I could concentrate, focus and make it three minutes without any distractions. Have no illusions, counting breath meditation is taming a wild horse that does not want to be tamed—your mind. But once you succeed, you and your horse can travel to outlooks you never thought possible.

An excellent use for counting breaths is calming anxiety. This is a take–it–anywhere meditation. You don't need mats, a special place, or a change of clothes. It really gives you an ability to achieve a feeling of mindfulness because you are holding the reins to your mind and thoughts and not the other way around. A necessary prerequisite for inner calm and healing is the ability to quiet down and relax the mind.

Consistency is the most important thing in meditation, not how well you do it. I practice counting breaths daily and have been for several years now. After about a year I worked myself up to ten minutes. Nowadays I don't time myself anymore, rather I can sense when I should stop. I totally focus on breathing, counting, and I am oblivious to the constant wandering thoughts that float by. You are not going to encounter God, reach sudden enlightenment, nirvana or satori by counting breaths, but you will gain a sense of personal prophecy—mindfulness!

"And Isaac went out to meditate in the field at the evening time."[32] The Bible's purpose is to teach us with every word, sentence, and crowns on its letters lessons we need in order to live a better life. While many commentators cite the above passage as the Biblical source for meditation, I think it teaches a more important lesson— there is a deep connection between nature and meditation.

Dr. Servan–Schreiber lived a year with stage–four glioblastoma. He writes about a Canadian woman he knew, Molly, who had been living with stage–four glioblastoma for a decade. He says her exceptional remission maybe owed to the fact that Molly chose after conventional treatment to live almost in complete isolation north of Toronto where every day she takes long walks on the banks of a lake.[33]

All of us have lost contact with nature. We live climate controlled in an artificial world of glass and steel where plants in buildings are made of plastic and parks grow AstroTurf. And in doing so, I believe we have lost one of life's greatest therapeutic agents—nature. I didn't always think this way but I absolutely do now. A traveler once asked William Wordsworth's servant to show him her master's study, she answered, "Here is his library, but his study is out of doors."

A few years ago I moved to Eilat, the Northern tip of the Red Sea. Eilat was our family's favorite vacation spot for many years. My oldest son after completing his compulsory army service lived here several years as a dive master conducting underwater tours for visiting tourists. My middle son years ago decided to live here as he said, "Because I feel like I am always on a vacation every day."

Jacques Yves Cousteau said, "The Sea, once it casts its spell, holds one in its net of wonder forever." And I thought the blue Mediterranean was breath taking—the crystal clear coral studded Rea Sea has no equal. Surrounding Eilat are ranges of mountains across in Jordon and behind our city. The mountains and the sea every day cast its net of inner calm over you.

Nature is meditation unto itself. The term Shinrin-yoku, making contact with and taking in the atmosphere of the forest or forest bathing, was coined by the Japanese Ministry of Agriculture, Forestry, and Fisheries in 1982. Forest bathing is intended to improve an individual's state of mental and physical relaxation.

The results of studies[34] performed on the physiological effects of Shinrin-yoku show that forest environments could lower concentrations of cortisol, lower pulse rate, lower blood pressure, increase parasympathetic nerve activity, and lower sympathetic nerve activity compared with people living in urban environments; providing valuable insights into the relationship between forests and human health. These studies focused on short-span exposures to stimuli: approximately 15 min of viewing and 15 min of walking. Imagine spending an hour forest bathing; how great you will feel!

Rabbi Nachman of Breslov, the grandson of Rabbi Israel Baal Shem Tov, advised his followers that it is best to seclude yourself and meditate in the meadows outside the city. "Go to a grassy field, for the grass will awaken your heart."[35] The 16th century Kabbalists in the holy city of Safed would go out in the open fields, dance and sing, prior to welcoming in the arrival of the Sabbath.

Maimonides' son, Rabbi Abraham Maimonides, was recognized as the greatest scholar in his community, succeeding his father as the head of the Egyptian Jews and being appointed court physician at the age of only eighteen in addition to being a mystic steeped in Kabbala.

"The main method of meditation, as outlined by Rabbi Abraham," Rabbi Kaplan writes, "involves the contemplation of nature. A person can contemplate the greatness of the sea, marveling at the many creatures that live in it. One can gaze at a clear night sky, allowing his mind to be completely absorbed by the glory of the stars."[36] I have taken Rabbi Abraham Maimonides' advice to heart.

I found a secluded spot past the last hotel on the beach where I try to go once a week just to sit on the rocks and look out at the water. Across the bay are no hotels, only mountains in the fore and mountain to the rear. There I collect broken bits of corals, sea shells and have a word with Mother Nature. To me it is the most peaceful and tranquil place on the planet.

Of course, the beach lies in the center of the Middle East on the border between Egypt and Israel, just across the bay from Jordon and a short swim to Saudi Arabia. But that's the beauty of Mother Nature; she doesn't give a damn about the politics of man. She remains serene no matter what man does. A lesson we should take to heart.

I once heard a story from Rabbi Issachar Frand of Baltimore:

> Someone was visiting a separate beach in Israel when he noticed an old man with a long white beard sitting, gazing endlessly at the sea. It became obvious that the man was all alone; there was no family or grandchildren in sight. Curiosity pushed the person to speak to the old man.
>
> "Excuse me, but I was wondering why you came to the beach alone?" The old man answered, "You see, I am a judge in a very famous rabbinical court and all day I have to search for minute details in the Jewish law to rule on cases that come before me. Doing so causes me at times to lose context of the larger picture. I come here to reacquaint myself with the broadness of God's world and our lives in it."

Have you ever fed a rainbow? I have. Opposite the last hotel on the beach is a pier where rainbows come to swim. There you can view a rainbow gallery of fish, each painted from the pallet of the Master Artist. And there you witness that God is not Henry Ford—you can have a Model T in any color as long as it is black.

One day I brought some bread to feed the fish and I was hooked forever. You cannot imagine the multitude of fish; excuse me, rainbows that came to feed. Weekly, I venture out to the pier, bread in hand, beckoning the snorkelers to come closer for a show the likes of which they will never see again. They say just looking at an aquarium is meditative. Imagine what an ocean full of fish, excuse me again, rainbows will do for you!

A century ago, economist and social critic Torstein Veblen coined the phrase "conspicuous consumption" in his classic work, *The Theory of the Leisure Class*. Our purchases and consumption of goods, Veblen said, are not items and things we need, intended for our enjoyment, rather by having them we impress others.[37] Economist

Jeffery D. Sachs likens this to an economic arms race that ends up in the proverbial "rat race."[38]

"There is no longer a workday, as our work and our capacity to do it anywhere expands into all hours of the clock. There is no longer a workweek for many of us, and no boundary between the week and the weekend. There is no longer a workplace—anyplace, airplanes, restaurants, and vacation homes, hotels, walking down the street, and a cell phone, e–mail. And internet portals."[39] So Jon Kabat–Zinn, Emeritus Professor of Medicine at the University of Massachusetts Medical School, fittingly describes the daily life for most all of us.

Linda Stone, a former vice–president at Microsoft, coined the phrase *continuous partial attention* to describe how many of us use our attention today:

> Continuous partial attention is motivated by a desire to be a live node on the network; a way of saying this is that we want to connect and be connected. We want to effectively scan for opportunity and optimize for the best opportunities, activities, and contacts, in any given moment. To be busy, to be connected, is to be alive, to be recognized, and to matter. We pay continuous partial attention in an effort not to miss anything. It is an always–on, anywhere, anytime, anyplace behavior that involves an artificial sense of constant crisis.[40]

We live today in a 24/7 always–on world where we feel over–whelmed, over–stimulation and a sense of being unfulfilled. Is there any salvation to living in a plugged in world?

The Bible says,[41] "Thus the heavens and the earth were finished, and all their host. And by the seventh day God ended His work which He had done and rested on the seventh day from all His work which He had done." The oblivious question comes to mind, if God is God why does He need to rest? I think the simple answer is

293

that God is setting an example for mankind. "If I, God, should rest, so should mankind!"

In Genesis there is a conundrum in the verse[42] that says, "And by the seventh day God finished His work which He had done and He rested on the seventh day from all his work." Rabbi Abraham Heschel explains[43] that surely we would expect the Bible to tell us that God finished his work on the sixth day and rested on the seventh. But what was it that God left until the seventh day to complete? Rabbi Heschel answers the puzzle by bringing a *Midrash*[44] that explains what God created on the Sabbath was—Tranquility, Ease, Peace, and Quiet.

Rabbi Joseph Soloveitchik explains the idea of the Sabbath. "The Torah demands temporary withdrawal from one's daily routine so that we can shake off the hypnotic influence which material possessions exert over us and face the truth that we are managing someone's estate, not our own."[45]

Tolstoy when he was questioning every aspect of religion wrote in his *A Confession and What I Believe*, "To remember the Sabbath, which is to devote one day to God. That was something I could understand."[46]

Stop and think for a moment. Why is it that all of humanity revolves around a seven–day work week? There have been a few attempts at modifying. France for nine and a half years from October 1793 to April 1802 used a 10–day week, called *décade*, the Paris Commune adopted the Revolutionary Calendar for 18 days in 1871. Between 1929 and 1931, the USSR changed from the seven–day week to a five–day week. In 1931, after its brief experiment with a five–day week, the Soviet Union changed to a six–day week. That calendar was abandoned June 1940 and the seven–day week reintroduced.

In the account of Creation, what was the first object made holy and sanctified in the world? The Bible says, "And God blessed the seventh day, and sanctified it." Rabbi Ovadiah Sforno, the 15th century Italian Talmudist and commentator, explains God sanctified the Sabbath by giving it an added soul setting it aside from the other days of the week to be *illuminated by the light of life* as the Book of Job[47] says.

The 12th century Spanish commentator, Rabbi Abraham Ibn Ezra, explains the sanctification as a blessing of increase; giving an increased strength and renewal of a man's body and his intellectual abilities on the Sabbath.

A Talmudic[48]tradition combines both opinions by saying God endows man with an additional soul during eve of the Sabbath. And that the Jewish separation ritual–*Havdalah*–that concludes the Sabbath with wine and spices in part is to bolster man as a compensation for the exit of his additional soul. As Rabbi Eliezer Berkovits points out, "The enjoyment of the Sabbath is neither spiritual nor material; it is wholly human. Body and spirit celebrate the Sabbath in communion."[49]

The Sabbath is truly a sanctuary in time. Notwithstanding the genocides of modern times, the most victimized people in history have been the Jews. Jews are an enigma, having survived while those civilizations that persecuted them have perished. Jews have survived because of the Sabbath. Achad ha–Am (Asher Ginsberg) was a Hebrew essayist and one of the foremost pre–state Zionist thinkers. Ginsberg rightly said, "More than the Jewish people has kept the Sabbath, the Sabbath has kept the Jewish people."

Rabbi Abraham Joshua Heschel was an internationally known twentieth century scholar, prophetic activist, and theologian. In his classic work, *The Sabbath*, he distills the essence of the Sabbath's meaning:

> The Sabbath is the day on which we learn the art of surpassing civilization.[50] It is a day on which we are called upon to share in what is eternal in time, to turn from the results of creation to the mystery of creations; from the world of creation to the creation of the world.[51] The seventh day is an armistice in man's cruel struggle for existence, a truce in all conflicts, personal and social, peace between

man and man, man and nature, and peace within man. [52] There are few ideas in the world of thought which contain so much spiritual power as the idea of the Sabbath.[53] What we are depends on what the Sabbath is to us.[54]

Victor Frankel, the founder of Logotherapy, says the real emptiness and ultimate poverty of meaning of man's existence come to the fore as soon as his vocational activity is halted for a certain period—on Sunday. "It is on Sunday when the tempo of the working week is suspended, that the poverty of meaning in every day urban life is exposed."[55] He called it the Sunday neurosis. "Labor without dignity causes misery," Rabbi Heschel says, "rest without spirit the source of depravity.[56]

Economist Jeffery D. Sachs answers the conundrum of how to battle conspicuous consumption. "Herein lies a least one reason the good Lord commanded that everybody take the Sabbath off. If we had to do so on our own, we'd have to worry whether our neighbor–competitor would do the same. Likely not, we'd both end up working through the weekend."[57]

It is not just the Jewish people who need a Sabbath rest. Dr. Matthew Sleeth, formerly an emergency room physician, is currently an author, speaker, and advocate for biblical mandate to care for the Earth. His book, *24/6: A Prescription for a Healthier, Happier Life*, is a firm advocate for Christians keeping Sunday as a day of rest. And in agreement with the Jewish sources I quoted, he says "Sabbath is a time to transition from human doings to human beings.[58]

Remember the Seventh–day Adventists of Loma Linda Blue Zone? Seventh–day Adventists while they share many of the doctrines of mainline Protestant churches, differ in their strict observance of Saturday, rather than Sunday, as their day of rest. Not only being vegetarians but being Sabbath observers contributes to their greater longevity: 9.5 years for men and 6.2 women years longer than non–Adventists.[59]

Randy Roberts, the pastor of Loma Linda University Church says, "Sabbath is meant to be a sanctuary in time for rest and rejuvenation, and I think it accomplishes that on a number of levels."[60]

Finally, the *Journal of Occupational Science* concludes:

> Sabbath is a day of rest, not for the purposes of regaining strength for the forthcoming week but rather for the sake of life providing opportunities for both physical and spiritual renewal; lessening the focus on doing, allowing more time for being.[61]

I would like to end with my personal feelings about the Sabbath. When I light the Sabbath candles, ushering in the solemn day of rest, at times I can actually feel the extra soul entering within me. I have tried to describe to people over the years what it feels like to have a weekly refuge from the trials and tribulations of life, but it really is impossible to explain.

The Sabbath is a time of peace you can always count on in a world where it is impossible to count on anything except on paying taxes and dying like the saying goes. In a mystical way, the Sabbath is a corridor between this world and the next, giving us a glimpse of things to come. The Sabbath *is* the spiritual interface of creation.

Rabbi Eliyahu Dessler, the renowned 20th century master of *Mussar* said, "There really is only one Sabbath, but we move through the weekly cycle and re–experience it week by week.[62]

The Sabbath is the most important of part of not only my achieving inner calm, but my ability to constantly maintain inner calm with equanimity—*manuchas hanefesh.*

Shabbat Shalom!

22

Telomeres

Imagine being centenarian looking half your age, playing outdoors with your great–grandchildren, dancing with much younger partners, enjoying new hobbies and pursuits, and, yes, still having a great sex life—all without having to worry about life–threatening conditions like cancer, heart disease, diabetes, chronic infections, dementia, poor eye sight, hearing loss, low energy, and other miserable conditions that plague too many older people. It may sound too good to be true, but it isn't.[1]

The Immortality Edge: Realize the Secrets of
Your Telomeres for a Longer, Healthier Life
Dr. Michael Fossel
Greta Blackburn
Dr. Dave Woynarowski

Everyone has a childhood image of what God looks like. For some it is the cartoon Father Time with his long white beard. For others, God is more a jovial Santa on whose knee we can sit, rattling off the wish lists of life. I must confess I have a totally different image. At times when I pray I think of George Burns.

The centenarian George Burns did achieve immortality by being unique in a career spanning Vaudeville, Radio, Television, Stage and Motion Pictures. George once said, "Retirement at sixty–five is ridiculous. When I was sixty–five I still had pimples."

But for me, his most memorable performance was as God in the 1977 classic comedy *Oh God!,* directed by Carl Reiner and co–

starring John Denver and Terri Garr. God, played by George Burns, appears to an assistant grocery store manager, played by John Denver, and selects him to be his messenger to the modern world.

Sitting in his VW Bug, Denver tells Burns if he is God, prove it by making it rain. But it only rains inside the VW Bug because God does not to want to ruin everyone's day outside. God openly admits to making two mistakes: the oversize avocado pit and the giraffe's long neck. That is my kind of God.

George Burns also made a fitting observation that applies to all I have written thus far in this book. "You know you're getting old when you stoop to tie your shoelaces and wonder what else you could do while you're down there." So, look down now at your shoelaces and I will explain what else you can do.

I wore my favorite college tennis shoes for at least twenty years. Together we went through generations of shoelaces. Those plastic tips on the ends of the shoelaces would at first crack, and then little by little pieces of the plastic would slowly break off until finally the plastic nib was completely gone. Trying to thread the shoelace without the plastic nib is virtually impossible. At that point in time the useful life of the shoelace comes to an end.

What I have just described by means of the analogy of shoelace nibs explains the most fascinating discovery I made in all my research—telomeres. Telomeres are a cells internal aging clock. Derived from the Greek nouns *telos*–end and *meros*–part, a telomere is a region of repetitive nucleotide sequences at each end of a chromatid. The genetic sequence of nucleotides in telomeres is TTAGGG which repeats approximately 2,500 times in humans.

So, like the plastic nibs on shoelaces, telomeres are the disposable buffers at the ends of chromosomes which are truncated during cell division. Their presence protects the genes on the chromosome from being curtailed instead of losing the DNA that matters. Over time, due to each cell division, the telomere ends become shorter until they are gone.

Alexis Carrel, the Nobel prize–winning surgeon, held the belief that all cells explanted in culture are immortal. In the early 1970s, a Russian theorist Alexei Olovnikov challenged this theory by suggesting that DNA sequences are lost every time a cell/DNA replicates until the loss reaches a critical level, at which point cell division ends.

The phenomenon of limited cellular division was first observed by Leonard Hayflick in 1961. Hayflick implicated telomere shortening as an aging process and discovered that cells tend to divide a set number of times—now called the Hayflick limit—and then stop. The upper Hayflick limit is 120 years, which is why I named my book *Until 120*.

Each time a cell divides; one or two copies of this sequence are not replaced. Eventually this protection of telomeres begins to run out and the chromosome ends begin to fray, at this point cell division ceases.[2]

In 1975–1977, Elizabeth Blackburn, working as a postdoctoral fellow at Yale University with Joseph Gall, discovered the unusual nature of telomeres with their simple repeated DNA sequences composing chromosome ends. Their work was published in 1978. Elizabeth Blackburn, Carol Greider, and Jack Szostak were awarded the 2009 Nobel Prize in Physiology or Medicine for the discovery of how chromosomes are protected by telomeres and the enzyme telomerase.[3]

Shortened telomeres are unmistakably associated with aging and most frequent aging related diseases like diabetes, cancer, cardiovascular and neurodegenerative diseases. It is becoming apparent that reversing telomere shortening through temporary activation of telomerase may be a potent means to slow aging and *could lengthen human life by extending the Hayflick limit.*

In writing this book, I effectively started with telomeres in mind and worked my way backward. As you will see, everything I have spoken about—childhood, self–esteem, anxiety, relationships, shame, stress, inflammation, diet and nutrition, exercise, aging, meditation, cancer and heart disease, etc—play an important role in the shortening process of telomeres. *Keeping your telomeres long is an essential step in reaching Until 120.*

A study in the *Journal of Gerontology:*

> Leukocyte [white blood cells] telomere length was associated with a characterization of age–related disease burden across multiple physiologic systems, which was comparable to, but independent of, its association with age. [4]

A study in the *Journal of Biosciences:*

> Telomerase dependent telomere damage is a key player in perpetrating age–associated decline in the functional capacities of an organ/tissue and disease progression related to stem cell functions. [5]

A study in *Experimental Gerontology:*

> The maintenance of long telomeres in centenarians underscores the role of the immune system in lifespan and longevity. [6]

A study in the *Journal of Gerontology: Biological Sciences:*

> Our results suggest that healthy centenarians have significantly longer telomeres than unhealthy centenarians have. [7]

A study in *Aging and Disease:*

> Individual–level interventions aimed at up–regulating telomerase and tumor suppression responses would have several applications. The most obvious would be to treat age–related diseases, such as cancer and reduce disease risk in susceptible individuals. [8]

A study in *Circulation Research*:

> Telomere dysfunction is emerging as an important factor in the pathogenesis of age–related cardiovascular disease. [9]

There are many dynamics that play their hand in shortening telomeres. As you might expect, stress is definitely one of them. Psychological responses to the anticipation of an acute stressor are associated with leukocyte telomere length, an index and potential mechanism of cellular aging; chronic stress may lead to higher threat appraisals and are associated with shorter leukocyte telomere length. [10]

In healthy women, psychological stress is associated with indicators of accelerated cellular and organismal aging: oxidative stress, telomere length, and telomerase activity in Peripheral Blood Mononuclear Cells. [11]

Experiencing chronic stress is associated with shortened telomere length in Peripheral Blood Mononuclear Cells; chronic stress is associated with altered T cell function and accelerated immune cell aging as suggested by excessive telomere loss. [12] Lower levels of Peripheral Blood Mononuclear Cells telomerase activity are associated with increased excretion of stress hormones and well established physiological and behavioral risk factors for cardio–vascular disease in a healthy sample. [13]

The stress of loneliness is also a factor. Social support in late life is positively associated with leukocyte telomere length and suggests that telomere erosion may be a mechanism through which social isolation influences disease vulnerability and premature death in later life. [14] Telomere length is associated with marital status, indicating that individuals who are married or have a partner have longer telomeres than individuals who are unmarried. [15]

Shorter relative leukocyte telomere length might act as a predisposing factor in the development of post–traumatic stress disorder (PTSD) after a severely traumatic event; telomere shortening may be an important marker for PTSD risk, with implications for early intervention and treatment.[16]

Chronic exposure to the psychobiological sequelae of childhood trauma could increase risk for PTSD and short leukocyte telomere length; even physically healthy young to middle–aged adults with PTSD and childhood trauma bear markers of cellular aging.[17] Shortened leukocyte telomere length and caregiver stress link to more remote stressful experiences in childhood, and suggest that childhood maltreatment could influence cellular aging.[18]

Midlife women reporting shorter sleep duration, poorer sleep quality, and longer sleep onset latencies more likely to report higher levels of perceived stress, had shorter leukocyte telomere length, independent of age, body mass index, race, and income, thus, providing preliminary evidence that leukocyte telomere length may reflect a potential biological mechanism linking sleep and age–related disease.[19]

High phobic anxiety may be associated with shorter leukocyte relative telomere lengths in middle–aged and older women.[20] Decreased perceived mental health is associated with shorter leukocyte telomere length in patients with chronic heart failure.[21]

Psychosocial factors are also important. Reduced telomere length has been correlated with psychosocial stress, lower socioeconomic status, lower educational attainment, current and long–term full–time work schedule and with early–life stress.[22]

Higher levels of educational attainment but not income were associated with longer leukocyte telomere length, which confers reduced risk for multiple diseases of aging. Blacks who obtained some education beyond high school had significantly longer leukocyte telomere length than any other group.[23] The rate of age–related telomere attrition was significantly associated with low income, housing tenure and poor diet.[24]

I formulated my new outlook on disease, focusing on inflammation, because chronic inflammation affects telomeres triggering them to shorten faster than a normal rate. And chronic inflammation, which characterizes cardiovascular disease and diabetes, may directly cause the shortening of telomeres, resulting in premature senescence contributing to disease.[25]

Remember natures' perfectly balanced hemp oil? Telomere length increased with decreasing omega–6 to omega–3 polyunsaturated fatty acids (PUFAs) ratios; omega–3 PUFA's anti–inflammatory and antioxidant properties provide one pathway for reductions in mortality; decreases in IL–6, an inflammation marker, were associated with telomere lengthening.[26]

A study of rheumatoid arthritis cases confirms the association of the disease with markedly reduced telomere length in peripheral white blood cells.[27] The chronic inflammatory burden in people with periodontitis could represent the driver of telomere shortening.[28]

Telomeres also figure widely in heart disease. Telomere length was positively associated with LDL and total cholesterol levels.[29] In the presence of chronic hypertension, a major risk factor for atherosclerotic lesions, shorter telomere length in white blood cells is associated with an increased predilection to carotid artery atherosclerosis.[30] Data show an inverse association between telomere length and risk of coronary heart disease, independent of conventional vascular risk factors.[31]

Short telomere length is an independent predictor of mortality in patients with coronary heart disease.[32] Cardiovascular disease risk factors that were negatively correlated to telomere length differed between genders. Telomere length seems to be coupled to an obesity phenotype but clearly only in women.[33]

And cancer too. Telomere attrition causes accelerated cell turnover, leading to premature aging symptoms and predisposition to cancer.

Similarly, defects in DNA repair machinery are often associated with premature aging and an elevated risk of cancer.[34]

Telomere shortening is an early event in the oncogenetic process and telomere erosion leads to genetic instability.[35] Several genetic and lifestyle factors were observed to influence telomere length. There is evidence for a linear association between influence telomere length and risk for colon cancer and a possible U–shaped association with rectal cancer.[36]

Barrett's esophagus patients who have short telomeres are at higher risk of developing esophageal adenocarcinoma, demonstrating the ability of leukocyte telomere length to predict cancer risk in a setting of chronic inflammation.[37]

Elderly cancer patients have significantly lower thymic output and shorter telomeres in their peripheral blood cells than age–matched non–cancer patients; immune senescence may hamper the ability of the immune system to prevent cancer initiation.[38]

Chronic obstructive pulmonary disease patients who have reduced telomere lengths in their peripheral blood leukocytes are at higher risk of total and cancer–related mortality. Accelerated aging is of particular relevance to cancer mortality in COPD.[39]

Migraine attacks impact significant stress on cellular function; telomeres are shorter in migraine patients and there is more variation in telomere length in migraine patients.[40]

By now I think you are getting the idea. The last paradigm shift Baby Boomers need to adopt for being healthy is nurturing their telomeres. The $64,000 question is can telomeres be lengthened? Is that really possible? It certainly is and there are many peer–reviewed studies to support not only nurturing telomeres but actually increasing their length. You understood me correctly; you can increase the length of telomeres. I think the implications of being able to increase telomere lengths are staggering.

A healthy lifestyle is associated with longer leukocyte telomere length, a marker of biological aging that may be a common mechanism underlying the etiology of multiple age related diseases.[41] The important thing to remember as I have been pointing out: life experiences, personal history, mindset and lifestyle are reflected in telomere length. For interventions to succeed, it is necessary to make a paradigm shift in your living. If you are willing to accept the challenge of altering certain lifestyle habits you might be able to lengthen your telomeres and benefit from its consequences.

I am sure you already guessed what are the lifestyle changes that have been associated with longer telomere lengths: good nutrition characterized by anti–inflammation, increasing omega–3 free fatty acids and antioxidants, eliminating animal protein and dairy, eating fruits and vegetables, an exercise routine, getting restful sleep, and eliminating stress by mediation.

Dr. Elizabeth Blackburn and Carol Greider showed that three months eating a plant–based diet along with moderate exercise and stress management increased telomere activity by almost 30 percent.[42] Dr. Dean Ornish published the results of his study in *Lancet Oncology* showing "that comprehensive lifestyle intervention including a low–fat vegan diet was associated with blood levels of telomerase increased by an average of 29 percent after 5 years of follow–up compared with controls."[43]

A typical study profile was based on dietary requirements of a low–fat vegan diet, plenty of fruits, vegetables, unrefined grains and legumes, soy, omega 3; moderate exercise walking 30 minutes a day, 6 days a week; stress management including gentle yoga based stretching, breathing, meditation or relaxation techniques for 1 hour a day, 6 days a week accompanied with 1 hour group support sessions, once per week.

Additionally, high dietary intake of vegetables and beta–carotene is positively associated with mean telomere length in blood lymphocytes, confirming the implication of oxidative damage in telomere erosion.[44] In women, vegetable intake was positively associated with leukocyte telomere length; men who ate the most butter and least fruits had significantly shorter telomeres; fat and vegetable intakes were associated with leukocyte telomere length.[45]

A significant inverse association between high intake of processed meat and shorter telomere length was observed.[46] Even sugar–sweetened soda consumption was associated with shorter telomeres.[47] Weight loss by caloric–restricted diets may contribute to the prevention of telomere shortening and DNA base damage, which are important initiating events in carcinogenesis.[48]

Greater adherence to the Mediterranean diet was significantly associated with longer leukocyte telomere length supporting the health benefits of adherence to the Mediterranean diet for promoting health and longevity.[49]

There is evidence for an association of high adherence to the Mediterranean diet and a slower rate of cellular ageing; that a lower rate of telomere shortening and higher telomerase activity might be involved in lifespan in populations consuming a traditional Mediterranean diet.[50]

Exercise is enormously important. Numerous studies implicate a telomere–protective phenotype induced by moderate levels of physical activity.[51] The stress relieving quality of exercise has been well documented. Vigorous physical activity appears to protect those experiencing high stress by buffering its relationship with telomere length.[52]

In a study of postmenopausal women, habitual physical exercise, defined as combined aerobic and anaerobic exercise for at least 60 minutes per session, more than three times a week, was associated with greater telomere length.[53]

Remember my favorite supplement CoQ_{10}? CoQ_{10} protects telomeres by slowing shortening. Some studies that used various forms of CoQ_{10} suggest that it can actually stop telomere shortening altogether.[54]

You can check your telomere age by a blood test that costs about $350. The book, *The Immortality Edge: Realizing the Secrets of Your Telomeres for a Longer, Healthier Life*[55] includes a telomere age questionnaire to give an approximation of your telomere age. Buying the book was much cheaper than having the blood test.

The seventy questions are based on known illnesses, conditions, and behaviors that correlate with telomere length. If you score less than 5,000, the book says, "Your telomere age is between eighty and one hundred years." That's pretty old for a Baby Boomer. The highest score is 8001 points or more. If your score is in this range, the book says, "Eureka! Your telomere age is less than thirty–five, and you're doing great. Let's keep it there for the next fifty years." I took the test. Drum roll—my score was 14,300!

Now is the time to take George Burns' advice and stoop down and look at your shoelaces. And while you are down there, consider how important as a Baby Boomer now is the critical time to make the telomere lengthening lifestyle changes. I know this is a hard decision to make. *Maybe looking at your grandchildren will help you decide!*

23

2070

"And God took the man and put him in the Garden of Eden, to work it and to watch over it."

Genesis 2:15.

The significant problems we face cannot be solved at the same level of thinking we were at when we created them.

Albert Einstein

We may not abdicate responsibility for the world we hand over to our children.

Rabbi Sir Jonathan Sacks[1]

No snowflake in an avalanche ever feels responsibility.

Voltaire

May 12, 2070. Today I celebrate my 119th birthday. Three years ago I surpassed the male longevity record set by Jiroemon Mimura of Japan at 116. And now I am only three years short of the maximum longevity record set by Jeanne Calment of France who died at the age of 122. But I am not going to be in the *Guinness Book of World Records* after all.

Living till the age of 120 is no longer considered special. There are hundreds worldwide who broke Mimura's record before me. Some have even made it until 120, but none have surpassed Calment's record. Anyway, longevity was only a personal goal for me at best. Now on the precipice of age 120, I am reminded of the old saying, "be sure what you wish for is really what you want because you may just end up getting it." The last half century has been a time I wish I had not seen!

Back when I wrote my book, *Until 120*, global climate warming effects were incessantly debated against the defense of freedom and a free market economy. Today, in the year 2070, absolutely no one denies the devastating consequences climate change has had for our planet. I am celebrating my birthday in a world that is +4° centigrade warmer than preindustrial levels.

What they said would never happen—happened. And despite all the hubris mitigations of geo–engineering the nations of the world in futile desperation tried, outside my window is an atmosphere saturated with carbon—550 ppm CO_2 equivalent. Theoretically, reaching this level means that even if emissions plummeted to zero, temperatures will continue to rise another century. *We are not at zero emissions even today!*

A +4°C world discriminates it effects. Oceans take longer to warm than land as northern latitudes reach temperatures in excess of +6°–+8°C and more. When it rains it pours, but in this case it melts. The Arctic sea lanes remain ice free all summer long, a boon for shipping using the elusive Northern Passage. But it unplugged the freezer causing an unstoppable meltdown of the Greenland and West Antarctica ice sheets. Global sea levels are currently one meter higher than they were 50 years ago and rising with each new tide.

And a higher sea level creates a higher storm surge with gargantuan devastation. Tsunami–type tidal waves embattle the worlds' coastal areas wielding powers the world has never seen before—ever! Of all cities, London's third–generation Thames surge barriers have held their own. However, the Big Apple's late entry saw subway sharks a common sight. Wall Street while bitterly contesting the truth of climate change effects to the very end was the first to relocate to higher ground.

Hurricanes are now common place in the South Atlantic Ocean swamping Rio de Janeiro while the European coasts of Spain and France now *batten down the hatches*. Though, it is still being debated, many believe it was a hurricane that hit the Greek Islands toppling the Parthenon.

The thirty–three countries that had land below sea level are now geographically redesigned with new coastlines further inland than ever imagined and their most vulnerable cities—Mumbai and Calcutta India, Dhaka Bangladesh, Guangzhou, Shanghai, Tianjin, and Shenzhen China, Ho Chi Minh City Vietnam, Osaka–Kobe, Tokyo and Nagoya Japan, Bangkok Thailand, Amsterdam Netherlands, Alexandria Egypt, Miami and New Orleans—are but a remake of the 1995 futuristic movie *Waterworld* starring Kevin Costner, Jeanne Tripplehorn, and Dennis Hopper.

Irony always looks as if to have the last laugh. After decades of battling terrorism as a growing response anti–infiltration walls were erected keeping migrants out—the building of Fortress Europe, Fortress America, Fortress India, etc. Reluctantly, after a rebirth of mid 21th century morality, nations finally opened their borders to the millions of climate refuges roaming northward. Now Amharic is often heard spoken in Siberia and Spanish is swiftly replacing French as Canada's second language.

Climate change *is* climate apartheid. The same third world nations that suffered the rape of colonialism, the inequity of globalization, starvation caused by the exploitation of native crops and cattle abroad, contributed zip to global warming were dealt a demoralizing sleight of hand. Their heavens closed, seeds lay sterile, rivers dried, thousands of thousands perished while civil war ruled the day.

The northern defrost brought forth upon us the hidden menace of the tundra—methane—the wild card of the apocalypse. Climate change was never a linear process. Methane and nitrous oxide are the two amplifying effects that hastened the greenhouse gas rise. Ominously, methane clathrates are beginning to melt bubbling their way to the surface from the ocean depths. "Wow unto me," says the Lord.

"I think that I shall never see a poem as lovely as a tree." Joyce Kilmer was unquestionably right, but generations hence may only have poems left to admire. America's Southwest, the Amazon Rain Forest, Sub–Saharan Africa and Australia have become an immense tinder box signaling an approaching Judgment Day. As trees and grasslands uncontrollably burn, carbon bellows upward in volcanic proportions, deforesting nature's ability to abate CO_2 and save our planet.

"Water, water everywhere and not a drop to drink," so wrote the English poet Samuel Taylor Coleridge in his *The Rime of the Ancient Mariner*. Today in 2070 there is not water everywhere. Our planet has been denuded of glaciers by global warming. The Himalayas, the Alps, Kilimanjaro, Patagonia, the Andes and even the great Glacier National Park and Alaska are laid bare where majestic white once crowned. And its effect has created cataclysmic global shortages of water.

The Ogallala, Central Valley and Southwest aquifers are running dry. Lawns are the dodo bird of Phoenix and Las Vegas. Vineyards of Napa Valley now grow in Washington State and Oregon and the best Bordeaux wines come from the English countryside. Asia's Ganges, Indus and Yangtze Rivers no longer quench the thirst of more than two billion people. *Oh, where are you, Gunga Din?*

Mockingly the world asks, "Where's the Beef?" Millions have starved to death reducing population levels well below replacement despite the warming northern latitudes' increased growing seasons. Potatoes in Iceland are just not enough to feed a starving planet.

We took the most productive fields to grow corn for distilling ethanol after the Saudi peak oil hoax was exposed when without warning Ghawar, Abqaiq and Berri oilfields went dry. Someone estimated that today every SUV tank of gas is filled at a cost of a thousand third–world deaths that could have been spared by growing grain instead of corn for ethanol.

Today my birthday wish is not to see another birthday. I have outlived my three sons and everyone I have ever known. My Facebook friends began to dwindle at an increasing rate until they were no more. Long ago my computer stopped singing the words,

"You've got mail." Now I sit alone quietly mourning the world that could have been, but never was.

The wisest of men, King Solomon, began *Ecclesiastes* by saying, "Vanities of vanities; all is vanity. What profit has man of all his labors wherein he labors under the sun?" The King is right, we could have chosen to make a better world, but alas we demurred. To truthfully answer the King, sadly in insincerity we preferred the profit above all else.

If you listen very closely, you can hear the earth cry as I can. I close my eyes for the last time, whilst King Solomon has the final word. "For God shall bring every work into judgment, with every secret thing, whether it be good, or it be evil!"

I am not a prophet, nor am I the son of a prophet. But I assert the silhouette scenario I have just described accurately portrays what our world will look like a half century from now. I base my belief on the same erudite research into global climate change as I have done for the contents of the previous chapters.

Rabbi Eliezer Berkovits said, "Mankind seems to have reached a dead–end street. All dreams have already been dreamt and found wanting. Man seems to have already had his future and stands now in a wasteland of history with his only wretched preoccupation how to save his skin from ultimate disaster."[2] Are we really facing immanent doom?

After WWII, the world found itself in a precarious position once the atomic bomb was used to end the war. Did man now possess the capacity for total–self–annihilation in unleashing the destructive capability within the atom? "I do not know what weapons will be used in the next war," Einstein said, "but the one after that will be fought with bows and arrows." Will Boomers ever in truth know how close we came during the 1962 Cuban Missile Crisis?

Karl Jaspers was a German psychiatrist and philosopher. In 1958 he tried to remedy the fears of many in his book, *The Future of*

Mankind. History is always plagued by uncertainty, disbelief, skepticism, hesitation, and distrust. "We can rely on the natural scientists' judgment of facts," Jaspers wrote, "What they tell us is reality, not speculation. An intelligent person cannot read their statements without sense of enormity; they have put the hand writing on the wall for all to see."[3]

What was true then, I deem true today. The average person in the street is left thinking that climate change is a questionable topic with no harmony of opinion. I see this first hand with my many conservative Facebook friends and the posts they inundate me with. But just how undivided is the scientific community on the truth that humans are the cause of global climate change and that climate change is not just a result of the natural cycles of the earth?

Naomi Oreskes in 2004[4] analyzed 928 abstracts published in refereed scientific journals between 1993 and 2003 and listed in the ISI database with the keywords 'global climate change.' Remarkably, *none* of the papers disagreed with the consensus scientific position that greenhouse gases are accumulating in Earth's atmosphere as a result of human activities, causing surface air temperatures and subsurface ocean temperatures to rise.

"Politicians, economists, journalists, and others may have the impression of confusion, disagreement, or discord among climate scientists," Oreskes writes, "but that impression is incorrect."[5] Deniers will always be deniers, whether tobacco, fat or climate change, I am afraid.

Since the beginnings of the Industrial Revolution mankind has turned to technology as its savior, mastering nature in an unparalleled manner. There is no denying that for most, but certainly not all, it has created the good life.

Rachel Carlson reminded us, "As man proceeds toward his announced goal of the conquest of nature, he has written a depressing record of destruction, directed not only against the earth he inhabits but against the life that shares it with him.[6] The question is whether any civilization can wage relentless war on life without destroying itself, and without losing the right to be called civilized."[7]

Is technology, then, the cardinal sin of industrialized man? I turn again to Karl Jaspers:

> Technology as such is by no means a process of total destruction. It gives man both chances. . . . It is still up to him to decide—by decisions of countless individuals—what will become of him. He can win technological mastery over natural forces, so he ought to do so—for this provides him with a steadily widening foundation of new potentialities. The technology he has produced does not threaten him as such; it is he who threatens himself with it. The situations it confronts him with are challenges for him. To cope with them, he must change. He will either change or he is unworthy of life and against his will, destroys himself by his technology.[8]

The 17th century views of Sir Francis Bacon, Descartes and theology all advanced the opinion that man must be master over a conquered nature. "And God said, 'Let us make mankind . . . and let them have dominion over the fish of the sea, over the birds of the air, over the cattle, and over all the earth.'"[9] "And God said to them, 'Be fruitful and multiply replenish the earth and subdue it.'"[10] *Never has a commandment been so fulfilled as "subdue it" has.*

The basis for this belief has roots growing back to the ancient world. Pagans worshiped nature and natural causes as deities. Greeks invented nature as a substitution of God. Not worshiping nature is what distinguished Judaism from pagan or pantheist religions. Judaism extolled a limited appreciation for nature as mere instrument of God but not to the point of natures' self–deification. Judaism swung the pendulum away from nature, never intending the severity of later interpretations.

Ancient Hebrew is a language written without punctuation. Where pauses and stops occur is largely based on custom and tradition; like most everything in Judaism. Thus you can read the aforementioned passage emphasizing the purpose and significance of "fruitful and multiply" is to "replenish the earth." Today we have seven billion individual testimonies on how well we have done with that interpretation. The rest of the passage, "and subdue it" is the source of theologians' insensitivity as man brings to bear his dominance over nature.

There is, I believe, another interpretation in the words of God. See what changing the pause does to the meaning. I read the verse as if, "be fruitful and multiply" is a self–contained thought of God. Next God declares that first we should "replenish the earth" and only then may we "subdue it." I believe God's intention is to interject the principle of sustainability into the world.

Rabbi Joseph Soloveitchik writes:

Man's domination of nature is not that of an alien autocrat over a people subjugated by force, but a loving father over his young son. Nature surrenders voluntarily to man's control and rule, she trusts man with her most guarded secrets. It is more cooperation than domination, more partnership than subordination. Let us watch out for moments of tension and conflict, when nature begins to hate man and to resent his presence, and as we will convince ourselves that man's sense of security and strength is nothing but a mirage. If nature refuses to be dominated, man is left helpless and weak.[11]

A *Midrash* conveys a warning God gave to the First Man Adam:

When the Holy One, blessed be He, created the first man, He took him and led him around all the trees of the Garden of Eden, and said to him, "Behold My works, how beautiful and admirable they are! Pay heed that you do not corrupt and destroy My universe. For if you corrupt it there is no one to repair it after you."[12]

God cares very much for His world. During times of war rules of humanity are often suspended in the heat of the battle. Yet, God warns man, "When you besiege a city for a long time, in making war against it, you shall not destroy its trees by forcing an axe against them . . . only the trees you know that are not food trees can you destroy and cut down."[13] Nahmanides in his commentary on this verse explains that not cutting food trees provides sustainability; after you defeat your enemy you will have provisions to live on.

Jewish sages learn another important teaching from commandant not to cut down fruit trees—*bal tashkit*—you shall not destroy. The Bible forbids wanton destruction of any kind. The 16th century Rabbi Aaron haLevi of Barcelona Spain in his work, *Sefer ha Hinnuch,* explains the reasoning as follows:

> The root reason for the precept is evident: for it is in order to train our spirits to love what is good and beneficial and to cling to it; and as a result, good fortune will cling to us, and we will move away from every evil thing and from every matter of destructiveness.[14]

Another *Mishnah* also speaks to sustainability:

> The world was created by means of ten utterances. What does this teach us—for it could indeed have been created by one utterance? It comes to tell us that God will exact severe penalty from the wicked who destroy the world which was created by ten utterances, *and to bestow rich reward upon the righteous who sustain the world that was created by ten utterances.*[15] [Emphasis added]

Judaism, however, teaches that we should not live an aesthetic life in reverence to nature. We are allowed to kill animals for food, for ritual sacrifice, utilize nature for commerce and the welfare of mankind, but within limits. The Jewish laws of *shehita*—kosher slaughtering, for example, are designed to minimize the pain an animal suffers being killed. God wants us to understand animals *do* feel pain.

Another prohibition in the Bible is "And whether it is a cow or a ewe, you shall not kill it and its young both on the same day."[16]

Maimonides explains, "This is a precautionary measure in order to avoid slaughtering the young in front of its mother. For in these cases animals feel very great pain, there being no difference regarding this pain between man and other animals." [17]

The Talmud[18] teaches that God did not create anything needlessly in the world. Everything has a purpose unto itself—everything. Therefore, Maimonides makes clear that, "it should not be believed that all things exist for the sake of the existence of man. On the contrary, all other beings too have been intended for their own sakes and not for something else." [19]

The laws of the Sabbath are in actuality meant to teach man that in order to achieve sustainability for himself, his animals, his family, his tools, and his lands; he must give each time necessary for rest, rejuvenation and replenishment.

The Bible makes this point again in a much broader milieu. "When you come to the land which I give you, then the land shall keep a Sabbath to the Lord. Six years you shall sow your field, six years you shall prune your vineyard, and gather its fruit, but the seventh year shall be a Sabbath of solemn rest for the land, a Sabbath for the Lord."[20]

Obliviously, the ramifications of this precept are to give the land time to replenish and rejuvenate; granting it the ability for self–sustainability in perpetuity. But there is, I believe, a more mystical reason implied.

Our earlier conundrum of if God is God, why does He need to rest, is answered because rest is a crucial element for the continuing sustainability of creation. God didn't chill out from the formation of the world by creating the Sabbath or take a 7th inning stretch in the middle; God does not need to rest. God wants his creations—the universe, planets, stars and our earth—to rest. By allowing them time to rest, the work of creation perpetuates itself. That is why the Bible says the Sabbath of the land *is* the Sabbath of the Lord.

So, as we see, God's message to us is that mankind has an awesome responsibility in the stewardship and sustainability of His planet. "Living is not a private affair of the individual," Rabbi Abraham Heschel said, "Living is what man does with God's time, what man does with God's world."[21]

The Jewish people have been long–suffering, uncomplaining, enduring, and unwearied while awaiting the Messiah to redeem us as promised by our sages and God. One can only imagine the intensity of that day when it finally arrives. However, Rabbi Yohanan ben Zakkai tells of an undertaking that takes precedent. "If you have a sapling in your hand and someone tells you that the Messiah has finally come, go and complete the task of planting the sapling, and then go and greet the Messiah!"[22] *WOW!*

A story in the Talmud[23] about Honi the circle maker teaches a final lesson on green Judaism's outlook on sustainability:

> One day Honi the circle maker was walking along when he saw an old man planting a carob tree. Honi asked him, "How many years does it take before a carob tree bears fruit?" The man replied, "Seventy years." "Do you really believe you will live another seventy years to eat its fruit?" asked Honi. The old man answered, "I found this world provided with carob trees, and as my forbearers planted them for me, so I too plant them for those who will come after me."

Back in college one day in the Student Center I overheard a group of people discussing a class they were taking. It sounded like an interesting subject, one I had never heard of before. So the next semester, I too enrolled in Ecology 101. Therein were nurtured my roots in environmentalism. Looking back now I can appreciate what a paradigm shift it made in my life.

One of the main texts we studied had just been published that year, *The Limits to Growth*, the report by The Club of Rome. The concept that growth had reached exponential capacity and would soon wreak havoc to our planet with untold ramifications was to say the least was hotly debated. Despite the immediate criticisms, the book has proved its validity in the long run. It was never intended as prediction, rather scenarios of what could happen.

More than anyone, Al Gore, the former next President of the United States, has promoted educating the peoples of the world to the reality of what global climate change means to humanity. His award winning 2006 film, *An Inconvenient Truth: A Global Warning*, was "a wakeup call that cuts through the myths and misconceptions to deliver the message that global warming is a real and present danger" and hailed as one of the most important films of our time.

Gore shared the 2007 Nobel Peace Prize with the United Nations Intergovernmental Panel on Climate Change, IPCC, "for their efforts to build up and disseminate greater knowledge about man–made climate change and to lay the foundations for the measures that are needed to counteract such change." Yet, there is actually *another* inconvenient truth about global warming which Gore did not address, and is only rarely spoken about, with even more serious ramifications.

The Rev. Thomas Robert Malthus was an 18th–19th English cleric and scholar. In his *An Essay on the Principle of Population*, he observed controversially that sooner or later population would ultimately be held in check by famine and disease. He placed long term economic stability above short–term expediency:

Assuming then my postulata as granted, I say, that the power of population is indefinitely greater than the power in the earth to produce subsistence for man. Population, when unchecked, increases in a geometrical ratio. Subsistence increases only in an arithmetical ratio. A slight acquaintance with numbers will show the immensity of the first power in comparison of the second. By that law of our nature which makes food necessary to the life of man, the effects of these two unequal powers must be kept equal. This implies a strong and constantly operating check on population from the difficulty of subsistence. This difficulty must fall somewhere and must necessarily be severely felt by a large portion of mankind.[24]

Today, Malthus is scoffed at. But in defense of *olde* Tom, how could he have known of the 20th century Green Revolution and the creation of ammonia and nitrogen based fertilizers? World food production has outpaced population with all of our techno–fixes. The real problem today, Tom, is we have run out of planet.

August 19, 2014 will go down in the annals of the history of our world as the day we overshot the earth's capacity, creating for the first time an ecological deficit, necessitating renewable ecological resources of more than 1.5 earths. And by mid–century we will require the equivalent of two full earths.

Economically speaking, we are spending our natural capital assets more rapidly than they are replenished. Greenhouse gases are emitted faster than they can be absorbed by our forests and oceans, tree numbers are dwindling, species are being forever lost, and our oceans' fisheries are collapsing. *We are overdrawn at the bank, people!*

President Lyndon Johnston in 1965 received the first scientific evidence of global warming and its potential threat to the planet. Fifty years later after Rio, Berlin, Kyoto, and Copenhagen at the Paris Climate Summit 2015, 196 nations of the world came together and signed a historic non–binding resolution that global warming was a real, unequivocal event and agreed to outline how each nation will achieve the goal of keeping temperature levels lower than +2°C and optimally under +1.5°C. Don't be duped, Boomers, there is no realistic way of achieving this goal despite the *greenwash* accolades you hear in the press.

And now for the other inconvenient truth! In 2006, CO_2 emission levels for the entire transportation sector were estimated to be 13% of the total. That year the United Nations Food and Agriculture Organization (FAO) released a report entitled *Livestock's Long Shadow*, that estimated that 7,516 million metric tons per year of

CO_2 equivalents (CO_2e), or 18 percent of annual worldwide greenhouse gases (GHGs) emissions, are attributable to cattle, buffalo, sheep, goats, camels, horses, pigs, and poultry.

Livestock was a bigger contributor to global warming more than the tailpipe emissions from all the world's cars, trucks, planes, trains, and ships combined! Where was the public outcry to administer emission standards for the steak we eat? Or fried chicken? Or pork chops? Or milk and eggs? Where was the Governator of California?

Just wait another moment. In 2009, Robert Goodland, the retired lead environmental adviser at the World Bank Group, and Jeff Anhang, a research officer and environmental specialist at the World Bank Group's International Finance Corporation, published a study in *World Watch* in which they challenged the United Nations Food and Agriculture Organization's report as flawed because it overlooked, unaccounted, and misallocated livestock–related contributions to GHG emissions—respiration by livestock, land use, and methane among others.[25]

When they recalculated livestock's contribution, their analysis showed that livestock and their byproducts actually account for at least 32,564 million tons of CO_2e per year, *or 51 percent of annual worldwide GHG emissions.* Since then, other estimates have place livestock's contribution around 30%.

Today, there is no denying that the production of animals and of crops for feed alone accounts for at least a third if not more of GHG emissions; is a primary source of methane and nitrous oxide, two of the most potent GHGs; and in terms of water, land and energy use it is highly resource–intensive.[26]

Worldwide demand for crops is increasing rapidly due to global population growth, increased biofuel production, and changing dietary preferences. Heightened demand for meat and dairy products is putting pressure on agricultural land; increased demand means increased GHG emissions.

Consumption of meat and dairy produce is expected to rise by 76 per cent and 65 per cent respectively by the middle of the century, driven by a rising population and a shift in dietary preferences towards protein–rich foods in developing nations. *The US uses 67% of its total calorie production for animal feed.* Because so much of the United States calorie production goes to animal feed, only 33% of the calories produced in the US are delivered to the food system. The US agricultural system alone could feed 1 billion additional people by shifting crop calories from livestock to direct human consumption. [27]

One recent study estimates feeding 9 billion people a Western diet with Western technologies in 2050 would require almost twice the amount of cropland currently under cultivation.[28] About 70% of the planet's agricultural land is already used for livestock production and an equal amount of our rainforests have been slashed and burned in order to raise livestock and feed. In fact, 30% of all terrestrial land on the planet is used for livestock.

Remember I called methane the wild card of the apocalypse? Methane has twenty–three times the global warming effect potential as carbon dioxide. Worldwide, approximately 40 percent of all methane produced by human activities is from livestock and their flatulence and manure. The average cow raised in a feedlot, belches out 117 pounds (53 kilograms) of methane per year. In the United States alone, livestock produce 89,000 pounds of excrement *every second*—over 5,340,000 pounds of excrement per minute—130 times as much as the entire human population of the country.[29]

Nitrous oxide—the ultimate greenhouse gas—is 310 times more powerful than carbon dioxide as a GHG. The livestock industry generates 65 percent of all human–related nitrous oxide; the offshoot from all our heavy use of nitrogen and ammonia based fertilizers to grow feed.

Fifty–five percent of our fresh water is being given to livestock. It takes only twenty to sixty gallons of water to produce one pound of vegetables, fruit, soybeans, or grain, but it takes over 5,000 gallons of water to produce one pound of meat.[30] On any given acre of land we can grow twelve to twenty times the amount in pounds of edible vegetables, fruit, and grain as we can in pounds of edible animal products.[31] Producing one calorie of animal protein requires more than ten times as much fossil fuel input and produces more than ten times as much CO_2 as does one calorie of plant protein.[32]

The Chatham House Report *Changing Climate, Changing Diets Pathways to Lower Meat Consumption* concluded in 2015:

> Left unchecked, current dietary patterns are incompatible with a two–degree pathway. If we are to avoid dangerous climate change, global yearly emissions must fall rapidly from today's levels of 49 GtCO2e to around 23 GtCO2e by 2050. If meat and dairy consumption continues to rise at current rates, the agricultural sector alone will soak up 20 of the 23 GtCO2e yearly limits in 2050, *leaving just 3 GtCO2e for the rest of the global economy.*[33] [Emphasis added]

The hand writing is on the wall and we don't need a Daniel to interpret it for us. The world cannot sustain itself with a meat–based diet. As Albert Einstein said, "Nothing will benefit human health and increase chances for survival of life on earth as much as the evolution of a vegetarian diet." Unless we accept the moral, *yes moral*, obligation of reducing our individual consumption of meat, then I am afraid that the Rev. Thomas Robert Malthus just might have the last laugh. *Buying a hybrid car, insulating your home, and changing light bulbs are just not enough!*

One last caveat! I must admit that the global warming deniers are right. No, they are not correct in their view of global warming as a hoax. Yet, they are right in why they refuse to believe in global warming and why they fight its truth so vehemently.

Who are the deniers? Honestly they are the salt of the earth Americans who champion freedom above all else. And there is absolutely nothing wrong with their values. They defend the constitution, the right to bear arms, and are willing to put their life on the line when needed.

As heirs to the Regan–Thatcherites' neo–liberalism view that only a free and independent market system, devoid of government intervention, can solve the worlds' ills, a free–market economy is exalted above all else, they hailed the fall of the Berlin Wall and communism as proof–positive.

The only problem is they are worshiping a false god. Despite the writings of Adam Smith, David Ricardo and James Mill, there never has been a true free market economy. More recently, the 2008 financial crisis showed what an unregulated market can do. The government bailout cost billions; adding insult to injury, those whose greed caused the debacle were rewarded with astronomical bonuses at the taxpayers' expense. A truly free market system would have dictated the banking industry should be allowed to fail, but the Chinese were standing in the wings ready to foreclose our T–Bills.

Sir Nicholas Stern is not a green left–wing environmentalist. Lord Stern was the chief economist and senior vice–president of the World Bank; second permanent secretary to Her Majesty's Treasury, chief economist of the European Bank of Reconstruction and Development, and is the Chair of Economics and Government at the London School of Economics. Stern said, "Greenhouse gas emissions constitute the greatest market failure the world has seen."

> At the heart of economic policy must be the recognition that the emission of greenhouse gases is a market failure. When we admit greenhouse gases we damage the prospects for others and, unless appropriate policy is in place, we do not bear the costs of the damage. Markets then fail in the sense that their main coordinating mechanism—prices—give the wrong signals. That is, prices . . . do not reflect the true cost to society of producing and using those goods.
>
> In the language of economists, the social cost of production and consumption exceeds the private cost, so that markets without policy

intervention will lead to too much of such goods being produced and consumed. By producing less of these products and more of others, we create economic gains that make everyone better off. Markets with uncorrected failures lead to inefficiency and waste.[34]

To solve global warming, we need to seek an end to the policy of the oil, gas, and coal industry's corporate colonialism—rape, pillage, plunder and leave. We must face up to perils that this strategy has brought upon us and stop believing energy doublespeak. Clean Coal is an oxymoron. Saying that we will build only new coal plants that will be carbon capture and sequestration ready is the same as saying, "I will respect you in the morning" and "the check is in the mail." *We must stop having a McDonald's day every day!*

Although Karl Jaspers was speaking to the threat of nuclear proliferation, I think his words are worth repeating:

> In the past, folly and wickedness had limited consequences; today they draw all mankind to perdition. Now, unless all of us live with and for one another, we shall all be destroyed. This new situation demands a corresponding answer. It is not enough to find new situations; we must change ourselves, our characters, our moral–political wills. . . . I do not think I am exaggerating. *Whoever goes on living as before has not grasped the menace.* [Emphasis added]

Viktor Frankl, the founder of Logotherapy, the Third Viennese School of Psychotherapy, lived the horrors of the holocaust—Theresienstadt, Auschwitz, and Dachau—until liberated by American soldiers. He understood the importance of freedom. In the camps he also realized that striving to find meaning in one's life is the primary motivational force in man.

"Freedom, however, is not the last word," Frankl says. "Freedom is only part of the story and half of the truth. Freedom is but the negative aspect of the whole phenomenon whose positive aspect is responsibleness. In fact, freedom is in danger of degenerating into mere arbitrariness unless it is lived in terms of responsibleness. That is why *I recommend that the Statue of Liberty on the East Coast be supplemented by a Statue of Responsibility on the West Coast.*[35]

Frankl's right. I think a Lady Responsibility is a noble idea. What better venue than Alcatraz Island; home to those who abnegated their societal responsibilities. Lady Liberty holds a torch in her right hand; Lady Responsibility should embrace a globe of our planet.

Emma Lazarus was a 19th century Jewish–American poet best known for her 1883 sonnet *The New Colossus* which is inscribed on a bronze plaque in the pedestal of the Statue of Liberty:

> *Give me your tired, your poor,*
> *Your huddled masses yearning to breathe free,*
> *The wretched refuse of your teeming shore.*
> *Send these, the homeless, tempest–tossed, to me:*
> *I lift my lamp beside the golden door."*

My choice for a bronze plaque inscription to do justice to Lady Responsibility's pedestal is one of my beloved quotes by Rabbi Abraham Heschel:

> *There is a realm of time*
> *Where the goal is not to have but to be,*
> *Not to own but to give,*
> *Not to control but to share,*
> *Not to subdue but to be in accord."*[36]

The long walk to responsibility lies ahead!

This page left intentionally blank

Epilogue

Do not go gentle into that good night,
Old age should burn and rave at close of day;
Rage, rage against the dying of the light.

Though wise men at their end know dark is right,
Because their words had forked no lightning they
Do not go gentle into that good night.

Good men, the last wave by, crying how bright
Their frail deeds might have danced in a green bay,
Rage, rage against the dying of the light.

Wild men who caught and sang the sun in flight,
And learn, too late, they grieved it on its way,
Do not go gentle into that good night.

Grave men, near death, who see with blinding sight
Blind eyes could blaze like meteors and be gay,
Rage, rage against the dying of the light.

And you, my father, there on that sad height,
Curse, bless, me now with your fierce tears, I pray.
Do not go gentle into that good night.
Rage, rage against the dying of the light.

Dylan Marlais Thomas was a popular 20th century Welsh poet and regular to the audiences of the BBC as voice of the literary scene. He also enjoyed a level of fame by his readings across the US. Dying at age 39, Thomas was plagued most of his life with alcoholism, which contributed to his epigrammatic life.

Thomas wrote *Do Not Go Gentle Into That Good Night* in 1947, fraught with severe alcoholism and an unhappy marriage, as an elegy to his father. The poem is an evocative message of struggling with death, surviving, and the will to live on. Sadly, all too well, Thomas knew its prose first hand, finding earning a living as a writer difficult; an identification I too can make.

Lifestyle is a set of attitudes, habits, behaviors or objects associated with a particular person or an affiliated group. Lifestyle can be healthy or unhealthy reflecting your choices, bring you happiness, or lead to sadness, illness and depression. Changes in lifestyle characteristically are associated with diet, physical activity, smoking, alcohol and/or drug use, take time and typically require support to accomplish.

Making a lifestyle change is certainly challenging, but rewards are as a rule always worth the effort. In essence, when you appreciably change your lifestyle, you become a different person—a Kafkaesque metamorphic transformation. To be successful, lifestyle changes necessitate being both revolutionary at initiation and evolutionary in due course.

I write these words, finishing my book, bearing witness that I am a wholly different person than I was prior to my angioplasty; feeling today like I just entered high school, drifting toward the new landscapes of life. Then I was shedding the feathers of adolescence as the clay of personality, character, and being were beginning to shape itself into adulthood, drying into the statue of myself I would carry through life.

My angioplasty gave me that often unappreciated second chance that is known so rarely in life, to remold myself into who *I* wanted to be rather than the way others had twisted me. As you read, I have learned a lot along the way, navigated crossroads in the darkest night, praying I chose the proper paths. In reflection I can say each time I look into a mirror and smile that frankly the effort paid off.

Physically, I feel sixteen again, mentally twenty–five but with one major variance. Yet, this time around at sixteen I bear with me more than a half century of life experience. And I owe it all to meeting my inner child. What would my life have been if I had met my inner child in high school between the football games, among the back seats on lover's lane, the higher drug induced worlds I explored or the lost days of hooky where life's precious time wasted away?

What motivated me to embrace the lifestyle changes I made with a tenacity I never before possessed? I made a vow as soon as I left the hospital after my angioplasty that never would my three sons gather around another hospital bed shedding tears over my illness—Alzheimer, diabetes, cancer, heart disease—that could easily have been prevented if only I had chosen to live in a different way. I promised myself they would never have to utter Dylan Thomas' refrain as he did for his father, beseeching me:

> *Do not go gentle into that good night.*
> *Rage, rage against the dying of the light.*

I chose Thomas's poem of all poems because I felt its message most fittingly places you at the end where my book began: the junction of choice where the *Two Roads Diverged in a Yellow Wood* of your life. Dylan Thomas challenges you presently to make your choice:

> ***Do you go gentle into that good night?***
> ***Or do you rage, rage against the dying of the light?***

Appendix

Frequently Asked Questions—FAQ

The man who asks a question is a fool for a minute, the man who does not ask is a fool for life.

Confucius

A wise man's question contains half the answer.

Solomon Ibn Gabirol

Let food be thy medicine and medicine be thy food.

Hippocrates

Life expectancy would grow by leaps and bounds if green vegetables smelled as good as bacon.

Doug Larson

A common feature of most web sites is a section called FAQ— frequently asked questions. Well, since I do not have a web site, I am including an appendix to answer questions I get. Honestly, there is only one question people ask me.

FAQ: Just what the hell *do you eat?*

Uri: I eat a whole food, plant and fungus based diet that is anti–inflammatory, anti–angiogenic, anti–oxidant and alkaline that boosts my immune system.

FAQ: Can you be more specific?

Uri: My diet consists of acetoxychavicol acetate, allicin, alpha–linolenic acid (ALA), anethole, anthocyanidins, apigenin, avenanthramides, beta–carotene, carnosic acid, carnosol, carvacrol, catechols, cineole, cinnamaladehyde, citral, citronella, cuminaldehyde, curcumin, diallyl sulfide, ellagic acid, epigallocatechin, ergothioneine, eugenol, flavonoids, garcinol, genistein, geraniol, geranyl acetate, gingerols, glucosinolates, isoflavones, isothiocyanates, limonene, linalool, linolenic acid, lupeol, lutein, lycopene, organosulphurs, orientin, phytoestrogens, phytosterols, piperine, polyphenols, proanthocyaninds, quercetin, resveratrol, rosmarinic acid, sequiterpenes, sesamin, sesamolin, sulforaphane, tartaric acid, thymol, ursolic acid, vicenin.

FAQ: Funny! We didn't mean that specific.

Uri: Honestly, I was not trying to be funny. I do not eat just healthy—I eat medicinally! After my angioplasty, I regained my health for the first time in my life by switching from the standard American diet (called the SAD diet for good reason) to the Mediterranean diet. I began reversing my coronary heart disease the moment I made the decision to change to a plant–based diet. A decade ago after reversing heart disease, I decided it was time to take on the Big C—cancer. The specifics I listed are the ammunition in my arsenal to defeat cancer.

FAQ: Okay then, where do you get your ammunition supply?

Uri: *veggies & fungus:* beets, broccoli, carrots, cauliflower, green chilies, green onions, kale, Nori seaweed, orange bell peppers, mushrooms (oyster, portobello, shitake, white), purple cabbage, red bell peppers, red chilies, red onions, shallots, tomatoes, yams.

   grains: black quinoa, black rice, brown basmati rice, kasha, oat bran, red quinoa, red rice, teff, wild rice.

beans: akuzi beans, black beans, black–eyed peas, cacao bean nibs, chick peas, green lentils, mung beans, red kidney, red lentils.

fruits: apricots, bananas, black currents, blackberries, cantaloupe, cherries, honey dew, Goji berries, kiwi, lemon, lime, mangos, Medjool dates, nectarines, oranges, papaya, passion fruit, peaches, pears, persimmons, pink grapefruit, plums, red apples, red grapes, strawberries, tangerines, watermelon, white grapes.

nuts & seeds: almonds, Brazil nuts, chia seeds, flax seeds, pumpkin seeds, sesame seeds (black, brown), edamame (soy), walnuts.

spices: allspice, amla, aniseed, basil, bay leaf, caraway, cardamom, chili peppers, cinnamon, cloves, coriander, cumin, fennel, fenugreek, galangal, garlic, ginger, green tea, hibiscus, kokum, lemon grass, marjoram, mint, mustard (yellow, black), onion, oregano, paprika, parsley, peppercorns (black, green, red), rosemary, sage, shallots, tamarind, thyme, turmeric.

drinks & brews: Hibiscus tea, Japanese sencha green tea, jasmine tea, lemon grass tea, pomegranate juice (100% pure juice), red cabernet sauvignon wine, water, white tea.

processed foods: organic apple vinegar, rice vinegar, Tabasco® pepper sauce, tofu, tomato paste (tomatoes 99%, 1% citric acid), unsweetened apple sauce.

Eating fruits, vegetables, mushrooms, spices, rice and beans full of phytochemicals, antioxidants, flavanols, lignans, phylates, etc is a non–toxic version of chemotherapy. Phytochemicals are the molecules in plants that defend against damage caused by insects, infection, microorganisms, etc. A category of phytochemicals responsible for the bright colors in fruits and vegetables called polyphenols absorb damaging free radicals. *Save the mitochondria!*

A new paradigm is surfacing in the treatment of cancer. The old maximum tolerated dose treatment protocols forced long rest periods which enabled the re–growth of tumor cells and promoted the growth of treatment resistant clones.

The new modality, metronomic chemotherapy, entails equally spaced low doses of various chemotherapeutic drugs without extended rest periods. Almost all of the items I have listed that are found in my kitchen have been proven in either laboratory tests, animal tests and/or human trials to prevent, arrest, and/or kill cancer.

I am sure that some of the items, such as the spice kokum, are unfamiliar. Rather than present the findings I have on each entry which probably would add another hundred pages to this book, I suggest you just Google a search with the phrase "health benefits of . . ." for the ones you don't know. And it will be well worth your time, I assure you, even for the ones you are familiar with.

A word of caution. There are significant side effects in using this approach to prevent cancer—so be warned. This same natural plant–spice based metronomic non–toxic chemotherapy will also reduce cholesterol, lower triglycerides, lower blood pressure, regulate insulin levels in diabetes, prevent Alzheimers and dementia, ease arthritis pain, reduce inflammation, increase the PH–alkaline level in urine and slow down the aging process.

FAQ: So, what does your average daily menu look like?

Uri: For starters, I eat rice and beans at every meal like millions of disease free people all over the world. In order for my diet to truly be metronomic, I eat the same things everyday—six days a week with the only exception being the Sabbath.

FAQ: Which of the items are most important?

Uri: You missed the point. I eat 90% of the items listed every day. I'll explain how by generally giving you my recipes and cooking procedures. For example: Tofu–Spice–Bean Rice. In my pantry I have containers filled with the following mixed together in equal proportions:

rice mix: brown basmati rice, red and black rice, occasionally adding wild rice
bean mix: akuzi beans, black beans, black–eyed peas, chick peas, green lentils, mung beans, red kidney, red lentils.
dried green spices: basil, bay leaf, coriander, lemon grass, marjoram, mint, oregano; and of course:— parsley, sage, rosemary, and thyme.
spice seeds: allspice, caraway, cardamom, cloves, coriander, cumin, fennel, fenugreek, mustard (yellow, black), peppercorns(black, green, red, white)
quinoa–kasha mix: black quinoa, red quinoa, and kasha.

Instead of plain water, I boil dried galangal, fresh ginger, and kokum in a large pot, after it cools, freezing the liquid in one liter containers. To make the Tofu–Spice–Bean Rice, I boil the galangal–ginger–kokum liquid. I soak the *bean mix* overnight in water, drain and rinse. In a coffee grinder, I freshly grind a tablespoon of each *spice seed;* makes about a cup. Once the water boils, I add the *rice mix*, *bean mix*, *green spices*, ground *spice seeds*, adding tofu cubes, fresh turmeric root, red onions, garlic, whole lemon, tamarind concentrate and used green tea leaves. I eat Tofu–Spice–Bean Rice three times a day; breakfast, lunch and supper!

FAQ: Okay, how do make the veggies?

Uri: Basically, I have two recipes: Three Alarm Tofu–Bean–Chili and Nuclear–Steamed Veggies.

First the Tofu–Bean–Chili. I start with the galangal–ginger–kokum liquid. I cut up red hot chilies, hot green chilies, red and orange bell peppers, Shitake mushrooms, whole lemon, fresh turmeric root, Nori seaweed, ginger, tomatoes, dried red chilies, red onions, garlic, and add whole cumin seeds, tofu cubes, *bean mix*, *dried green spices*, freshly ground *spice seeds*, hot paprika, tomato paste, tamarind concentrate and used green tea leaves.

Nuclear–Steamed Veggies: cut up broccoli, shallots, cauliflower, purple cabbage, green onions. I keep these pre–cut in a large jar in the fridge.

For breakfast, I mix the Tofu–Spice–Bean Rice and Three Alarm Tofu–Bean–Chili in a large glass bowl and nuke it. At the table I sprinkle on brown and black sesame seeds, pumpkin seeds, cacao bean nibs, amla, and freshly ground flax seeds, dousing it with either rice vinegar or organic apple vinegar. I eat until I feel full, usually about half the bowl. (You can only feel that you are getting full on a plant–based diet.) I save the rest and re–heat it for lunch.

Supper consists of Tofu–Spice–Bean Rice and Nuclear–Steamed Veggies. I put the Tofu–Spice–Bean Rice in the same large glass bowl and spread the cut veggies on top of the rice. I nuke it for a few minutes. The moisture of the rice mix helps steam the veggies.

Using a microwave instead of steaming the veggies over water retains almost all of the nutrients. Again, at the table I sprinkle on brown and black sesame seeds, pumpkin seeds, cacao bean nibs, amla, freshly ground flax seeds and dousing it with organic apple vinegar.

FAQ: What about the fruit?

Uri: I make a Blender–Smoothie with as many of the fruits listed based upon seasonal availability. It makes a very large amount which I freeze in three–cup containers. I pour pomegranate juice in the blender until it covers the blades. Then I start adding cut up fruit, berries, dates, Brazil nuts, walnuts, and almonds; pouring each blend into a very large bowl. When I finish, I whisk the mixture and fill the containers. In the afternoon, every afternoon, I'll have a three–cup container of Blender–Smoothie.

FAQ: You mentioned you ate differently for the Sabbath.

Uri: For the Sabbath I make a Tofu–Quinoa Pilaf. As before I start with the galangal–ginger–kokum liquid, adding tofu cubes, *bean mix, quinoa–kasha mix, dried green spices*, fresh turmeric root, ground peppercorns, red onions, garlic, whole lemon, yams, tamarind concentrate and used green tea leaves. My Sabbath meals consist of Tofu–Quinoa Pilaf instead of the Tofu–Spice–Bean Rice topped with the Nuclear–Steamed Veggies (of course, I do not use the microwave on the Sabbath.

FAQ: How do you wash it all down?

Uri: As with the recipes above, I do not use plain water to make my tea. In a large pot I boil lemon grass leaves, cinnamon quills, and sliced ginger, when cooled, freezing the mixture in one liter containers. I do not use tea bags; rather I blend Japanese Sencha green tea, jasmine tea, and white tea leaves in a glass container.

There are studies that have convinced me that cold steeping is the best way to make tea. In a one liter bottle, I pour in the lemon grass–cinnamon–ginger liquid, adding a tablespoon of the tea mix and a teaspoon of ground hibiscus flowers. Either I allow the bottle to stand at room temperature for two to four hours or I place it in the fridge over night. Before drinking, I filter out the tea leaves and add them, as you saw, to my cooked dishes as an additional spice.

Every day, without exception, I drink two to three liters of the tea drink, a glass of 100% pomegranate juice in the morning and one glass of red cabernet sauvignon wine usually with supper.

FAQ: We suppose you have eliminated snack foods.

Uri: On the contrary, I make the healthiest snacks around. Like so many, I make kale chips. I dust kale leaves with onion and garlic powder and bake them at a low temperature. Boy, are the ever so tasty. And I make my own no–salt pickled beets with just water and vinegar in equal amounts, fresh dill, chopped onions, coriander seeds and a few whole peppercorns.

But my favorites are sun–baked tomatoes and sun–baked onion chips I dry myself. Eilat is located at latitude: 29°33'N which means that officially we have an arid desert climate with 360 sun–days a year. In the winter, temperatures can reach in the 70's F and most of the summer it stays between 100°–112°F; at times reaching 122°F. In fact, there is so much sun if you look closely you can almost see droplets of vitamin D in the air.

I built my own vegetable dryer which I put on my roof, using it virtually year round. I cut vine–ripened tomatoes in quarters with the seeds and spread them on the rack. After a few days, I turn them. It never takes more than a week to get mouthwatering sun–dried tomatoes that do melt in your mouth. If you close your eyes, you can taste pizza.

But my favorite is sun–dried red onion chips. I quarter red onions, separating each layer. I dry them same as with the tomatoes. The sun's heat caramelizes the onions resulting in a crispy, sweet tasting onion chip.

I have big jars of sun–baked tomatoes and sun–baked onion chips in my pantry. A friend of mine suggested I sell them. Not a chance, they are that good; I'll keep them for myself. Make your own unless you live in a place like Scotland at latitude of 51°N.

FAQ: You seem to spend all day in your kitchen with all the extra preparation time.

Uri: I have a motto in my kitchen: *extra time = extra life!* Actually, I only cook twice a month. You see, to me the kiss of death is opening the fridge and saying, "Now, what are we in the mood for?" I have eaten the same things I have explained for a decade and have never grown tired of it. It is all fast food. I may spend a few extra minutes in the kitchen, but I more than make it up by just nuking everything when I am hungry. It takes me only five minutes at each meal to prepare my food!

FAQ: We noticed you do not eat wheat products. Whole grains are healthy, aren't they? Do you have celiac disease?

Uri: Without going in to great detail, I'll just say I weigh in on the side that feels gluten is not that good for you. I chose the phrase "I weigh in" for a reason. When I stopped eating wheat products, twenty pounds literally fell off of me and has never returned.

I have read that gluten affects immunity in mice and is able to induce cellular changes both in animals predisposed to disease and in healthy animals;[1] that withdrawal of wheat flour from a mouse's diet was sufficient to prevent diabetes in non–obese diabetic NOD mice;[2] there is low risk of developing a colon cancer in celiac patients with a strict adherence to a gluten–free diet[3] and a guten–free diet during fetal and early postnatal life reduces development of diabetes.[4]

You asked about celiac disease. In the 1950's celiac disease was a rare condition affecting 1 in 8,000. Today its prevalence in the United States is 1 in 141.[5] Why? Glyphosate, the active ingredient in the herbicide, Roundup®used in wheat and other crops, is the most important causal factor in the celiac disease epidemic.[6] *Think about this next time you eat GMOS.*

So, I make my own oat bran–teff bread using only ground flax seeds, unsweetened apple sauce, baking powder, water and with ground aniseed which is ten times sweeter than sugar and gives the bread a snappy licorice taste.

FAQ: But isn't whole–wheat bread healthy?

Uri: Yes, it is in a way. A study in the *American Journal of Clinical Nutrition*[7] did conclude that developing a simple habit as substituting whole–wheat bread for white bread when making a sandwich may have long–term health benefits. If you are not going to change from a Western diet to a plant–based diet, by all means, eat whole–wheat.

FAQ: We are confused.

Uri: Most people are. When they think of wholegrains, they only think of whole–wheat. A study in the

Proceedings of the Nutrition Society[8] showed that wholegrain foods are considered amongst the healthiest food choices that are available and that there exists a growing body of epidemiological data showing strong evidence for protection against cardiovascular disease, type 2 diabetes and some cancers. This is why I eat wholegrain foods three times a day–everyday. Wholegrains are rice, oats, quinoa, teff, wild rice, kasha, etc, which I eat, not just whole–wheat bread and pasta.

FAQ: It really is just the gluten.

Uri: I am not totally convinced that gluten is bad. There are studies that show beneficial effects. All my life I have lived with the following rule: *when it doubt–leave it out.*

    Ultraman Rich Roll in May 2010 with his ultra–colleague Jason Lester accomplished an unprecedented feat of staggering endurance many said was not possible. Something they called the EPIC5 CHALLENGE—a odyssey that entailed completing five ironman–distance triathlons on 5 islands of Hawaii in under a week. Commencing on Kauai, they travelled to Oahu, Molokai and Maui before finishing on the Big Island, following the Ironman World Championship's course of on the Kona coast. Rich said,[9] "The less gluten I consumed, the better I felt, slept, and performed athletically." I agree with *Ultraman.*

FAQ: You don't really expect people to eat like you!

Uri: Recently, my son Jonathan said he was going to buy me a white lab coat to wear in the kitchen while preparing my food. I took it as a great compliment. This book has been about what I have done and what I have learned. If you take anything away, please let it be that as a Baby Boomer, you should change to a plant–based diet as soon as you can, whatever way you can. King Solomon wrote in Ecclesiastes *that to everthing there is a season and a time for every purpose under heaven.* This is the final season of our lives to make lifestyle changes. Make it a happy, healthy purposeful time by switching to fruits and vegtables instead of animal products.

FAQ: You certainly think out of the box when it comes to eating. Any final quirks you would like to share with us?

Uri: We dig our gaves each day with our forks. I take it more than just a metaphor. Instead of a fork, I eat using chopsticks. I have seen studies that show the smaller the amount of food you take in, the fuller you feel and allows your metabolism and digestion more time to function normally. However, I only use stainless steel chopsticks because in China they sacrfice 600,000 trees a year just to supply the country with chopsticks. *Save the Planet!*

FAQ: Last question. If we wanted to meet out our inner child, where would we begin?

Uri: Years ago, when I was counseling clients, I recorded a workshop where I introduced people to their inner child. I have musically enhanced the recording which you can listen to free. Type this URL:

soundcloud.com/user-551518680

Have a great time meeting your inner child!

References

(Note: The initials KP stand for the position on a Kindle reader.)

Preface

1. Raskin, U., *Cracks in the Wall*, Brooklyn: Tamar Books/Mesorah Publications, 1994; Raskin, U., *The Scribe*, Jerusalem: Jerusalem Publications, 2005; Raskin, U., *El Escriba* (Spanish Translation), Mexico City: Jerusalem de Mexico, 2008; Raskin, U., The Peddler, *Horizons Jewish Family Journal*, Fall 1997;14:51–55; Raskin, U., The Game, *Horizons Jewish Family Journal*, 1998;16:94–100; Raskin, U., The Candy Man, *Horizons Jewish Family Journal*, 1999;21:62–67; Raskin, U., The Unknown Soldier, *Horizons Jewish Family Journal*, 2002;31:122–127.

1. Chanukah 1998

1. Josephus, Trans. Williamson, G.A., *The Jewish War*, Middlesex: Penguin Books, 1959, p. 223.
2. Ibid., p. 229.
3. I was able to secure my records from University Hospital in Augusta, Georgia.

2. Boomers

1. May, R., *Man's Search for Himself: How We Can Find a Center of Strength Within Ourselves to Face and Conquer the Insecurities of This Trouble Age*, New York : W.W. Norton & Company, 1953, p. 19.
2. Kuhn, T.S., *The Structure Of Scientific Revolutions*, Chicago: University of Chicago Press, 1996, p. 52–3.
3. Robbins, J., *Healthy At 100*, New York: Random House, 2006, p. 225.
4. Schulz, M., *Awakening Intuition*, New York: Three Rivers Press, 1998, p. 245.

5. Lynch, J., *A Cry Unheard: The Medical Consequences of Loneliness*, Baltimore: Bancroft Press, 2000, p. 111–2.

6. Ornish, D., *Love & Survival*, New York: Harper Perennial, 1998, p. 33.

7. Lynch, J., *A Cry Unheard: The Medical Consequences of Loneliness*, p. 92.

8. Mc Taggart, L., The Intention Experiment: Using Thoughts to Change Your Life and the World, New York: Free Press, 2007, p 135.

9. Ornish, D., *Love & Survival*, p.36.

10. Dossey, L., *Reinventing Medicine: Beyond Mind–Body to a New Era of Healing*, New York: Harper Collins, 1999, p.176.

11. Guarneri, Mimi, *The Heart Speaks: A Cardiologist Reveals the Secret Language of Healing*, New York: Touchstone, 2006, KP, 1706–1708.

12. Attwood, C., *Dr. Attwood's Low Fat Prescription for Kids*, New York: Penguin Books, 1995, p. xx.

13. Bohm, D. and Peat, D., *Science, Order and Creativity*, London: Routledge, 2000, p. 237.

14. Ibid., p. 216.

3. Survival and Change

1. Gonzales, L., *Deep Survival*, New York: W.W. Norton, 2005, p. 232.

2. Sheehy, G., *New Passages: Mapping Your Life Across Time*, New York: Ballantine Books, 1995, p. 258.

3. Survival, *Army Field Manual FM 21–76*, 1970, p. 12.

4. Ibid., p. 13.

5. Ibid., p. 19.

6. Ibid., p. 25.

7. Babylonian Talmud, Tractate Eruvin, 53b.

8. Siebert, A., *The Resiliency Advantage*, San Francisco: Berrett–Koehler Publishers Inc., 2005, p.71.

9. Ibid., p. 247.

10. Ibid., p. viii.

11. Ibid., p. 30.

12 Gonzales, L., *Deep Survival*, p.199.

13. Ibid., p.204.

14. Watzlawick, P., et al., *Change*, New York: W.W. Norton, 1974.

15. Ibid., p. 22.

16. Ibid., p. 83.

17. Schwartz, J. and Begley, S., *The Mind and the Brain: Neuroplasticity and the Power of Mental Force*, New York: Harper Perennial, 2002, p.179.

18. Schwartz, J. and Gladding, R., *You Are Not Your Brain: The 4–Step Solution for Changing Bad Habits, Ending Unhealthy Thinking, and Taking Control of Your Life*, New York: Avery, 2011, p. xii.

19. Bohm, D. and Peat, D., *Science, Order and Creativity*, London: Routledge, 2000, p. 22.

20 Schwartz, J. and Begley, S., *The Mind and the Brain: Neuroplasticity and the Power of Mental Force*, p. 15.

21. Siegel, D., *The Mindful Therapist: A Clinician's Guide to Mindsight and Neural Integration*, New York: W.W. Norton, 2010, p. 218.

22. Noe, Alva, *Out of Our Heads: Why You Are Not Your Brain, and Other Lessons from the Biology of Consciousness*, New York: Hill and Young, 2009, KP, 809–10.

23. Peli, P., *Soloveitchik on Repentance: The Thought and Oral Discourses of Rabbi Joseph B. Soloveitchik*, New York: Paulist Press, 1984, p. 175.

24. Ibid., p. 56.

25. Maimonides Mishnah Torah, Hilchos Teshuvah, 1:1.

26. Maimonides Mishnah Torah, Hilchos Teshuvah, 2:1.

4. Childhood

1. Piaget, J. and Inhelder, B., *The Psychology of the Child*, New York: Basic Books, 1969, p. xi.

2. Sullivan, H., *The Interpersonal Theory of Psychiatry*, New York: W.W. Norton & Company, 1953, p. 382.

3. Brazelton, T. and Greenspan, S., *The Irreducible Needs Of Children: What Every Child Must Have to Grow, Learn, and Flourish*, Cambridge MA: Da Capo Press, 2000, p. x.

4. Erikson, E., *Childhood and Society*, New York: W.W. Norton, 1963, p. 295.

5. Ibid., p. 295.

6. Ibid., p. 291.

7. Mishnah, Chapters of the Fathers, 5:20.

8. Erikson, E., *Childhood and Society*, New York: W.W. Norton, 1963.

9. Vaillant, G., *Adaptation to Life*, Cambridge MA: Harvard University Press, 1997, p. 207.

10. Harris, J., *The Nurture Assumption: Why Children Turn Out the Way They Do*, New York: Free Press, 1998, p. xx.

11. Ibid., p. 135.

12. Erikson, E., *Childhood and Society*, p. 268.

13. Ibid., p. 269.

14. Wilber, K., *Integral Psychology*, Boston: Shambhala Publications, 2000, p. 28.

15. Bradshaw, J., *Healing the Shame That Binds You*, Deerfield Beach, FL: Health Communications, 1988, p. 29.

16. Siebert, A., *The Survivor Personality*, New York: A Perigee Book, 1994, p.75

17. Eliot, L., *What's Going On In There: How the Brain and Mind Develop in the First Five Years of Life*, p. 32.

18. Ibid., p. 5.

19. Wilber, K., *Integral Psychology*, p. 39–40.

20. Pennebaker, J., *Opening Up: The Healing Power of Expressing Emotions*, New York: Guilford Press, 1990, p. 20.

21. Eliot, L., *What's Going On In There: How the Brain and Mind Develop in the First Five Years of Life*, p. 136.

22. Firestone, R., *Creating a Life of Meaning and Compassion*, Washington, DC: American Psychological Association, 2003, p. 33.

23. Wilber, K., *Integral Psychology*, p. 94.

24. Verny, T. with Kelly, J., *The Secret Life of the Unborn Child*, New York: Dell, 1981, p. 19.

25. Ibid., p. 25.

26. Lipton, B., *The Biology of Belief*, Santa Rosa, CA: Elite Books, 2005, p. 173.

27. Sapolsky, R., *Why Zebras Don't Get Ulcers: The Acclaimed Guide to Stress, Stress-Related Diseases, and Coping*, New York: St. Martin's Griffin, 1998, p. 289.

28. Nathanielsz, P., *Life in the Womb: the Origin of Health and Disease*, Ithaca, New York: Promethean Press, 1999, p. 120.

29. Eliot, L., *What's Going On In There: How the Brain and Mind Develop in the First Five Years of Life*, p. 174.

30. Ibid., p. 194.

31. Ibid., p. 176.

32. Carey, N., *The Epigenetics Revolution: How Modern Biology is Rewriting Our Understanding of Genetics, Disease, and Inheritance*, New York: Columbia University Press, 2012, p. 112.

33. Nathanielsz, P., *Life in the Womb: the Origin of Health and Disease*, p. 1.

34. Ibid., p. 143.

35. Ibid., p. 140.

36. Ibid., p. 93.

37. Goodman, S., *9 Steps for Reversing or Preventing Cancer*, Franklin Lakes NJ: New Page Books, 2004, p. 60.

38. Kaptchuk, T., *The Web That Has No Weaver: Understanding Chinese Medicine*, Chicago: Contemporary Books, 2000, p. 4.

39. Friedman, H., *The Self Healing Personality*, Lincoln NE: iUniverse, 2000, p. 20.

40. Benson, H., *Timeless Healing: The Power and Biology of Belief*, London: Simon & Schuster, 1998, p. 22.

41. Babylonian Talmud, Tractate Yoma 83a.

42. Proverbs 14:10.

43. May, R., *Man's Search for Himself: How We Can Find a Center of Strength Within Ourselves to Face and Conquer the Insecurities of This Trouble Age*, New York: W.W. Norton & Company, 1953, p. 95.

5. Shame and Self–Esteem

1. Twerski, A., *Angels Don't Leave Footprints: Discovering What's Right with Yourself*, New York: Shaar Press, 2001, p. 133.

2. Paul, M., *Inner Bonding: Becoming a Loving Adult to Your Inner Child*, San Francisco CA: Harper Collins Publishers, 1992, p. 46.

3. Erikson, E., *Childhood and Society*, New York: W.W. Norton, 1963, p. 252.

4. Soloveitchik, J., *Family Redeemed: Essays on Family Relationships*, Jersey City: Ktav Publishing House, 2000, p. 80.

5. Ibid., p. 83.

6. Twerski, A., *Angels Don't Leave Footprints: Discovering What's Right with Yourself*, p. 184.

7. Brown, B., *Daring Greatly: How the Courage to Be Vulnerable Transforms the Way We Live, Love, Parent, and Lead*, New York: Gotham Books, 2012, p. 69.

8. Brown, B., *The Gifts of Imperfection: Your Guide to a Wholehearted Life*, Center City MN: Hazelden, 2010, p. 41.

9. Firestone, R., Firestone, L., Catlett, J., *Conquer Your Critical Inner Voice*, Oakland: New Harbinger Publications, 2002, p. 34.

10. Mate, G., *In the Realm of Hungry Ghosts: Close Encounters with Addiction*, Berkeley, CA: North Atlantic Books, 2010, p. 147.

11. Ibid., p. 116.

12. Soloveitchik, J., *Family Redeemed: Essays on Family Relationships*, p. 80.

13. Erikson, E., *Childhood and Society*, p. 253.

14. Whitfield, C., *Healing The Child Within*, Deerfield Beach, FL: Health Communications, 1989, p. 46.

15. Bradshaw, J., *Healing the Shame That Binds You*, Deerfield Beach, FL: Health Communications, 1988, p. 44.

16. Twerski, A., *Angels Don't Leave Footprints: Discovering What's Right with Yourself*, p. 39.

17. Ibid., p. 69.

18. Overstreet, B., *Understanding Fear in Ourselves and Others*, New York: Collier Books, 1951, p. 25.

19. Goleman, D., *Emotional Intelligence: Why It Can Matter More Than IQ*, London: Bloomsbury Publishing, 1985, p. 100.

20. Berne, P. and Savary, L., *Building Esteem in Children*, New York: The Crossroad Publishing Company, 2000, p. xv.

21. Twerski, A., Angels Don't Leave Footprints: Discovering What's Right with Yourself, p. 123.

22. Berne, P. and Savary, L., *Building Esteem in Children*, p. xiv.

23. Becker, E., *The Birth and Death of Meaning*, NY: The Free Press, 1971, p.3.

24. Twerski, A., *Angels Don't Leave Footprints: Discovering What's Right with Yourself*, p. 124.

25. Berne, P. and Savary, L., *Building Esteem in Children*, p. xvi.

26. Bradshaw, J., *Healing the Shame That Binds* You; Firestone, R., *The Fantasy Bond*; Whitfield, C., *Healing The Child Within*.

27. Brown, B., *The Gifts of Imperfection*, p. 50.

28. Brown, B., *Daring Greatly: How the Courage to Be Vulnerable Transforms the Way We Live, Love, Parent, and Lead*, p. 33.

29. Ibid., p 12.

30. Ibid., p 34.

31. Mate, G., *In the Realm of Hungry Ghosts*, p. 41.

32. Brown, B., *Daring Greatly: How the Courage to Be Vulnerable Transforms the Way We Live, Love, Parent, and Lead*, p. 33.

33. http://www.ted.com/talks/brene_brown_listening_to_shame

34. http://www.ted.com/talks/brene_brown_on_vulnerability

6. Addictions and Emotions

1. Shoshana, A., *The Complete Mesillat Yesharim in Two Versions: Dialogue and Thematic*, Cleveland: Ofeq Institute, 2007, p. 129.

2. Ornish, D., *Eat More, Weigh Less*, New York: Harper Perennial, 1993, p. 66.

3. Siegel, B., *The Art of Healing: Uncovering Your Inner Wisdom and Potential for Self–Healing*, Novato CA: New World Library, 2013, KP, 2745.

4. Forward, S., *Toxic Parents*, New York: Bantam Book, 2002, p. 182.

5. Kessler, D., *The End of Overeating: Taking Control of the Insatiable American Appetite*, New York: Rodale, 2009, p. 37.

6. Nuland, S., *How We Die: Reflections of Life's Final Chapter*, New York: Vintage Books, 1993, p. 133.

7. Ibid., p. 131.

8. Gearhardt, et al., 'Can Food be Addictive? Public Health and Policy Implications,' *Addiction*, 2011; 106(7):1208–1212.

9. Moss, M., *Salt Sugar Fat: How the Food Giants Hooked Us*, New York: Random House, 2013, p. 4.

10. Ibid., p. 132.

11. Barnard, N., *Breaking the Food Seduction: The Hidden Reasons Behind Food Carvings*, New York: St. Martin's Griffin, 2003, p. 63.

12. Babylonian Talmud, Tractate Ta'anit, 13b.

13. Ibid., p. 42.

14. Eliot, L., *What's Going On In There: How the Brain and Mind Develop in the First Five Years of Life*, New York: Bantam Books, 2000, p. 182.

15. Barnard, N., *Breaking the Food Seduction: The Hidden Reasons Behind Food Carvings*, p. 51.

16. Ibid., p. 50.

17. Erikson, E., *Childhood and Society*, New York: W.W. Norton, 1963, p. 61.

18. Kessler, D., *The End of Overeating: Taking Control of the Insatiable American Appetite*, p. 62.

19. Ibid., p. 61.

20. Olsen, Christopher M., 'Natural Rewards, Neuroplasticity, and Non–Drug Addictions,' *Neuropharmacology*, 2011; 61(7):1109–1122.

21. Ibid., p. 37.

22. Davis, W., *Wheat Belly*, New York: Rodale, 2011, p. 166.

23. Parylak, et al., 'The dark side of food addiction," *Physiology & Behavior,* 2011; 104(1): 149–156.

24. Barnard, N., *Breaking the Food Seduction: The Hidden Reasons Behind Food Carvings,* p. 32.

25. Moss, M., *Salt Sugar Fat: How the Food Giants Hooked Us,* p.148.

26. Ibid., p. xvii.

27. Ibid., p. 123.

28. Mate, G., *In the Realm of Hungry Ghosts: Close Encounters with Addiction,* Berkeley, CA: North Atlantic Books, 2010, p. 142.

29. Ibid., p. 141.

30. Alexander, B., *The Globalization of Addiction: A Study in Poverty of the Spirit,* New York: Oxford University Press, 2008.

31. Ibid., p. 86.

32. Ibid., p. 99.

33. Ibid., p. 129.

34. Ibid., p. 62.

35. Colbert, T., *Broken Brains or Wounded Hearts: What Causes Mental Illness,* Santa Ana CA: Kevco Publishing, 1996, p. 154.

36. Mate, G., *In the Realm of Hungry Ghosts,* p. 14.

37. Ornish, D., *Eat More, Weigh Less,* p. 66.

38. Siegel, B., *The Art of Healing: Uncovering Your Inner Wisdom and Potential for Self–Healing,* KP, 2590/94.

39. Mate, G., *In the Realm of Hungry Ghosts,* p. 38.

40. Ibid., p. 33.

41. Epstein, G., *Healing Visualizations: Creating Health Through Imagery,* New York: Bantam Books, 1989, p. 41.

42 Baik, Ja–Hyun, 'Dopamine signaling in food addiction: role of dopamine D2 receptors,' *Journal of Biochemistry and Molecular Biology,* 2013; 46(11): 519–526.

43. Meule, et al., 'The psychology of eating,' *Frontiers in Psychology,* 2013; 4: Article 215.

44. Kessler, D., *The End of Overeating: Taking Control of the Insatiable American Appetite*, p. 50.

45. Ibid., p. 54.

46. Ibid., p. 37–38.

47. Noble, E., *Primal Connections: How Our Experiences from Conception to Birth Influence Our Emotions, Behavior, and Health*, New York: Simon and Schuster, 1993, p. 132.

48. Twerski, A., *Angels Don't Leave Footprints: Discovering What's Right with Yourself*, New York: Shaar Press, 2001, p. 69.

49. Schulz, M., *Awakening Intuition*, New York: Three Rivers Press, 1998, p. 214.

50. Firestone, R., *Creating a Life of Meaning and Compassion*, Washington, DC: American Psychological Association, 2003, p.114.

51. Ramachandran, V.S. and Blakeslee, S., *Phantoms in the Brain: Probing the Mysteries of the Human Mind*, New York: Quill, 1998, p. 133.

52. Firestone, R., *The Fantasy Bond: Structure of Psychological Defenses*, Santa Barbara CA: The Glendon Association, 1987, p 35.

53. Borysenko, J., *Minding the Body, Mending the Mind*, Cambridge MA: Da Capo Press, 2007, p. 3.

54. Cameron–Bandler, L and Lebeau, M., *The Emotional Hostage: Rescuing Your Emotional Life*, FuturePace: San Rafael CA, 1986, p. 4.

55. Levine, P., *In an Unspoken Voice: How the Body Releases Trauma and Restores Goodness*, Berkeley CA: North Atlantic Books, 2010, p. 312.

56. Whitfield, C., *Healing The Child Within*, Deerfield Beach, FL: Health Communications, 1989, p. 78.

57. Kabat–Zinn, J., *Full Catastrophe Living: Using the Wisdom of Your Body and Mind to Face Stress, Pain, and Illness*, New York: Bantam Dell, 1990, p. 205.

58. Sarno, J., *The Mindbody Prescription: Healing the Body, Healing the Pain*, New York: Warner Books, 1998, p. xxvii.

59. Schulz, M., *Awakening Intuition*, p. 113.

60. Janov, A., *The New Primal Scream*, Franklin Lakes NJ: Career Press, 2007, p. 110.

61. Sarno, J., *The Mindbody Prescription*, p. 44.

62. Lipton, B., *The Biology of Belief*, Santa Rosa, CA: Elite Books, 2005, p. 67.

63. Pert, C., *Molecules of Emotion*, New York: Scribner, 2003, p. 147.

64. Schulz, M., Awakening Intuition, p. 90.

65. Ibid., p. 273.

66. Ibid., p. 183.

67. Peat, F.D., *Synchronicity: the Bridge Between Matter and Mind*, New York: Bantam Books, 1987, p. 62.

68. Noble, E., *Primal Connections: How Our Experiences from Conception to Birth Influence Our Emotions, Behavior, and Health*, p. 187.

7. Psyche—Soma

1. Sarno, J., *The Divided Mind: The Epidemic of Mindbody Disorders*, New York: Regan Books, 2006, p. 113.

2. Twerski, A., *Angels Don't Leave Footprints: Discovering What's Right with Yourself*, New York: Shaar Press, 2001, p. 133.

3. Janov, A., *Primal Healing: Access the Incredible Power of Feelings to Improve Your Health*, Franklin Lakes NJ: Career Press, 2007, p. 217.

4. Numbers, 21:4–9.

5. Babylonian Talmud, Tractate Rosh Hashanah, 29 b.

6. Babylonian Talmud, Tractate Pesachim, 56a.

7. Babylonian Talmud, Tractate Bava Metziva, 85b.

8. Rosenthal, R., and Jacobson, L., *Pygmalion in the Classroom: Teacher Expectation and Pupils' Intellectual Development*, Norwalk, CT: Crown House Publishing Company, 1992, p. 15.

9. Le Fanu, J., *The Rise and Fall of Modern Medicine*, London: Abacus, 1999, p. 249.

10. Benson, H., *The Wellness Book: the Comprehensive Guide to Maintaining Health and Treating Stress–Related Illness*, New York: Birch Lane Press, 1992, p. 9.

11. Heffernan, M., *Willful Blindness: Why We Ignore the Obvious at Our Peril*, New York: Walker & Company, 2011, p. 185.

12. Siegel. B., *The Art of Healing: Uncovering Your Inner Wisdom and Potential for Self–Healing*, Novato CA: New World Library, 2103, KP, 2913/16.

13. Rosenthal, R., and Jacobson, L, *Pygmalion in the Classroom: Teacher Expectation and Pupils' Intellectual Development*, p. 165.

14. Benson, H., *The Wellness Book: the Comprehensive Guide to Maintaining Health and Treating Stress–Related Illness*, p. 9.

15. Rosenthal, R., and Jacobson, L. *Pygmalion in the Classroom: Teacher Expectation and Pupils' Intellectual Development*, p. 25.

16. Friedman, H., *The Self Healing Personality*, Lincoln: iUniverse, 2000, p. 117.

17. Sherman, et al., 'Academic Physicians Use Placebos in Clinical Practice and Believe in the Mind–Body Connection,' *Journal of General Internal Medicine*, 2007; 23 (1): 7 –10.

18. Kermen, et al., 'Family Physicians Believe the Placebo Effect Is Therapeutic But Often Use Real Drugs as Placebos,' *Family Medicine*, 2010; 42(9):636–42.

19. Howick, et al., 'Placebo Use in the United Kingdom: Results from a National Survey of Primary Care Practitioners,' *PLoS ONE*, 2103; 8(3): e58247.

20. Hrobjartsson, A. and Norup, M., 'The use of placebo interventions in medical practice: a national questionnaire of Danish clinicians,' *Evaluation & the Health Professions*, 2003; 26 (2): 153–165.

21. Nitzan, et al., 'Questionnaire survey on use of placebo,' *British Medical Journal*, 2004; 329:944–6.

22. Sherman, et al., 'Academic Physicians Use Placebos in Clinical Practice and Believe in the Mind–Body Connection,' *Journal of General Internal Medicine*, 2007; 23 (1): 7 –10.

23. Alexander, F. and Selesnick, S., *The History of Psychiatry: An Evaluation of Psychiatric Though and Practice from Prehistoric Times to the Present*, New York: Harper and Row, 1966, p. 392.

24. Borysenko, J., *Minding the Body, Mending the Mind*, Cambridge MA: Da Capo Press, 2007, p. 6; Benson, H., *The Relaxation Response*, New York: William Morrow, 1975, p. 49.

25. Pelletier, K., *Mind as Healer, Mind as Slayer*, New York: Delta Seymour Lawrence Books, 1992, p. 7.

26 Schulz, M., *Awakening Intuition*, New York: Three Rivers Press, 1998, p. 94.

27. Sarno, J., *The Mindbody Prescription: Healing the Body, Healing the Pain*, New York: Warner Books, 1998, p. xiii.

28. Sarno, J., *The Divided Mind: The Epidemic of Mindbody Disorders*, p. 51.

29. Goodman, S., *9 Steps for Reversing or Preventing Cancer*, Franklin Lakes NJ: New Page Books, 2004, p. 58.

30. Guarneri, Mimi, *The Heart Speaks: A Cardiologist Reveals the Secret Language of Healing*, New York: Touchstone, 2006, KP 815–816.

31. Erikson, E., *Childhood and Society*, New York: W.W. Norton, 1963, p. 33.

32. Goff, S. with Bennett, H., *The Holographic Mind: The Three Levels of Human Consciousness and How They Shape Our Lives*, New York: Harper Collins, 1993, p. 206.

33. Whitfield, C., *Co–Dependence: Healing The Human Condition*, Deerfield Beach FL: Health Communications, 1991, p. 77.

34. Levine, P., *In an Unspoken Voice: How the Body Releases Trauma and Restores Goodness*, Berkeley CA: North Atlantic Books, 2010, p. 276.

35. Salanter, Y., Trans. Miller, D., *Ohr Yisroel*, Southfield, Mi: Targum Press, 2004, p. 380.

36. Kabat–Zinn, J., *Full Catastrophe Living: Using the Wisdom of Your Body and Mind to Face Stress, Pain, and Illness*, New York: Bantam Dell, 1990, p. 216.

37. Morris, S. and Nguyen, C., 'Blastomycosis,' *University of Toronto Medical Journal*, 2004; 81(3): 172–175.

38. 'Blastomycosis,' *Manitoba Communicable Disease Management Protocol*, September 2007: 1–7.

39. Sarno, J., *The Divided Mind: The Epidemic of Mindbody Disorders*, p. 309.

40. Ibid., p. 309.

41. Ibid., p. 48.

42. Sarno, J., *The Mindbody Prescription*, p. xiii.

43. Ibid., p. 8.

44. Ibid., p. xxvii.

45. Ibid., p. xxi.

46. Sarno, J., *The Mindbody Prescription*, p. 134.

47. Ibid., p. 60.

48. Ibid., p. 64.

49. Jenson, M. et al., 'Magnetic Resonance Imaging of the Lumbar Spine in People without Back Pain,' *New England Journal of Medicine*, 1994; 331:69–73.

50. Sarno, J., *The Mindbody Prescription*, p. 96.

51. James, W., *Varieties of Religious Experience*, Charleston: BibiloBazaar, 2007, p. 14.

8. Attitude

1. Peale, N., *The Power of Positive Thinking*, New York: Wing Books, 1994, p. 170.

2. Rosenthal, R., and Jacobson, L., *Pygmalion in the Classroom: Teacher Expectation and Pupils' Intellectual Development*, Norwalk, CT: Crown House Publishing Co., 1992, p. 24.

3. Kabat–Zinn, J., *Full Catastrophe Living: Using the Wisdom of Your Body and Mind to Face Stress, Pain, and Illness*, New York: Bantam Dell, 1990, p. 216.

4. Ibid., p. 210.

5. Dossey, L., *Reinventing Medicine: Beyond Mind–Body to a New Era of Healing*, New York: Harper Collins, 1999, p. 176.

6. Guarneri, Mimi, *The Heart Speaks: A Cardiologist Reveals the Secret Language of Healing*, New York: Touchstone, 2006, KP, 1256–1258.

7. Rosenthal, R., and Jacobson, L., *Pygmalion in the Classroom: Teacher Expectation and Pupils' Intellectual Development*, p.121.

8. Ibid., p. 34.

9. Ibid., p. 8.

10. Ibid., p. 14.

References

11. Mc Taggart, L., *The Intention Experiment: Using Thoughts to Change Your Life and the World*, New York: Free Press, 2007, p. xxii.

12. Ibid., p. 165.

13. Mc Taggart, L., *The Field: The Quest for the Secret Force of the Universe*, New York: Harper Collins, 2008, p. 176.

14. Lipton, B., *The Biology of Belief*, Santa Rosa, CA: Elite Books, 2005, p. 30.

15. Siegel, B., *The Art of Healing: Uncovering Your Inner Wisdom and Potential for Self-Healing*, Novato CA: New World Library, 2013, KP, 530–32.

16. Bolte, J., *My Stroke of Insight: A Brain Scientist's Personal Journey*, New York: Viking, 2008, p. 146.

17. Frankl, V., *Man's Search for Meaning*, New York: Touchstone Book, 1984, p. 116.

18. Peli, P., *Soloveitchik on Repentance: The Though and Oral Discourses of Rabbi Joseph B. Soloveitchik*, New York: Paulist Press, 1984, p. 172.

19. Bohm, D., *Wholeness and the Implicate Order*, London: Routledge Classics, 1980, KP, 575–77.

20. Bohm, D. and Peat, D., *Science, Order and Creativity*, London: Routledge, 2000, p. 236.

21. Ibid., p. 93.

22. Ibid., p. 236.

23. Ibid., p. 236.

24. Talbot, M., *The Holographic Universe: A Remarkable Theory of Reality*, New York: Harper Perennial, 1991, p. 4.

25. Mc Taggart, L., *The Field: The Quest for the Secret Force of the Universe*, p. 136.

26. Bohm, D. and Peat, D., *Science, Order and Creativity*, p. 105.

27. Ibid., p. 236.

28. Ibid., p. 223.

29. Ibid., p. 107.

30. Ibid., p. 239.

9. *Судьба*

1. Rossman, M., *Guided Imagery for Self–Healing: An Essential Resource for Anyone Seeking Wellness*, Navato, CA: H J Kramer, 2000, p. 208.

2. Twerski, A., *Like Yourself and Others Will Like You*, Englewood NJ: Prentice–Hall, 1978, p. 131.

3. Lipton, B., *The Biology of Belief*, Santa Rosa, CA: Elite Books, 2005, p. 166.

4. Goodman, S., *9 Steps for Reversing or Preventing Cancer*, Franklin Lakes NJ: New Page Books, 2004, p.102.

5. Svirsky, E., *Connection: Emotional and Spiritual Growth Through Experiencing God's Presence*, Jerusalem: Institute of Psycho–Spiritual Therapy, 2004, p. 35.

6. Ibid.

7. Carmell, A., *Strive for Truth: Selected Writings of Rabbi Eliyahu Dessler, Part One*, Jerusalem: Feldheim Publishers, 1978, p. 122.

8. Ibid., p. 235.

9. Lopian, E., *Lev Eliyahu*, Jerusalem, 1975, p. 1.

10. Rossman, M., *Fighting Cancer from Within: How to Use the Power of Your Mind for Healing*, New York: Henry Holt and Company, 2003, p. 102.

11. Siegel, B., *The Art of Healing: Uncovering Your Inner Wisdom and Potential for Self–Healing*, Novato CA: New World Library, 2013, КР, 671–672.

12. Simonton, C., *Getting Well Again*, New York: Bantam Books, 1992, p. 140.

13. Yoo, et al., 'Efficacy of progressive muscle relaxation training and guided imagery in reducing chemotherapy side effects in patients with breast cancer and improving their quality of life,' *Support Care Cancer*, 2005 Oct; 13(10):826–33.

14. Kwekkeboom, et al., 'Patients' Perceptions of the Effectiveness of Guided Imagery and Progressive Muscle Relaxation Interventions Used for Cancer Pain,' *Complementary Therapies Clinical Practice*, 2008; 14(3):185–194.

15. Ramachandran, V.S. and Blakeslee, S., *Phantoms in the Brain: Probing the Mysteries of the Human Mind*, New York: Quill, 1998, p. 58.

16. Freeman, et al., 'Mind–body imagery among Alaska breast cancer patients: a case study,' *Alaska Med*, 2006; 48(3):74–84.

17. Schlesinger, et al., 'Relaxation Guided Imagery Reduces Motor Fluctuations in Parkinson's Disease,' *Journal of Parkinson's Disease*, 2014, March 31.

18. Epstein, G., *Healing Visualizations: Creating Health Through Imagery*, New York: Bantam Books, 1989, p. 6.

19. Benson, H., *Timeless Healing: The Power and Biology of Belief*, London: Simon & Schuster, 1998, p. 21.

20. Twerski, A., *Angels Don't Leave Footprints: Discovering What's Right with Yourself*, New York: Shaar Press, 2001, p. 149.

21. Siegel, B., *The Art of Healing: Uncovering Your Inner Wisdom and Potential for Self–Healing*, KP, 698–699.

10. Inner Child

1. Twerski, A., *Generation to Generation: Personal Recollections of a Chassidic Legacy*, New York: CIS Publishers, 1989, p. 2–3.

2. Adler, A., *Understanding Life*, Center City MN: Hazelden Foundation, 1947, p. 59.

3. Pelletier, K., *Sound Mind, Sound Body: A New Model for Lifelong Health*, New York: Fireside, 1994, p. 55.

4. Bradshaw, J., *Healing the Shame That Binds You*, Deerfield Beach, FL: Health Communications, 1988, p. 136.

5. Bradshaw, J., *Home Coming: Reclaiming and Championing Your Inner Child*, New York: Bantam Books, 1990, p. 57.

6. Miller, A., *The Drama of the Gifted Child*, New York: Basic Books, 1997, p. 4.

7. Breggin, P., *The Heart of Being Helpful: Empathy and the Creation of a Healing Presence*, New York: Springer Publishing Co., 1997, p. 93.

8. Soloveitchik, J., *Vision and Leadership: Reflections on Joseph and Moses*, Jersey City: Ktav Publishing House, 2013, p. 76–7.

9. Genesis 23:1.

10. Soloveitchik, J., *And From There You Shall Seek*, Jersey City: Ktav Publishing House, 2008, p. 187.

11. Piaget, J., *The Language and Though of the Child*, New York: New American Library, 1974, p. 139.

12. Colbert, T., *Broken Brains or Wounded Hearts: What Causes Mental Illness*, Santa Ana CA: Kevco Publishing, 1996, p. 156.

13. Firestone, R., *The Fantasy Bond: Structure of Psychological Defenses*, Santa Barbara CA: The Glendon Association, 1987, p. 35.

14. Peck, M., *The Road Less Traveled By: A New Psychology of Love, Tradition, Values and Spiritual Growth*, New York: Touchstone, 1978, p. 58.

15. Friday, N., *My Mother, Myself: The Daughter's Search for Identity*, New York: Dell Publishing Co. Inc., 1977, p. 20.

16. Ibid., p. 84.

17. Personal notes from Rabbi Shlomo Wolbe's Talk, given at the Lehman Mussar Center, Jerusalem, May 16, 2001.

18. Miller, A., *The Truth Will Set You Free*, New York: Basic Books, 2001, p. 97.

19. Ibid., p. 133.

20. Ibid., p. 124.

21. Yalom, I., *The Gift of Therapy*, New York: Harper Collins Publishers Inc., 2003, p.107.

22. Agnon, S.Y., *Days of Awe*, New York: Schocken Books, 1965, p. 22.

23. Real, T., *I Don't Want to Talk About It: Overcoming the Secret Legacy of Male Depression*, New York: Simon & Schuster, 1997, p. 24.

11. Reframing

1. Brown, et al., 'Adverse Childhood Experiences and the Risk of Premature Morbidity,' *American Journal of Preventative Medicine*, 2009; 37(5):389–396.

2. Nathanielsz, P., *Life in the Womb: the Origin of Health and Disease*, Ithaca, New York: Promethean Press, 1999, p. 256.

3. Janov, A., *The New Primal Scream*, London: Abacus Books, 1990, p. 156.

References

4. Lussana, et al., 'Prenatal exposure to the Dutch famine is associated with a preference for fatty foods and a more atherogenic lipid profile,' *American Journal of Clinical Nutrition*, 2008; 88:1648–52.

5. Simmons, Rebecca A., 'Developmental Origins of Diabetes: The Role of Oxidative Stress,' *Best Practice Research Clinical and Metabolism*, 2012; 26(5):701–708.

6. Mathew, et al., 'Developmental origins of adult diseases,' Indian *Journal of Endocrinology and Metabolism*, 2004; 16(4):532– 541.

7. Barker, D., 'Fetal origins of coronary heart disease,' *British Medical Journal*, 1995; 311:171–174.

8. Nguyen, et al., 'Effectiveness of community–based comprehensive healthy lifestyle promotion on cardiovascular disease risk factors in a rural Vietnamese population: a quasi– experimental study,' *BMC Cardiovascular Disorders*, 2012; 12(56).

9. Bercovich, et al., 'Long– Term Health Effects in Adults Born during the Holocaust,' *Israel Medical Association Journal*, 2014; 16:203–207.

10. Nathanielsz, P., *Life in the Womb*, p. 93.

11. Brown, D. et al., Adverse Childhood Experiences and Premature Death, *American Journal of Preventative Medicine*, 2009; 37(5): 389–396.

12. Janov, A., *The New Primal Scream*, p. 279.

13. Goff, S. with Bennett, H., *The Holographic Mind: The Three Levels of Human Consciousness and How They Shape Our Lives*, New York: Harper Collins, 1993, p. 114.

14. Noble, E., *Primal Connections: How Our Experiences from Conception to Birth Influence Our Emotions, Behavior, and Healt*h, New York: Simon and Schuster, 1993, p. 37.

15. Eliot, L., *What's Going On In There: How the Brain and Mind Develop in the First Five Years of Life*, New York: Bantam Books, 2000, p. 338.

16. Sagan, C., *The Dragons of Eden: Speculations on the Evolution of Human Intelligence*, New York: Random House, 1977, p. 156.

17. Babylonian Talmud, Tractate Shabbos 127b.

18. Langer, E., *Mindfulness*, Cambridge MA: Da Capo Press, 1989, p. 138.

19. Bandler, R. and Grinder, J., *Reframing: Neuro–linguistic Programming and the Transformation of Meaning*, Moab UT: Real People Press, 1982, p. 1.

20. Borysenko, J., *Minding the Body, Mending the Mind*, Cambridge MA: Da Capo Press, 2007, p. 156.

21. Bandler, R. and Grindler, J., *Frogs into Princes: Neuro Linguistic Programming*, Moab UT: Real People Press, 1979, p. 138.

22. Borysenko, J., *Minding the Body, Mending the Mind*, p. 152.

23. Noble, E., *Primal Connections: How Our Experiences from Conception to Birth Influence Our Emotions, Behavior, and Health*, p. 101.

24. Bandler, R. and Grindler, J., *Frogs into Princes*, p. 169.

25. Bandler, R. and Grindler, J., *Reframing: Neuro–linguistic Programming and the Transformation of Meaning*, p. 124.

26. Egloff, et al., 'Traumatization and chronic pain: a further model of interaction,' *Journal of Pain Research*, 2013; 6:765–770.

13. Personality

1. Ganzfried, S. Trans. Goldin, H., *Code of Jewish Law: A Compilation of Jewish Laws and Customs*, New York: Hebrew Publishing Company, 1963, p. 106.

2. Friedman, H., *The Self Healing Personality*, Lincoln NE: iUniverse, 2000, p. 20.

3. Martin, P., *The Sickening Mind: Brain, Behavior, Immunity and Disease*, London: Flamingo, 1997, p. 200–1.

4. Mate, G., *When the Body Says No: Exploring the Stress–Disease Connection*, Hoboken NJ: John Wiley & Sons, 2003, p. 125.

5. Martin, P., *The Sickening Mind*, p. 200–1.

6. Mate, G., *When the Body Says No*, p. 125.

7. Martin, P., *The Sickening Mind*, p. 223.

8. Mate, G., *When the Body Says No*, p. 125.

9. Guex, P., *An Introduction to Psycho–Oncology*, London: Routledge, 1989, p.1.

10. Martin, P., *The Sickening Mind*, p. 219.

References

11. Lambley, P., *The Psychology of Cancer*, London: Futrua Publications, 1987, p. 10.

12. Siegel, B., *The Art of Healing: Uncovering Your Inner Wisdom and Potential for Self-Healing*, Novato CA: New World Library, 2013, KP, 3173–75.

13. 'Psychological attributes of women who develop breast cancer: A controlled study', *Journal of Psychosomatic Research*, 1975; 19(2):147–153.

14. Sapolsky, R., *Why Zebras Don't Get Ulcers: The Acclaimed Guide to Stress, Stress-Related Diseases, and Coping*, New York: St. Martin's Griffin, 1998, p. 174.

15. LeShan, L., *You Can Fight For Your Life: Emotional Factors in the Treatment of Cancer*, New York: M. Evans & Company, 1976, p 64.

16. Ibid., p. 2.

17. LeShan, L., *Cancer As A Turning Point*, New York: Plume, 1994, p. 119.

18. Ibid. p. 13.

19. Ibid., p. 15.

20. Lambley, P., *The Psychology of Cancer*, p. 37.

21. Ibid., p. 69.

22. Ibid., p. 32.

23. Ibid.

24. Servan-Schreiber, D., *Anti-Cancer: A New Way of Life*, New York: Viking Penguin, 2008, p. 136.

25. Siebert, A., *The Survivor Personality*, New York: A Perigee Book, 1994, p.167.

26. Siegel, B., *Love, Medicine & Miracles*, New York: Quill, 1986, p. 105.

27. Friedman, H., *The Self Healing Personality*, 2000, p. 80.

28. Denollet, John, 'DS14: Standard Assessment of Negative Affectivity, Social Inhibition, and Type D Personality,' *Psychosomatic Medicine*, 2005; 67:89–97.

29. Mols, F. and Denollet, J., 'Type D personality in the general population: a systematic review of health status, mechanisms of disease, and work-related problems,' *Health and Quality of Life Outcomes*, 2010; 8:9.

30. Mommersteeg, et al., 'Type D personality is associated with increased metabolic syndrome prevalence and an unhealthy lifestyle in a cross–sectional Dutch community sample,' *BioMed Central Public Health*, 2010; 10:714.

31. Denollet, J., 'Personality and risk of cancer in men with coronary heart disease,' *Psychological Medicine*, 1998; 28(4), 991–995.

32. Pedersen, S. and Denollet, J., 'Validity of the Type D personality construct in Danish post–MI patients and healthy controls,' *Journal of Psychosomatic Research*, 2004; 57:265–272.

33. Williams, et al., 'Type–D personality mechanisms of effect: The role of health–related behavior and social support,' *Journal of Psychosomatic Research*, 2008; 64: 63–69.

34. Denollet, J, et al., 'Personality as independent predictor of long term mortality in patients with coronary heart disease,' *Lancet*, 1996; 347(8999): p. 417–421.

35. Pedersen, et al, and Denollet, J., 'Is Type D Personality Here to Stay? Emerging Evidence Across Cardiovascular Disease Patient Groups,' *Current Cardiology Reviews*, 2006; 2: 205–213.

36 Costa, PT., Jr. and McCrae, RR., *The NEO personality inventory manual*, Psychological Assessment Resources, Odessa, FL: 1992.

37. McCrae, R. and Costa, P., 'Reinterpreting the Myers–Briggs Type Indicator From the Perspective of the Five–Factor Model of Personality,' *Journal of Personality*, 1989; 57(1):17–40.

38. Psalm 55:7–7.

39. Chapman, et al., 'Personality and Longevity: Knowns, Unknowns, and Implications for Public Health and Personalized Medicine,' *Journal of Aging Research*, 2011, Article ID 759170.

40. Martin, et al., 'Personality and longevity: findings from the Georgia Centenarian Study,' *AGE*, 2006; 28: 343–352.

41. Masui, et al., 'Do personality characteristics predict longevity? Findings from the Tokyo Centenarian Study,' *AGE*, 2006; 28: 353–361.

References

42. Andersen, S.L., et al., 'Personality factors in the Long Life Family Study,' *Journals of Gerontology, Series B: Psychological Sciences and Social Sciences*, 2013; 68(5):739–749.

43. Ibid.

44. Martin, et al., "Engaged Lifestyle, Personality, and Mental Status Among Centenarians," *Journal of Adult Development*, 2009; 16 (4):199–208.

45. Tiainen, et al., "Personality and Dietary Intake – Findings in the Helsinki Birth Cohort Study," *PLoS ONE* 8(7): e68284.

46. Ibid.

47. Goodman, S., *9 Steps for Reversing or Preventing Cancer*, Franklin Lakes NJ: New Page Books, 2004, p. 80.

48. Brazelton, T. and Greenspan, S., *The Irreducible Needs Of Children: What Every Child Must Have to Grow, Learn, and Flourish*, Cambridge MA: Da Capo Press, 2000, p. 82.

49. Whitfield, C., *Memory and Abuse: Remembering and Healing the Effects of Trauma*, Deerfield Beach FL: Health Communications, 1995, p. 262.

50. Mate, G., *When the Body Says No*, p. 246.

51. Horney, K., *Our Inner Conflicts*, New York: W.W. Norton & Company, 1972, p. 183.

52. Herman, J., *Trauma and Recovery: The Aftermath of Violence*, New York: Basic Books, 1997, p. 52.

53. Seligman, M., *What You Can Change and What You Can't: The Complete Guide to Successful Self-Improvement*, New York: Vintage Books, 2007, p. 45.

54. Friedman, H., *The Self Healing Personality*, p. 22.

55. Siegel, D., *Mindsight: The New Science of Personal Transformation*, New York: Bantam Books, 2011, p. 41.

56. Harris, J., *The Nurture Assumption: Why Children Turn Out the Way They Do*, New York: Free Press, 1998, p. 137.

57. Friedman, Howard S., 'Long–Term Relations of Personality and Health: Dynamisms, Mechanisms, Tropisms,' *Journal of Personality*, 2000; 68:6:1089–1107.

58. Genesis, 15: 1–7.

59. Babylonian Talmud, Tractate Shabbos 156a.

60. Frankl, V., *Man's Search for Meaning*, New York: Touchstone Book, 1984, p. 133.

61. Friedman, H., *The Self Healing Personality*, p. 37.

62. Peli, P., *Soloveitchik on Repentance: The Though and Oral Discourses of Rabbi Joseph B. Soloveitchik*, New York: Paulist Press, 1984, p. 173.

14. Character

1. Jung, C., *Four Archetypes*, Princeton: Princeton University Press, 1992, p. 119–120.

2. Vilna Gaon, Trans, Singer, Y. and Ackerman, C., *Even Sheleimah*, Jerusalem: Targum Press, 1994, p. 17.

3. Warren, R., *The Purpose Driven Life: What On Earth Am I Here For?* Grand Rapids: Zondervan, 2012, p. 172.

4. Ibid., p. 176.

5. Berkovits, E., *Crisis and Faith*, New York: Sanhedrin Press, 1976, p. 74.

6. Wolbe, S., *Pathways: A Brief Introduction to the World of Torah*, Jerusalem: Feldheim Publishers, 1983, p. 99.

7. Twerski, A., *Angels Don't Leave Footprints: Discovering What's Right with Yourself*, New York: Shaar Press, 2001, p. 9.

8. Salanter, Y., Trans. Miller, D., *Ohr Yisroel*, Southfield, Mi: Targum Press, 2004, p. 308.

9. Maimonides Mishnah Torah, Hilchot Deot, 1:2.

10. Maimonides Mishnah Torah, Hilchot Deo, 1:1.

11. Maimonides Mishnah, Chapters of the Fathers, 2:10.

12. Luzzatto, M., *The Path of the Just*, Jerusalem: Feldheim Publishers, 1980, p.19.

13. Warren, R., *The Purpose Driven Life*, p. 46.

14. Ibid., p. 195.

15. Carmell, A., *Strive for Truth: Selected Writings of Rabbi Eliyahu Dessler, Part Two*, Jerusalem: Feldheim Publishers, 1985, p. 142.

References

16. Maimonides, Introduction to Eight Chapters, p. 15.

17. Twerski, A., *Angels Don't Leave Footprints: Discovering What's Right with Yourself*, p. 125.

18. Heschel, A. J., *God In Search of Man*, New York: Farrar, Straus and Giroux, 1955, p. 384.

19. Zohar 47a.

20. Carmell, A., *Strive for Truth: Selected Writings of Rabbi Eliyahu Dessler, Part One*, Jerusalem: Feldheim Publishers, 1978, p. 73.

21. Warren, R., *The Purpose Driven Life*, p. 128.

22. Carmell, A., *Strive for Truth: Selected Writings of Rabbi Eliyahu Dessler, Part Three*, Jerusalem: Feldheim Publishers, 1989, p. 211.

23. Shoshana, A., *The Complete Mesillat Yesharim in Two Versions: Dialogue and Thematic*, Cleveland: Ofeq Institute, 2007, p. 35.

24. Karelitz, A. Y., Trans. Goldstein, Y., *Faith and Trust*, Am Asefer, 2008, p 47–48.

25. Lopian, E., *Lev Eliyahu*, Jerusalem, 1975, p. 87.

26. Karelitz, A. Y., *Faith and Trust*, p. 150.

27. Salanter, Y., *Ohr Yisroel*, p. 331.

28. Karelitz, A. Y., *Faith and Trust*, p. 68.

29. Wheelis, A., *How People Change*, New York: Harper Perennial, 1972, p. 101.

30. Maimonides, Mishnah Torah, Hilchot Deot, 2:7.

31. Karelitz, A. Y., *Faith and Trust*, p. 194.

32. Salanter, Y., *Ohr Yisroel*, p. 181.

33. Babylonian Talmud, Tractate Shabbos, 88B:

34. Rabbi Shlomo Wolbe, *Aleh Shor: Vaad 9*, Jerusalem.

35. Personal notes from Rabbi Shlomo Wolbe's Talk, given at the Lehman Mussar Center, Jerusalem, November 4, 1998.

36. Personal notes from Rabbi Shlomo Wolbe's Talk, given at the Lehman Mussar Center, Jerusalem, November 3, 1999.

37. Carmell, A., *Strive for Truth: Selected Writings of Rabbi Eliyahu Dessler, Part Three*, p. 121.

38. Ibid., p. 235.

39. Proverbs, 27:19.

40. Karelitz, A. Y., *Faith and Trust*, p. 124.

41. Maimonides Introduction to Eight Chapters, p. 31.

42. Wolbe, S., Pathways: *A Brief Introduction to the World of Torah*, p. 69.

15. Relationships

1. Sacks, J., *The Great Partnership: Science, Religion, and the Search For Meaning*, New York: Schocken Books, 2011, p. 4.

2. Chapman, G., *The 5 Love Languages: The Secret of Love That Lasts*, Chicago: Northfield Publishing, 2010, p. 40.

3. Ornish, D., *Love & Survival*, New York: Harper Perennial, 1998, p. 1.

4. Genesis 2:18.

5. Sacks, J., *The Great Partnership: Science, Religion, and the Search For Meaning*, p. 176.

6. Hirsch, S. R., Trans. Hirschler, G., *The Psalms*, New York: Philipp Feldheim, 1960, p. 239.

7. Zohar 186b.

8. Mishnah, Chapters of the Fathers, 4:14.

9. Mishnah, Chapters of the Fathers, 2:5.

10. Babylonian Talmud, Tractate Ta'anit, 22a.

11. Mishnah, Chapters of the Fathers, 3:13.

12. Buber, M., *On Judaism*, New York: Schocken Books, 1967, p. 208.

13. Leviticus 19:18.

14. Buber, M., *On Judaism*, p. 212.

15. Mlodinow, L., *Subliminal: How Your Unconscious Mind Rules Your Behavior*, New York: Vintage Books, 2012, p. 84.

16. Lieberman, M., *Social: Why Our Brains Are Wired to Connect*, New York: Crown Publishers, 2013, p. 65.

17. Mlodinow, L., *Subliminal: How Your Unconscious Mind Rules Your Behavior*, p. 83.

18. Lieberman, M., Social: *Why Our Brains Are Wired to Connect*, p. 93.

19. Twerski, A., *Angels Don't Leave Footprints: Discovering What's Right with Yourself*, p. 69.

20. Lieberman, M., *Social: Why Our Brains Are Wired to Connect*, p. 232.

21. Levy, B. and Wagner, D., 'Cognitive control and right ventrolateral prefrontal cortex: reflexive reorienting, motor inhibition, and action updating,' *Annals of the New York Academy of Sciences*, 2011; 1224(1): 40–62.

22. Lieberman, M., *Social: Why Our Brains Are Wired to Connect*, p. 234.

23. Ibid., p. 231.

24. Valliant, G., *Aging Well*, New York: Little Brown and Company, 2002, p. 13.

25. Personal notes from Rabbi Shlomo Wolbe's Talk, given at the Lehman Mussar Center, Jerusalem, November 3, 1999.

26. Lieberman, M., *Social: Why Our Brains Are Wired to Connect*, p. 248.

27. Sapolsky, R., *Why Zebras Don't Get Ulcers: The Acclaimed Guide to Stress, Stress–Related Diseases, and Coping*, New York: St. Martin's Griffin, 1998, p. 164.

28. Lynch, J., *A Cry Unheard: The Medical Consequences of Loneliness*, Baltimore: Bancroft Press, 2000, p. 24.

29. Valliant, G., *Aging Well*, p. 217.

30. Guarneri, Mimi, *The Heart Speaks: A Cardiologist Reveals the Secret Language of Healing*, New York: Touchstone, 2006, KP, 174–176.

31. Martin, P., *The Sickening Mind: Brain, Behavior, Immunity and Disease*, London: Flamingo, 1997, p. 160.

32. Whitfield, C., *Healing The Child Within*, Deerfield Beach, FL: Health Communications, 1989, p. 49.

33. Ornish, D., *Love & Survival*, p. 63.

34. Lynch, J., *A Cry Unheard*, p. 111.

35. Ornish, D., *Love & Survival*, p. 14.

36. Ibid., p. 216.

37. Ibid., p. 139.

38. Becker, E., *The Birth And Death Of Meaning*, New York: The Free Press, 1971, p. 52.

39. Brazelton, T., and Greenspan, S., *The Irreducible Needs Of Children: What Every Child Must Have to Grow, Learn, and Flourish*, Cambridge MA: Da Capo Press, 2000, p. 5.

40. Firestone, R., *The Fantasy Bond: Structure of Psychological Defenses*, Santa Barbara CA: The Glendon Association, 1987, p. 54–5.

41. Hendrix, H., *Getting The Love You Want*, New York: Henry Holt & Company, 1988, p. 64.

42. Ibid., p. 65.

43. Ibid., p. 69.

44. Ibid., p. 17.

45. Ibid., p. 88.

46. Wallerstein, J., and Kelly, J., *Surviving the Breakup*, New York: Basic Books, 1979, p 14

47. Ornish, D., *Love & Survival*, p. 40.

48. Chapman, G., *The 5 Love Languages*, p. 33.

16. Divorce, Marriage, Love

1. Breggin, P., *The Heart of Being Helpful: Empathy and the Creation of a Healing Presence*, New York: Springer Publishing Co., 1997, p. 32.

2. Friday, N., *My Mother, Myself: The Daughter's Search for Identity*, New York: Dell Publishing Co. Inc., 1977, p. 276.

3. Twerski, A., *Angels Don't Leave Footprints: Discovering What's Right with Yourself*, New York: Shaar Press, 2001, p. 355.

4. My source is an article I read on the internet but have lost the citation. Sorry!

5. "That's The Way I've Always Heard It Should Be" written by Carly Simon, Jacob Brackman.

6. Ridley, M., *The Agile Gene: How Nature Turns on Nurture*, New York: Perennial, 2003, p. 48.

7. Berkovits, E., *Crisis and Faith*, NY: Sanhedrin Press, 1976, p. 31.

8. Sacks, J., *The Dignity of Difference: How to Avoid: The Clash of Civilizations*, London: Continuum, 2003, p. 155

References

9. Berkovits, E., *Crisis and Faith*, p. 59.

10. Soloveitchik, J., *Family Redeemed: Essays on Family Relationships*, Jersey City: Ktav Publishing House, 2000, p. 48.

11. Mishnah, Chapters of the Fathers, 5:16.

12. Second Samuel 8:20.

13. Buber, M., Trans. Kaufmann, W., *I and Thou*, New York: Charles Scribner's Sons, 1970, KP, 826/27.

14. Frankl, V., *The Doctor & The Soul: From Psychotherapy to Logotherapy*, New York: Vintage Books, 1973, p. 151.

15. Hellman, L., *The Little Foxes*, New York: Dramatists Play Service Inc., 1969, p. 65.

16. Ibid., p. 77.

17. Wallerstein, J, and Lewis, J., 'The Unexpected Legacy of Divorce: Report of a 25–Year Study,' *Psychoanalytic Psychology*, 2004; 21(3):353–370.

18. Wallerstein, J., and Kelly, J., *Surviving the Breakup*, New York: Basic Books, 1979, p 14.

19. Siegel, D., *The Mindful Therapist: A Clinician's Guide to Mindsight and Neural Integration*, New York: W.W. Norton, 2010, p. 35.

20. Wallerstein, J., and Kelly, J., *Surviving the Breakup*, p. 19.

21. Babylonian Talmud, Tractate Gittin, 90b.

22. Wallerstein, J., and Kelly, J., *Surviving the Breakup*, p 14.

23. Ibid., p. 209.

24. Ibid., p. 211.

25. Ibid., p. 211.

26. Ibid., p. 16.

27. Ornish, D., *Love & Survival*, NY: Harper Perennial, 1998, p. 84.

28. Buber, M., *For The Sake of Heaven: A Chronicle*, New York: Meridian Books, 1958, p. 120.

29. Besdin, Abraham, *Reflections of the Rav: Lessons in Jewish Thought*, Jerusalem: Alpha Press, 1979, p. 122.

30. Soloveitchik, J., *Family Redeemed*, p. 32.

31. Ibid., p. 68.

32. Berkovits, E., *Crisis and* Faith, p. 76.

33. Soloveitchik, J., *Vision and Leadership: Reflections on Joseph and Moses*, Jersey City: Ktav Publishing House, 2013, p. 182.

34. Sacks, J., *The Dignity of Difference*, p. 151.

35. Ibid., p. 151.

36. Curtis, K & Ellison, C., 'Religious heterogamy and marital conflict,' *Journal of Family Issues*, 2002; 23(4):551–576.

37. Carmell, A., *Strive for Truth: Selected Writings of Rabbi Eliyahu Dessler, Part One*, Jerusalem: Feldheim Publishers, 1978, p. 213.

38. Ibid., p. 214.

39. *Jewish Action*, Summer, 2010, p. 29.

40. *National Marriage Project*, Feb 2009, marriage.rutgers.edu

41. Why Arranged Marriages Work: An Interview With Dr. Robert Epstein by Jack LaValley, January 16, 2012.

42. Ibid.

43. Brown, B., *Daring Greatly: How the Courage to Be Vulnerable Transforms the Way We Live, Love, Parent, and Lead*, New York: Gotham Books, 2012, p. 34.

44. Ibid., p. 33.

45. Reid, C., McKinney, P., Epstein, R., *A Vulnerability Theory of Emotional Bonding: Preliminary Experimental Support for a New Quantitative Theory*, Paper presented at the 95th annual meeting of the Western Psychological Association, Las Vegas, NV April 2015.

46. Buber, M., *On Judaism*, New York: Schocken Books, 1967, p. 210.

47. Buber, M., Trans. Kaufmann, W., *I and Thou*, KP, 984–85.

48. Sullivan, H., *Conceptions of Modern Psychiatry*, Washington, DC: William Alanson White Psychiatric Foundation, 1941, p. 20.

49. May, R., *Man's Search for Himself: How We Can Find a Center of Strength Within Ourselves to Face and Conquer the Insecurities of This Trouble Age*, New York: W.W. Norton & Company, 1953, p. 206.

50. Peck, M., *The Road Less Traveled By: A New Psychology of Love, Tradition, Values and Spiritual Growth*, New York: Touchstone, 1978, p. 81.

51. Frankl, V., *The Doctor & The Soul*, p. 132.

52. Warren, R., *The Purpose Driven Life: What On Earth Am I Here For?* Grand Rapids: Zondervan, 2012, p. 130.

53. Carmell, A., *Strive for Truth: Selected Writings of Rabbi Eliyahu Dessler, Part One*, p. 126.

54. Genesis 24: 66–67.

55. Nelson, Portia, *There's a Hole in My Sidewalk*, Hillsboro, Oregon: Beyond Words Publishing, 1993.

17. Doctored

1. Babylonian Talmud, Tractate Ta'anit, 21b.

2. Babylonian Talmud, Tractate Megillah, 14a.

3. Exodus 23:25–26.

4. Nahmanides Commentary, Leviticus, 26:11.

5. Ibid.

6. Babylonian Talmud, Tractate Berachos, 60a.

7. Exodus 21:19.

8. Chapter 8 Psyche—Soma

9. Babylonian Talmud, Tractate Megillah, 25a; Babylonian Talmud, Tractate Niddah, 16b.

10. Babylonian Talmud, Tractate Cullin, 7b.

11. Angel, M., *The Essential Pele Yoetz by Rabbi Eliezer Papo: An Encyclopedia of Ethical Jewish Living*, New York: Sepher–Hermon Press, 1991, p 204.

12. Babylonian Talmud, Tractate Bava Basra, 144b, Tractate Kesubos, 30a.

13. Babylonian Talmud, Tractate Kiddushin, 82a.

14. Lieberman, M., *Social: Why Our Brains Are Wired to Connect*, New York: Crown Publishers, 2013, p 224.

15. Starfield, Barbara, 'Is US Health Really the Best in the World?' *Journal of the American Medical Association*, 2000; 284(4):483–485.

16. Null, G., 'Death by Medicine', *Journal of Orthomolecular Medicine*, 2005; 20(1):21–34.

17. Starfield, Barbara, 'Is US Health Really the Best in the World?'

18. Kaptchuk, T., *The Web That Has No Weaver: Understanding Chinese Medicine*, Chicago: Contemporary Books, 2000, p 41.

19. www.bloomberg.com/rank/2014.

20. Bale, B. and Doneen, A., *Beat The Heart Attack Gene: The Revolutionary Plan to Prevent Heart Disease, Stroke, and Diabetes*, New York: Wiley, 2014.

21. Mlodinow, L., *Subliminal: How Your Unconscious Mind Rules Your Behavior*, New York: Vintage Books, 2012, p. 198.

22. Milch, C. et al, 'Voluntary Electronic Reporting of Medical Errors and Adverse Events—An Analysis of 92,547 Reports from 26 Acute Care Hospitals', *Journal of General Internal Medicine*, 2006; 21:165–170.

23. Hutchinson, W., *Preventable Diseases*, New York: Curtis Publishing Company, 1909, KP, 5.

24. Selye, H., *The Stress of Life*, New York: McGraw Hill, 1984, p 11.

25. Maimonides, M., *Regimen of Health*, 1198, KP, 157/58.

26. Hutchinson, W., Preventable Diseases, KP, 31.

27. www.ted.com/talks/abraham_verghese_a_doctor_s_touch/transcript?

28. Zipes, D. et al., *Braunwald's Heart Disease: A Textbook of Cardiovascular Disease, 7th Edition, Volume 1*, Philadelphia: Elsevier Saunders, 2005, p. 63.

29. John P. Geyman, 'The Corporate Transformation of Medicine and Its Impact on Costs and Access to Care', *Journal of the American Board of Family Practice*, 2003:16(5):443–455.

30. Frenkel, M. and Borkana, J., 'An approach for integrating complementary–alternative medicine into primary care,' *Family Practice*, 2003; 20(3):324–332.

31. Siegel, Bernie, 'The Key to Reducing Quackery Lies in Healing Patients and Treating Their Experience,' *Oncology (Williston Park)*, 2012 Aug; 26(8):760, 762.

32. Kubler–Ross, E., *On Death and Dying: What the Dying Have to Teach Doctors, Nurses, Clergy and Their Own Families*, New York: Macmillan Publishing Co., 1969, p. 11.

33. Horrigan, B., et al, 'Integrative Medicine in America—How Integrative Medicine Is Being Practiced in Clinical Centers Across the United States,' *Global Advances in Health and Medicine*, 2012; 1(3):18–94.

34. Wang, J and Xiong, X., 'Current Situation and Perspectives of Clinical Study in Integrative Medicine in China,' *Evidence–Based Complementary and Alternative Medicine*, 2012, Article ID 268542.

35. Jacques, Martin, *When China Rules the World*, New York: Penguin Press, 2009, p. 409.

36. Adams, et al., 'Status of nutrition education in medical schools,' *American Journal of Clinical Nutrition*, 2006; 83(4): 941S–944S.

37. Vickers, et al., 'Unconventional approaches to nutritional medicine,' *British Medical Journal*, 1999; 319(14): 19–22.

38. Maimonides, M., *Regimen of Health*, 1198, KP, 218.

39. 'Diet, nutrition, and the prevention of chronic diseases,' Report of a World Health Organization Study Group, Geneva, *World Health Organization*, 1990, WHO Technical Report Series, No. 797.

18. Big Parma

1. Bates, D. et al., 'Incidence of Adverse Drug Effects and Potential Drug Effects: Implications for Prevention,' *Journal of the American Medical Association*, 1995; 274:29–34.

2. Gandhi, T. et al., 'Adverse Drug Events in Ambulatory Care,' *New England Journal of Medicine*, 2003; 348:1556–64.

3. Forster, A. et al., 'Adverse Drug Events Occurring Following Hospital Discharge,' *Journal of General Internal Medicine*, 2005; 20:317–323.

4. Spector, N. et al., 'Aging, Cancer, and Longevity: The Uncertain Road,' *Current Aging*, 2013; 6:89–9.

5. Angell, Marcia, 'Is academic medicine for sale?' *New England Journal of Medicine*, 2000; 342(20):1516–8.

6. Keller MB, McCullough JP, Klein DN, et al., 'A comparison of nefazodone, the cognitive behavioral–analysis system of

psychotherapy, and their combination for the treatment of chronic depression,' *New England Journal of Medicine*, 2000; 342:1462–70.

7. *The New York Review of Books*, July 15, 2004.

8. Timothy S. Jost, 'Oversight of Marketing Relationships Between Physicians and the Drug and Device Industry: A Comparative Study,' *American Journal of Law and Medicine*, 2010; 36: 326–342.

9. John P. Geyman, 'The Corporate Transformation of Medicine and Its Impact on Costs and Access to Care,' *Journal of the American Board of Family Medicine*, 2003:16(5):443–455.

10. McCartney, M., 'Clinical Trials: Leaping to Conclusion,' *British Medical Journal*, 2008; 336:1213–1214.

11. Montori, V. et al., 'Randomized trials stopped early for benefit,' *Journal of the American Medical Association*, 2005; 294:2203–2209.

12. David Christmas, 'Has the pharmaceutical industry commandeered evidence based medicine?' *Scottish Universities Medical Journal*, 2014; 3 (supp1):s19s25.

13. Sachs, Jeffery D., *The Price of Civilization: Reawakening American Virtue and Prosperity*, New York: Random House, 2011, p. 130.

14. Gøtzsche PC., 'Big Pharma often commits corporate crime, and this must be stopped,' *British Medical Journal*, 2012; 345:e8462.

15. Hamilton, Kirk, 'Heart Disease: Risk and Lipids in 2011. What Do We Really Know? An Interview with William Castelli, MD,' Staying Healthy Today Radio, Feb. 18, 2011, www.prescription2000.com.

16. Rose, Geoffrey, 'Sick individuals and sick populations,' *International Journal of Epidemiology*, 2001; 30: 427–432.

17. Accad, et al., 'Is Jupiter Also a God of Primary Prevention?' *Texas Heart Institute Journal*, 2010; 37(1).

18. Ornish, Dean, 'Low–Fat Diets,' *New England Journal of Medicine*, 1998, 338(2):127.

19. Ridker, et al., 'Rosuvastatin to Prevent Vascular Events in Men and Women with Elevated C–Reactive Protein,' *New England Journal of Medicine*, 2008; 359:2195–2207.

20. Ibid., p. 2205–2206.

21. July 30, 2015.

22. *Press Release–AstraZeneca Global, Crestor Demonstrates Dramatic CV Risk Reduction in a Large Statins Outcome Study*, November 9, 2008, Reference code: wf5392.

23. Kones, Richard, 'Rosuvastatin, inflammation, C–reactive protein, JUPITER, and primary prevention of cardiovascular disease–a perspective,' *Drug Design, Development and Therapy*, 2010:4.

24. Ibid., p. 395.

25. Ray, et al., 'Statins and All Risk Mortality in High–Risk Primary Prevention,' *Archives of Internal Medicine*, 2010; 170(12):1024–1031.

26. Lorgeril, et al., 'Cholesterol lowering, Cardiovascular Diseases, and the Rosuvastatin Jupiter Controversy,' *Archives of Internal Medicine*, 2010; 170(12):1032–1036.

27. 'Therapeutics Initiative, University of British Columbia. Do statins have a role in primary prevention?' An update, *Therapeutics Letter #* 77, March–April 2010.

28. Accad, et al., 'Is Jupiter Also a God of Primary Prevention?' Texas Heart Institute Journal, 2010; 37(1).

29. de Grey, A., *The Mitochondrial Free Radical Theory of Aging*, Austin: R.G. Landes Company, 1999, p 10.

30. Lane, N. Power, *Sex, and Suicide: Mitochondria and the Meaning of Life*, Oxford: Oxford University Press, 2005.

31. Cullen, Heidi, *The Weather of the Future: Heat waves, Extreme Storms, and Other Sources from a Climate Changed Planet*, New York: HarperCollins, 2010, p. 95.

32. Neustadt, et al., 'Medication–induced mitochondrial damage and disease,' *Molecular Nutrition & Food Research*, 2008; 52: 780–788.

33. Wallis, T., *Minding My Mitochondria: How I Overcame Secondary Progressive Multiple Sclerosis (MS)*, Iowa City: TZ Press, L.L.C., 2010.

34. de Grey, A., *The Mitochondrial Free Radical Theory of Aging*, Austin: R.G. Landes Company, 1999.

35. Guha, et al., 'Mitochondrial retrograde signaling induces epithelial–
mesenchymal transition and generates breast cancer stem cells,'
Oncogene 4, 2013; 467.

36. Boland, et al., 'Mitochondrial dysfunction in cancer,' Molecular and
Cellular Oncology, 2013; 3(292).

37. Isidoro, et al., 'Breast carcinomas fulfill the Warburg hypothesis and
provide metabolic markers of cancer prognosis,' *Carcinogenesis*, 2005;
26(12):2095–2104.

38. Formentini, et al., 'The Mitochondrial Bioenergetic Capacity of
Carcinomas,' *International Union of Biochemistry and Molecular Biology
Life*, 2010; 62(7):554–560.

39. Rosca, et al., 'Mitochondria in heart failure,' *Cardiovascular Research*,
2010; 88:40–50.

40 Lee, et al., 'The Failure of Mitochondria Leads to Neuro–
degeneration: Do Mitochondria Need A Jump Start?' *Advanced Drug
Delivery Reviews*, 2009 November 30; 61(14): 1316–1323.

41. Wallis, T., *Minding My Mitochondria: How I Overcame Secondary Progressive
Multiple Sclerosis (MS)*, p. 33.

42. Neustadt, et al. 'Medication–induced mitochondrial damage and
disease,' *Molecular Nutrition & Food Research*, 2008; 52: 780–788.

43. Marcoff, et al., 'The Role of Coenzyme Q10 in Statin–Associated
Myopathy: A Systematic Review,' *Journal of the American College of
Cardiology*, 2007; 49(23).

44. Deichmann, et al., 'Coenzyme Q10 and Statin–Induced
Mitochondrial Dysfunction,' *The Ochsner Journal*, 2010; 10:16–21.

45. Cooney, et al., 'Low plasma coenzyme Q10 levels and breast cancer
risk in Chinese women,' *Cancer Epidemiology, Biomarkers & Prevention*,
2011; 20(6):1124–1130.

46. Premkumar, et al., 'Effect of Coenzyme Q10, Riboflavin and Niacin
on Serum CEA and CA 15–3 Levels in Breast Cancer Patients
Undergoing Tamoxifen Therapy,' *Biological & Pharmaceutical Bulletin*,
2007; 30(2):367–370.

47. Rusciani, et al., 'Low plasma coenzyme Q10 levels as an independent prognostic factor for melanoma progression,' *Journal of the American of Dermatology*, 2006; 54(2):234–41.

48. Gao, et al., 'Effects of coenzyme Q10 on vascular endothelial function in humans: a meta–analysis of randomized controlled trials,' *Atherosclerosis*, 2012; 221(2):311–6.

49. Kaya, et al., 'Correlations between Oxidative DNA Damage, Oxidative Stress and Coenzyme Q10 in Patients with Coronary Artery Disease,' *International Journal of Medical Sciences*, 2012; 9(8):621–626.

50. Lee, et al., 'The Relationship between Coenzyme Q10, Oxidative Stress, and Antioxidant Enzymes Activities and Coronary Artery Disease,' *Scientific World Journal*, 2012; Article ID 792756.

51. Nahas, Richard, 'Complementary and alternative medicine approaches to blood pressure reduction: An evidence–based review,' *Canadian Family Physician*, 2008; 54:1529–33.

52. Lee, et al., 'Coenzyme Q10 inhibits glutamate excitotoxicity and oxidative stress–mediated mitochondrial alteration in a mouse model of glaucoma,' *Investigative Ophthalmology and Vision Science*, 2014; 55(2):993–1005.

53. Lee, et al., 'Effects of coenzyme Q10 supplementation on inflammatory markers (high–sensitivity C–reactive protein, interleukin–6, and homocysteine) in patients with coronary artery disease,' *Nutrition*, 2012; 28(7–8):767–72.

54. Cocchi, et al., 'Coenzyme Q10 levels are low and associated with increased mortality in post–cardiac arrest patients,' *Resuscitation*, 2012; 83(8):991–995.

55. Lee, et al., 'Coenzyme Q10 ameliorates oxidative stress and prevents mitochondrial alteration in ischemic retinal injury,' *Apoptosis*, 2014; 19:603–614.

56. Matthews, et al., 'Coenzyme Q10 administration increases brain mitochondrial concentrations and exerts neuroprotective effects,' *Protocols of the National Academy of Science*, 1998 Jul; 95:8892–8897.

57. Spindler, et al., 'Coenzyme Q10 effects in neurodegenerative disease,' *Neuropsychiatric Disease and Treatment*, 2009; 5:597–610.

58. Briggs, et al., 'A statin a day keeps the doctor away: comparative proverb assessment modeling study,' *British Medical Journal*, 2013; 347:f7267.

59. Hamilton, Kirk, Heart Disease: Risk and Lipids in 2011. What Do We Really Know? An Interview with William Castelli, MD, Staying Healthy Today Radio, Feb.18, 2011, www.prescription2000.com

60. Malhotra, Aseem, 'Saturated fat is not the major issue,' *British Medical Journal*, 2013; 347:f6340.

61. Kones, Richard, 'Rosuvastatin, inflammation, C–reactive protein, JUPITER, and primary prevention of cardiovascular disease–a perspective,' *Drug Design, Development and Therapy*, 2010:4.

62. Jenkins, et al., 'Effects of a Dietary Portfolio of Cholesterol–Lowering Foods vs Lovastatin on Serum Lipids and C–Reactive Protein,' *Journal of the American Medical Association*, 2003; 290(4):502–510.

63. Wahawisan, et al., 'Statin Therapy: When to Think Twice,' Journal of Family Practice, 2013; 62(12):726–732.

64. Ebrahim, et al., 'Statins for the primary prevention of cardiovascular disease,' British *Medical Journal*, 2014; 348:g280.

64. Kones, Richard, 'Rosuvastatin, inflammation, C–reactive protein, JUPITER, and primary prevention of cardiovascular disease–a perspective,' Drug Design, Development and Therapy, 2010:4.

64. McDougall, et al., 'Long term statin use and risk of ductal and lobular breast cancer among women 55–74 years of age,' Cancer Epidemiology Biomarkers Prevention, 2013; 9: 1529–1537.

19. Fat Lies

1. Gregory, D., *Dick Gregory's Natural Diet for Natural Folks Who Eat: Cookin' with Mother Nature*, New York: Harper & Row, 1973, p. 5.

2. Campbell, C., and Campbell II, T., *The China Study*, Dallas TX: Ben Bella Books, 2006, p.23.

3. Roll, R., *Finding Ultra: Rejecting Middle Age, Becoming One of the World's Fittest Men, and Discovering Myself,* New York: Crown Archtype, 2012, p. 99.

4. Ward, Peter, *The Flooded Earth: Our Future in a World Without Ice Caps*, New York: Basic Books, 2010, p. 45.

5. Festinger, L., *A Theory of Cognitive Dissonance*, Stanford: Stanford University Press, 1957.

6. Gary Taubes, 'What If It's All Been a Big fat lie?' *New York Times*, July 7, 2002.

7. Fleming, Richard M., 'The Effect of High–, Moderate–, and Low–Fat Diets on Weight Loss and Cardiovascular Disease Risk Factors,' *Preventive Cardiology*, 2002; 5:110–118.

8. Wrangham, R., *Catching Fire: How Cooking Made Us Human*, New York: Basic Books, 2009, p.7.

9. Ibid., p. 9.

10. Weiss, et al., 'The broad spectrum revisited: Evidence from plant remains,' *Proceedings of the National Academy of Sciences*, 2004; 101(26):9551–9555.

11. Wrangham, R., *Catching Fire: How Cooking Made Us Human*, p. 57.

12. Revedina, et al., 'Thirty thousand–year–old evidence of plant food processing,' *Proceedings of the National Academy of Sciences*, 2010; 107(44):18815–18819.

13. Jabr, Ferris., *How to Really Eat Like a Hunter Gatherer Why the Paleo Diet Is Half Baked*, www.scientificamerican.com / article/why–paleo–diet–half–baked–how–hunter–gatherer–really–eat/

14. Smith, et al., 'Unrestricted Paleolithic diet is associated with unfavorable changes to blood lipids in healthy subjects,' International *Journal of Exercise Science*, 2014; 7:128–139.

15. Konstantinov, et al., 'Nikolai N. Anichkov and His Theory of Atherosclerosis,' *Texas Heart Institute Journal*, 2006; 33:417–23.

16. Keys, A., *Eat Well and Stay Well*, NY: Doubleday, 1959, p. 132.

17. Ibid., p. 14.

18. http://blogs.bmj.com/bmj/2015/04/28/neal–d–barnard–and–angela–eakin–yes–cholesterol–matters/

19. 'Fat Under Fire: New findings or shaky science?' *Nutrition Action Newsletter*, May, 2004, p. 3–7.

20. Chowdhury, et al., 'Association of dietary, circulating, and supplement fatty acids with coronary risk,' *Annals of Internal Medicine*, 2014; 160(6):398–406.

21. Posted online March 19, 2014 by *The Nutrition Source*.

22. Herman, Jeff, 'Saving U.S. Dietary Advice from Conflicts of Interest, *Food and Drug Law Journal*, 2010; 65(2): 285–361.

23. Ibid., p. 288–289.

24. Ibid., p. 295–296.

25. Ibid.

26. Ibid.

27. Ibid., p. 308.

28. Genesis 1:29.

29. Soloveitchik, Joseph, *The Emergence of Ethical Man*, Jersey City: Katav Publishing House, Inc., 2005, p. 75.

30. Culi, Y. Trans. Kaplan, A., *The Torah Anthology MeAm Lo'ez: Genesis*, New York: Maznaim Publishing Company, 1977, p. 318.

31. Babylonian Talmud, Tractate Pesachim, 42a.

32. Babylonian Talmud, Tractate Avodah Zarah, 29a, Tractate Berachos, 57b.

33. Daniel, 1: 1–16.

34. Midrash Rabbah, Ecclesiastes, 16:1.

35. Barnard, N., *Dr. Neal Barnard's Program for Reversing Diabetes: The Scientifically Proven System for Reversing Diabetes Without Drugs*, New York: Rodale, 2007, p. 24–25.

36. Campbell, C. with Jacobson, H., *Whole: Rethinking the Science of Nutrition*, Dallas TX: BenBella Books, 2013, p. 137.

37. Campbell, C., and Campbell II, T., *The China Study*, p. 59.

38. Fraser, G., *Diet, Life Expectancy, and Chronic Disease: Studies of Seventh–day Adventists and Other Vegetarians*, New York: Oxford University Press, 2003, p. 270.

39. Doll, R. and Peto, R., *The Causes of Cancer*, New York: Oxford University Press, 1981, p. 1226.

40. Carson, Rachel, *Silent Spring*, New York: Fawcett Crest, 1962, p. 162.

41. Rose, Geoffrey, 'Sick individuals and sick populations,' *International Journal of Epidemiology*, 2001; 30: 427–432.

42. Book of Job, 2:7.

43. Babylonian Talmud, Tractate Bava Basra, 144b, Tractate Kesubos, 30a.

44. Seaman, DR, 'The diet–induced proinflammatory state: a cause of chronic pain and other degenerative diseases?' *Journal of Manipulative and Physiolological Therapeutics*, 2002; 25(3):168–79.

45. Willcox, et al., 'Centenarian Studies: Important Contributors to Our Understanding of the Aging Process and Longevity,' *Current Gerontology and Geriatrics Research*, 2010; Article ID 484529.

46. de Grey, A., *The Mitochondrial Free Radical Theory of Aging*, Austin: R.G. Landes Company, 1999, p.36.

47. Bale, B. and Doneen. A., *Beat The Heart Attack Gene: The Revolutionary Plan to Prevent Heart Disease, Stroke, and Diabetes*, New York: Wiley, 2014, KP, 2458–60.

48. Fossel, M. et al., *The Immortality Edge: Realize the Secrets of Your Telomeres for a Longer, Healthy Life*, New York: John Wiley & Sons, 2011, p. 31.

49. Guarneri, Mimi, *The Heart Speaks: A Cardiologist Reveals the Secret Language of Healing*, New York: Touchstone, 2006, KP, 804–806.

50. Brodov, et al. 'Is Immigration Associated with an Increase in Risk Factors and Mortality among Coronary Artery Disease Patients? A Cohort Study of 13,742 Patients,' *Israel Medical Association Journal*, 2002 May; 4:326–330.

51. Servan–Schreiber, D., *Not the Last Goodbye: On Life, Death, Healing and Cancer*, New York: Viking Penguin, 2011, p.65.

52. Brodov, et al., 'Is Immigration Associated with an Increase in Risk Factors and Mortality among Coronary Artery Disease Patients? A Cohort Study of 13,742 Patients,' *Israel Medical Association Journal*, 2002 May; 4:326–330.

53. Esselstyn, C. Prevent and Reverse Hearth Disease, New York: The Penguin Group, 2007.

54. Luo, et al., 'Nut consumption and risk of type 2 diabetes, cardiovascular disease, and all–cause mortality: a systematic review and meta–analysis,' *American Journal of Clinical Nutrition*, 2014; 100:256–69.

55. Grosso, et al., 'Nut consumption on all–cause, cardiovascular, and cancer mortality risk: a systematic review and meta–analysis of epidemiologic studies,' American Journal of Clinical Nutrition, 2015; 101:783–93.

56. Ros, Emilio, 'Health Benefits of Nut Consumption,' Nutrients, 2010; 2:652–682.

57. van den Brandt, P. and Schouten, L., 'Relationship of tree nut, peanut and peanut butter intake with total and cause–specific mortality: a cohort study and meta–analysis,' International Journal of Epidemiology, 2015, Vol. 44, No. 3 1038–1049.

58. Tuso, et al., 'Nutritional Update for Physicians: Plant–Based Diets,' *The Permanente Journal*, 2013; 17(2):61–66.

59. Clarys, et al., 'Comparison of Nutritional Quality of the Vegan, Vegetarian, Semi–Vegetarian, Pesco–Vegetarian and Omnivorous Diet,' *Nutrients*, 2014; 6:1318–1332.

60. Yngve, Agneta, 'A Historical Perspective of the Understanding of the Link between Diet and Coronary Heart Disease,' *American Journal of Lifestyle Medicine*, 2009; 3(1 Suppl): 35S–38S.

61. haLevi, Aaron, *Sefer haHinnuch*, Jerusalem: Feldheim Publishers, 1992, p. 61.

62. Sung, et al., 'Cancer and diet: How are they related?' *Free Radical Research*, 2011; 45(8): 864–879.

63. Bazzano, et al., 'Diet and Nutrition in Cancer Survivorship and Palliative Care,' *Evidence–Based Complementary and Alternative Medicine*, 2013; Article ID 917647.

64. Bhupathiraju, et al., 'Greater variety in fruit and vegetable intake is associated with lower inflammation in Puerto Rican adults,' *American Journal of Clinical Nutrition*, 2011; 93:37–46.

65. Ibid.

66. Bruckdorfer, K. Richard, 'Antioxidants and CVD,' *Proceedings of the Nutrition Society*, 2008; 67: 214–222.

67. Esmaillzadeh, et al., 'Fruit and vegetable intakes, C–reactive protein, and the metabolic syndrome,' *American Journal of Clinical Nutrition*, 2006; 84:1489–7.

68. Middleton, et al., 'The Effects of Plant Flavonoids on Mammalian Cells: Implications for Inflammation, Heart Disease, and Cancer,' *Pharmacological Reviews*, 2000; 52:673–751.

69. Sharman, et al., 'Weight loss leads to reductions in inflammatory biomarkers after a very– low–carbohydrate diet and a low–fat diet in overweight men,' *Clinical Science*, 2004: 107: 365–369.

70. Morrison, Wallace B., 'Inflammation and Cancer: A Comparative View,' *Journal of Veterinary Internal Medicine*, 2012; 26:18–31.

71. Rayburn, E. et al., 'Anti–Inflammatory Agents for Cancer Therapy,' Molecular and Cellular *Pharmacology*, 2009; 1(1):29–43.

72. Ibid.

73. Anand, et al., 'Cancer is a Preventable Disease that Requires Major Lifestyle Changes,' *Pharmaceutical Research*, 2008; 25(9).

74. Colotta, et al., 'Cancer–related inflammation, the seventh hallmark of cancer: links to genetic instability,' *Carcinogenesis*, 2009; 30(7):1073–1081.

75. Coussens, et al., 'Inflammation and cancer,' *Nature*, 2002; 420(6917):860–867.

76. Davidsson, et al., 'Prostate Cancer and Inflammation: the Role of miRNAs, *European Medical Journal Oncology*, 2013; 1:56–60.

77. Eiró, et al., 'Inflammation and cancer,' *World Journal of Gastrointestinal Surgery*, 2012; 4(3):62–72.

78. Grivennikov, et al., 'Immunity, Inflammation, and Cancer,' *Cell*, 2010: 140:883–899.

79. Iyengar, et al., 'Obesity and Inflammation: New Insights .into Breast Cancer Development and Progression,' *American Society of Clinical Oncology*, 2013 ASCO Educational Book, 46–51.

80. Kinoshita, et al., 'Cancer and Inflammation: Suppress Inflammation, Suppress Cancer?' *Journal of Translational Medical Epidemiology*, 2013; 1:1004.

81. Liu, et al., 'Src as the link between inflammation and cancer,' *Frontiers in Psychology*, 2014; 4: Article 416.

82. Lu, et al., 'Inflammation, a Key Event in Cancer Development,' *Molecular Cancer Research*, 2006; 4:221–233.

83. Mantovani, Alberto, 'Inflammation and Cancer: The Macrophage Connection,' *Medicina* (Buenos Aries), 2007; 67(11):32–34.

84. Rakoff–Nahoum, Seth, 'Why Cancer and Inflammation?' *Yale Journal of Biology and Medicine*, 2006; 79:123–130.

85. Ramos–Nino, Maria E., 'The Role of Chronic Inflammation in Obesity–Associated Cancers,' *International Scholarly Research Network Oncology*, 2013: Article ID 697521.

86. Valavanidis, et al., 'Pulmonary Oxidative Stress, Inflammation and Cancer: Respirable Particulate Matter, Fibrous Dusts and Ozone as Major Causes of Lung Carcinogenesis through Reactive Oxygen

Species Mechanisms,' *International Journal of Environmental Research and Public Health*, 2013; 10:3888–3907.

87. Pierce, et al., 'Elevated biomarkers of inflammation are associated with reduced survival among breast cancer patients,' *Journal of Clinical Oncology*, 2009 May: Epublication.

88. Cliff, et al., 'The Coronary Arteries in Cases of Cardiac and Noncardiac Sudden Death,' *American Journal of Pathology*, 1988; 132(2):319–329.

89. Ferris–Tortajada, et al., 'Dietetic factors associated with prostate cancer: Protective effects of Mediterranean diet,' *Actas Urologicas Espanolas*, 2012; 36(4):239–245.

90. Koenig, et al., 'C–reactive protein and coronary artery disease–what is the link?' *Nephrology Dialysis Transplantation*, 1999: 14:2798–2800.

91. Kritchevsky, et al., 'Inflammatory markers and cardiovascular health in older adults,' *Cardiovascular Research*, 2005; 66:265–275.

92. Ridker, Paul M., 'Prevention of Cardiovascular Disease High–Sensitivity C–Reactive Protein: Potential Adjunct for Global Risk Assessment in the Primary,' *Circulation*, 2001; 103:1813–1818.

93. Gottlieb, Scott, 'Free radical damage pinpointed in Alzheimer's disease,' *British Medical Journal*, 1998; 317:1616.

94. Nägga, et al., 'Cerebral inflammation is an underlying mechanism of early death in Alzheimer's disease: a 13–year cause–specific multivariate mortality study,' *Alzheimer's Research & Therapy*, 2014; 6:41–49.

95. Álvarez–Arellano, Lourdes and Maldonado–Bernal, Carmen, 'Helicobacter pylori and neurological diseases: Married by the laws of inflammation,' *World Journal of Gastrointestinal Pathophysiology*, 2014; 5(4):400–404.

96. Fuster–Matanzo, et al., 'Role of Neuroinflammation in Adult Neurogenesis and Alzheimer Disease: Therapeutic Approaches,' *Mediators of Inflammation*, 2013; Article ID 260925: 9 pages.

97. Wilcock, Donna M., 'Neuroinflammation in the Aging Down Syndrome Brain; Lessons from Alzheimer's Disease,' *Current Gerontology and Geriatrics Research*, 2012; Article ID 170276.

98. Lathe, et al., 'Atherosclerosis and Alzheimer – diseases with a common cause? Inflammation, oxysterols, vasculature,' *BMC Geriatrics*, 2014; 14:36.

20. Timeless Aging

1. Robbins, J., *Healthy at 100: The Scientifically Proven Secrets of the World's Healthiest and Longest–Lived Peoples*, New York: Random House, 2006.

2. Buettner, D., *The Blue Zone: Lessons for Living Longer from the People Who've Lived the Longest*, Washington D.C.: National Geographic, 2008.

3. Deslandes, Andrea, 'The biological clock keeps ticking, but exercise may turn it back,' *Arquivos de Neuro–Psiquiatria*, 2013; 71(2):113–118.

4. Li, et al., 'Lifestyle of Chinese centenarians and their key beneficial factors in Chongqing, China,' *Asian Pacific Journal of Clinical Nutrition*, 2014; 23(2):309–314.

5. Cox, et al., 'Increasing longevity through caloric restriction or rapamycin feeding in mammals: common mechanisms for common outcomes?' *Aging Cell*, 2009; 8:607–613.

6. Frazer, et al., 'Ten Years: Is it a matter of choice?' *Archives of Internal Medicine*, 2001; 161:1645–1652.

7. Hodge, et al., 'Dietary patterns as predictors of successful ageing,' *Journal of Nutrition Health and Aging*, 2014; 18(3):221–7.

8. Robbins, *Healthy at 100*, p. 36–7.

9. Ibid., p. 18–19.

10. Willcox, et al., 'They Really Are That Old: A Validation Study of Centenarian Prevalence in Okinawa,' *Journal of Gerontology: Biological Sciences*, 2008; 63A (4):338–349.

11. Willcox, et al., 'The Okinawan Diet: Health Implications of a Low–Calorie, Nutrient–Dense, Antioxidant–Rich Dietary Pattern Low in

Glycemic Load,' *Journal of the American College of Nutrition*, 2009; 28(4):500S–516S.

12. Tokudome, et al., 'The Mediterranean Diet vs. the Japanese Diet, *European Journal of Clinical Nutrition*, 2004; 58:1323.

13. Buettner, D., *The Blue Zone*, p. 86.

14. Willcox, et al., 'Caloric Restriction, the Traditional Okinawan Diet and Healthy Aging: The Diet of the World's Longest–Lived People and Its Potential Impact on Morbidity and Life Span,' *Annals of the New York Academy of Sciences*, 2007; 1114:434–455.1

15. Ibid.

16. Breitbart, et al., 'Aging and the Human Immune System,' *Israel Medical Association Journal*, 2000; 2:703–707.

17. Selye, H., *The Stress of Life*, New York: McGraw Hill, 1984, p. 431–3.

18. de Grey, A., *The Mitochondrial Free Radical Theory of Aging*, Austin: R.G. Landes Company, 1999, p. 1.

19. de Grey, A. with Rae, M., *Ending Aging: The Rejuvenation Breakthroughs That Could Reverse Human Aging in Our Lifetime*, New York: St. Martin's Griffin, 2007, p. 201.

20. Tosato, et al., 'The aging process and potential interventions to extend life expectancy,' *Clinical Interventions in Aging*, 2007; 2(3):401–412.

21. Willcox, et al., 'Caloric restriction and human longevity: what can we learn from the Okinawans?' *Biogerontology*, 2006; 7: 173–177.

22. Willcox, et al., 'Caloric Restriction, the Traditional Okinawan Diet and Healthy Aging: The Diet of the World's Longest–Lived People and Its Potential Impact on Morbidity and Life Span,' *Annals of the New York Academy of Sciences*, 2007; 1114:434–455.

23. Bratic, et al., 'The role of mitochondria in aging,' *The Journal of Clinical Investigation*, 2013; 123(3).

24. de Grey, A. with Rae, M., *Ending Aging: The Rejuvenation Breakthroughs That Could Reverse Human Aging in Our Lifetime*, p. 54.

25. Ibid.

26. Weiss, et al., 'Caloric restriction: powerful protection for the aging heart and vasculature,' *American Journal of Physiology–Heart and Circulatory Physiology*, 2001; 301(4):H1205–H1219.

27. Ahmet, et al., 'Effects of Calorie Restriction on Cardioprotection and Cardiovascular Health,' *Journal of Molecular Cellular Cardiology*, 2011; 51(2):263–271.

28. Olivo–Marston, et al., 'Effects of Calorie Restriction and Diet–Induced Obesity on Murine Colon Carcinogenesis, Growth and Inflammatory Factors, and MicroRNA Expression,' *PLOS ONE*, 2014; 9(4):e94765.

29. Guarente, L., 'Sirtuins in Aging and Disease,' *Cold Spring Harbor Symposia on Quantitative Biology*, 2007; 72:483–488.

30. Klein, N., *This Changes Everything*, London: Penguin Books, 2104, p. 279.

31. Abramson, Z. and Touger, E., *Maimonides Mishneh Torah: Hilchot De'ot*, New York: Moznain Publishing Company, 1989, p.74, 4:14–15.

32. Maimonides, M., *Regimen of Health*, 1198, KP, 57–58.

33. Sternberg, E., *Healing Spaces: The Science of Place and Well–Being*, Cambridge MA: Harvard University Press, 2009, p. 115.

34. Ibid., p. 120.

35. Robbins, J., *Healthy At 100*, p. 194.

36. Willcox, et al., 'Caloric Restriction, the Traditional Okinawan Diet, and Healthy Aging,' *Annals of the New York Academy of Sciences*, 2007; 1114:434–455.

37. Fossel, M. et al., *The Immortality Edge: Realize the Secrets of Your Telomeres for a Longer, Healthy Life*, New York: John Wiley & Sons, 2011, p. 80.

38. Servan–Schreiber, D., *Anti–Cancer: A New Way of Life*, New York: Viking Penguin, 2008, p. 18.

39. Pereira, et al., 'Sedentary Behavior and Biomarkers for Cardiovascular Disease and Diabetes in Mid–Life: The Role of Television–Viewing and Sitting at Work,' *PLoS ONE* 7(2): e31132.

40. Vik, et al., 'Associations between eating meals, watching TV while eating meals and weight status among children, ages 10–12 years in eight European countries: the ENERGY cross–sectional study,' *International Journal of Behavioral Nutrition and Physical Activity*, 2013, 10:58.

41. Power, et al., 'Obesity and risk factors for cardiovascular disease and type 2 diabetes: Investigating the role of physical activity and sedentary behavior in mid–life in the 1958 British cohort,' *Atherosclerosis*, 2014; 233: 363e369.

42. Walton, Robert P., *Marihuana: America's New Drug Problem*, J. B. Lippincott, Philadelphia, 1938, 86–157.

43. Kogan, N. and Mechoulam, R., 'Cannabinoids in health and disease,' *Dialogues in Clinical Neuroscience*, 2007; 9(4):413–430.

44. Bar–Sela, et al., 'The Medical Necessity for Medicinal Cannabis: Prospective, Observational Study Evaluating the Treatment in Cancer Patients on Supportive or Palliative Care,' *Evidence–Based Complementary and Alternative Medicine,* 2013; Article ID 510392.

45. Waissengrin, et al., 'Patterns of use of medical cannabis among Israeli cancer patients: a single institution experience,' *Journal of Pain Symptom Management*, 2015; 49(2):223–230.

46. Webb, Charles and Webb, Sandra, 'Therapeutic Benefits of Cannabis: A Patient Survey,' *Hawaii Journal of Medicine & Public Health*, 2014; 73(4):109–111.

47. Thomas, et al., 'Association Between Cannabis Use and the Risk of Bladder Cancer: Results From the California Men's Health Study,' *Urology*, 2015; 85(2):388–393.

48. Bifulco, et al., 'Cannabinoids and cancer: pros and cons of an antitumor strategy,' *British Journal of Pharmacology*, 2006; 148:123–135.

49. Bifulco, et al., 'Endocannabinoids as emerging suppressors of angiogenesis and tumor invasion (Review),' *Oncology Reports*, 2007; 17:813–816.

50. Calvaruso, et al., 'Cannabinoid–associated cell death mechanisms in tumor models,' *International Journal of Oncology*, 2012; 41:407–413.

21. Inner Calm

1. LaShan, L., *How To Meditate: A Guide to Self–Discovery*, New York: Back By Books, 1974, p. 36.

2. Kabat–Zinn, J., *Coming to Our Senses: Healing Ourselves and the World Through Mindfulness*, New York: Hyperion, 2005, p. 11.

3. Servan–Schreiber, D., *Not the Last Goodbye: On Life, Death, Healing and Cancer*, New York: Viking Penguin. 2011, p. 61–2.

4. Servan–Schreiber, D., *Anti–Cancer: A New Way of Life*, New York: Viking Penguin, 2008.

5. Servan–Schreiber, D., *Not the Last Goodbye*, p. 66.

6. Ibid., p. 67.

7. Ibid., p. 78.

8. Book of Psalms, 16:8.

9. Schochet, J., *Tzava'at Harivash: The Testament of Rabbi Baal Shem Tov*, New York: Kehot Publication Society, 1998, p. 4.

10. Hirsch, S. R. Trans. Hirschler, G., *The Psalms*, New York: Philipp Feldheim, 1960, p. 107–108.

11. Psalm 23: 4.

12. Shoshana, A., *The Complete Mesillat Yesharim in Two Versions: Dialogue and Thematic*, Cleveland: Ofeq Institute, 2007, p. 311.

13. Babylonian Talmud, Tractate Berchos 33 a.

14. Langer, E., *Mindfulness*, Cambridge MA: Da Capo Press, 1989, p. 22.

15. Ibid., p.26.

16. Ibid., p. 25.

17. Ibid., p. 50.

18. Ibid., p. 118.

19. Siegel, D., *The Mindful Therapist: A Clinician's Guide to Mindsight and Neural Integration*, New York: W.W. Norton, 2010, p.1.

References

20. Ibid., p. 31.

21. Langer, E., *Mindfulness*, p. 131.

22. Ibid., p. 138.

23. Kaplan, A., *Jewish Mediation: A Practical Guide*, New York: Schocken Books, 1985, p.3.

24. Ibid., p. 5.

25. Ibid., p. 6.

26. Ibid., p. 8.

27. Shoshana, A., *The Complete Mesillat Yesharim in Two Versions: Dialogue and Thematic*, p. 317.

28. Shaarey Kedushah, p.15b.

29. Servan–Schreiber, D., *Not the Last Goodbye*, p. 96.

30. Genesis 2:7.

31. Book of Job 32:8.

32. Genesis 24:62.

33. Servan–Schreiber, D., Not the Last Goodbye, p. 63.

34. Park, et al., 'The physiological effects of Shinrin-yoku, taking in the forest atmosphere or forest bathing,' *Environmental Health and Preventive Medicine*, 2010; 15:18–26.

35. Kaplan, A., *Rabbi Nachman's Wisdom*, Brooklyn: Breslov Research Institute, 1973, p. 364.

36. Kaplan, A., *Meditation and the Bible*, Boston: Weiser Books.1978, p. 6.

37. Veblen, Thorstein, *The Theory of the Leisure Class: An Economic Study of Institutions*, New York: Macmillan, 1902, p. 68–101.

38. Sachs, Jeffery D., *The Price of Civilization: Reawakening American Virtue and Prosperity*, New York: Random House, 2011, p. 135.

39. Kabat–Zinn, J., Coming to Our Senses, p. 158.

40. Creative Commons, Wikipedia.

41. Genesis 2:1–2.

42. Genesis 2:2.

43. Heschel, A. J., *Between Man and God: An Interpretation of Judaism*, New York: Free Press, 1997, p. 220.

44. Genesis Rabbah 10:9.

45. Soloveitchik, J., *Vision and Leadership: Reflections on Joseph and Moses*, Jersey City: Ktav Publishing House, 2013, p. 137.

46. Tolstoy, L., *A Confession and What I Believe*, London: Oxford University Press, 1921.

47. Book of Job, 33:30.

48. Babylonian Talmud, Tractate Beitzah, 16a.

49. Berkovits, E., *Crisis and Faith*, New York: Sanhedrin Press, 1976, p. 64.

50. Heschel, A. J., *The Sabbath*, New York: Farrar, Straus and Giroux, 2005, p. 28.

51. Ibid., p.10.

52. Ibid., p. 28.

53. Ibid., p.101.

54. Ibid., p. 89.

55. Frankl, V., *The Doctor & The Soul: From Psychotherapy to Logotherapy*, New York: Vintage Books, 1973, p. 127.

56. Ibid., p.18.

57. Sachs, Jeffery D., *The Price of Civilization: Reawakening American Virtue and Prosperity*, p. 135.

58. Sleeth, M., *24/6: A Prescription for a Healthier, Happier Life*, Carol Stream IL: Tyndale House Publishers, 2012, p. 157.

59. Fraser, G., *Diet, Life Expectancy, and Chronic Disease: Studies of Seventh–day Adventists and Other Vegetarians*, New York: Oxford University Press, 2003, p. 270.

60. Buettner, D., *The Blue Zone: Lessons for Living Longer from the People Who've Lived the Longest*, Washington D.C.: National Geographic, 2008, p. 149.

61. Smith–Gabai, H. and Ludwig, F., 'Observing the Jewish Sabbath: A Meaningful Restorative Ritual for Modern Times,' *Journal of Occupational Science*, 2011; 18:4: 347–355.

62. Carmell, A., *Strive for Truth: Selected Writings of Rabbi Eliyahu Dessler, Part Two*, Jerusalem: Feldheim Publishers, 1985, p.21.

22. Telomeres

1. Fossel, M. et al., *The Immortality Edge: Realize the Secrets of Your Telomeres for a Longer, Healthy Life*, New York: John Wiley & Sons, 2011, p. 2

2. Allen, T. and Cowling, G., *The Cell: A Very Short Introduction*, Oxford: Oxford University Press, 2011, p. 108.

3. Creative Common, Wikipedia.

4. Sanders, et al., 'Leukocyte Telomere Length Is Associated With Noninvasively Measured Age–Related Disease: The Cardiovascular Health Study,' *Journal of Gerontology Series A: Biological Sciences and Medical Sciences*, 2012; 67A (4):409–416.

5. Saeed, et al., 'Stem cell function and maintenance – ends that matter: Role of telomeres and telomerase,' *Journal of Biosciences*, 2013; 38: 641–649.

6. Effros, Rita B., 'Telomere/telomerase dynamics within the human immune system: effect of chronic infection and stress,' *Experimental Gerontology*, 2011; 46(2–3):135–140.

7. Terry, et al., 'Association of Longer Telomeres With Better Health in Centenarians,' *Journal of Gerontology: Biological Sciences*, 2008; 63A (8):809–812.

8. Hartwig, et al., 'Up–Regulating Telomerase and Tumor Suppressors: Focusing on Anti–Aging Interventions at the Population Level,' *Aging and Disease*, 2014; 5(1):17–26.

9. Antonio L. Serrano, A. and Andrés, V., 'Telomeres and Cardiovascular Disease: Does Size Matter?' *Circulation Research*, 2004; 94:575–584.

10. O'Donovan, et al., 'Stress appraisals and cellular aging: A key role for anticipatory threat in the relationship between psychological stress and telomere length,' *Brain Behavior and Immunity*, 2012; 26(4):573–579.

11. Epel, et al., 'Accelerated telomere shortening in response to life stress,' *Proceedings of the National Academy of Sciences*, 2004, 101(49):17312–17315.

12. Damjanovic, et al., 'Accelerated Telomere Erosion Is Associated with a Declining Immune Function of Caregivers of Alzheimer's Disease Patients,' *Journal of Immunology*, 2007; 179(6):4249–4254.

13. Epel, et al., 'Cell aging in relation to stress arousal and cardiovascular disease risk factors,' *Psychoneuroendocrinology*, 2006; 31:277–287.

14. Carroll, et al., 'Low Social Support Is Associated With Shorter Leukocyte Telomere Length in Late Life: Multi–Ethnic Study of Atherosclerosis (MESA),' *Psychosomatic Medicine*, 2013; 75(2).

15. Mainous, et al., 'Leukocyte telomere length and marital status among middle–aged adults,' *Age and Ageing*, 2011; 40:73–78.

16. Malan, et al., 'Investigation of telomere length and psychological stress in rape victims,' *Depress Anxiety*, 2010; 28(12):1081–5.

17. O'Donovan, et al., 'Childhood Trauma Associated with Short Leukocyte Telomere Length in Post–Traumatic Stress Disorder,' *Biological Psychiatry*, 2011; 70(5):465–471.

18. Tyrka, et al., 'Childhood Maltreatment and Telomere Shortening: Preliminary Support for an Effect of Early Stress on Cellular Aging,' *Biological Psychiatry*, 2010; 67(6):531–534.

19. Prather, et al., 'Shorter Leukocyte Telomere Length in Midlife Women with Poor Sleep Quality,' *Journal of Aging Research*, 2011; Article ID 721390.

20. Okereke, et al., 'High Phobic Anxiety Is Related to Lower Leukocyte Telomere Length in Women,' *PLoS ONE*, 2012; 7(7):e40516.

21. Huzen, et al., 'Telomere length and psychological well–being in patients with chronic heart failure,' *Age Aging*, 2010; 39(2):223–7.

22. Price, et al., 'Telomeres and Early–Life Stress: An Overview,' *Biological Psychiatry*, 2013; 73(1):15–23.

23. Adler, et al., 'Educational Attainment and Late Life Telomere Length in the Health, Aging and Body Composition Study,' *Brain Behavior and Immunity*, 2013; 27(1):15–21.

24. Shiels, et al., 'Accelerated Telomere Attrition Is Associated with Relative Household Income, Diet and Inflammation in the pSoBid Cohort,' *PLoS ONE*, 2011; 6(7):1–7.

25. Salpea, et al., 'The Effect of Pro–Inflammatory Conditioning and/or High Glucose on Telomere Shortening of Aging Fibroblasts,' *PLoS ONE*, 8(9): e73756.

26. Kiecolt–Glaser, et al., 'Omega–3 Fatty Acids, Oxidative Stress, and Leukocyte Telomere,' *Brain Behavior and Immunity*, 2013; 28:16–24.

27. Steer, et al., 'Reduced telomere length in rheumatoid arthritis is independent of disease activity and duration,' *Annals of Rheumatic Disease*, 2007; 66:476–480.

28. Steffens, et al., 'Telomere length and its relationship with chronic disease—New perspectives for periodontal research,' *Archives of Oral Biology*, 2012 Nov 29.

29. Shiels, et al., 'Accelerated Telomere Attrition Is Associated with Relative Household Income, Diet and Inflammation in the pSoBid Cohort, *PLoS ONE*, 2011; 6(7):1–7.

30. Benetos, et al., 'Short Telomeres Are Associated With Increased Carotid Atherosclerosis in Hypertensive Subjects,' *Hypertension*, 2004; 43:182–185.

31. Haycock, et al., 'Leukocyte telomere length and risk of cardiovascular disease: systematic review and meta–analysis,' *British Medical Journal*, 2014; 349:g4227.

32. Krauss, et al., 'Physical Fitness and Telomere Length in Patients with Coronary Heart Disease: Findings from the Heart and Soul Study,' *PLoS ONE*, 2011; 6(11).

33. Nordfjäll, et al., 'Telomere Length Is Associated With Obesity Parameters but With a Gender Difference,' *Obesity*, 2008; 16: 2682–2689.

34. Kong, et al., 'Telomere shortening in human diseases,' *Federation of European Biochemical Societies Journal*, 2013; 280:3180–3193.

35. Bertorelle, et al., 'Telomeres, telomerase and colorectal cancer,' *World Journal of Gastroenterology*, 2014; 20(8):1940–1950.

36. Pellatt, et al., 'Genetic and lifestyle influence on telomere length and subsequent risk of colon cancer in a case control study,' *International Journal of Molecular Epidemiology Genetics*, 2012; 3(3):184–194.

37. Risques, et al., 'Leukocyte Telomere Length Predicts Cancer Risk in Barrett's Esophagus,' *Cancer Epidemiology, Biomarkers & Prevention*, 2007; 16:2649–2655.

38. Falci, et al., 'Immune senescence and cancer in elderly patients: Results from an exploratory study,' *Experimental Gerontology*, 2013; 48:1436–1442.

39. Lee, et al., 'The Relationship between Telomere Length and Mortality in Chronic Obstructive Pulmonary Disease (COPD),' *PLoS ONE*, 2012 Apr; 7(4):e35567.

40. Ren, et al., 'Shorter telomere length in peripheral blood cells associated with migraine in women,' *Headache*, 2010; 50(6):965–72.

41. Sun, et al., 'Healthy Lifestyle and Leukocyte Telomere Length in U.S. Women,' *PLoS ONE*, 2012; 7(5): e38374.

42. Stone, G., *The Secrets of People Who Never Get Sick*, New York: Workman Publishing, 2011, p. 85.

43. Ornish, et al., 'Effect of comprehensive lifestyle changes on telomerase activity and telomere length in men with biopsy–proven low–risk prostate cancer: 5–year follow–up of a descriptive pilot study,' *Lancet Oncology*, 2013, 14(11):1112–1120.

44. Marcon, et al., 'Diet–related telomere shortening and chromosome stability,' *Mutagenesis*, 2012; 27(1):49–57.

45. Tiainen, et al., 'Leukocyte telomere length and its relation to food and nutrient intake in an elderly population,' *European Journal of Clinical Nutrition*, 2012; 66(12):1290–4.

46. Nettleton, et al., 'Dietary patterns, food groups, and telomere length in the Multi–Ethnic Study of Atherosclerosis (MESA),' *American Journal Clinical Nutrition*, 2008; 88(5):1405–1412.

47. Leung, et al., 'Soda and Cell Aging: Associations between Sugar–Sweetened Beverage Consumption and Leukocyte Telomere Length in Healthy Adults from the National Health and Nutrition

Examination Surveys,' *American Journal of Public Health*, 2014; 104(12):2425–2431.

48. O'Callaghan, et al., 'Weight Loss in Obese Men Is Associated with Increased Telomere Length and Decreased Abasic Sites in Rectal Mucosa,' *Rejuvenation Research*, 2009; 12(3):169–176.

49. Crous–Bou, et al., 'Mediterranean diet and telomere length in Nurses' Health Study: population based cohort study,' *British Medical Journal*, 2014; 349:g6674.

50. Boccardi, et al., 'Mediterranean Diet, Telomere Maintenance and Health Status among Elderly,' *PLoS ONE*, 8(4):e62781.

51. Ludlow, et al., 'Do Telomeres Adapt to Physiological Stress? Exploring the Effect of Exercise on Telomere Length and Telomere–Related Proteins,' *BioMed Research International*, 2013, Article ID 601368.

52. Puterman, et al., 'The Power of Exercise: Buffering the Effect of Chronic Stress on Telomere Length,' *PLoS ONE*, 2010; 5(5):e10837.

53. Kim, et al., 'Habitual physical exercise has beneficial effects on telomere length in postmenopausal women,' *Menopause*, 2012; 19(10):1109–15.

54. Fossel, M. et al., *The Immortality Edge: Realize the Secrets of Your Telomeres for a Longer, Healthy Life*, New York: John Wiley & Sons, 2011, p. 61.

55. Ibid., 122–130.

22. 2070

1. Sacks, J., *The Dignity of Difference: How to Avoid The Clash of Civilizations*, London: Continuum, 2003, p. 88.

2. Berkovits, Eliezer, *Crisis and Faith*, New York: Sanhedrin Press, 1976, p. 165.

3. Jaspers, Karl, Trans. E.B., *The Future of Mankind*, Ashton, Chicago, The University of Chicago Press, 1958, p. 3.

4. Oreskes, Naomi, 'The Scientific Consensus on Climate Change,' *Science*, 2004; 306: 1686.

5. Ibid.

6. Carson, Rachel, *Silent Spring*, New York: Fawcett Crest, 1962, p. 83.

7. Ibid., p. 95.

8. Jaspers, Karl, *The Future of Mankind*, p. 194.

9. Genesis 1:19.

10. Genesis 1:28.

11. Soloveitchik, Joseph, *The Emergence of Ethical Man*, Jersey City: Katav Publishing House, Inc., 2005, p 60.

12. Midrash Rabbah, Ecclesiastes, 7: 14:2–3.

13. Deuteronomy 20:19.

14. haLevi, Aaron, *Sefer haHinnuch*, Jerusalem: Feldheim Publishers, 1992, p. 145.

15. Mishnah, Chapters of the Fathers, Chapter 5.

16. Leviticus 22:17.

17. Pines, Shlomo, *Moses Maimonides: The Guide of the Perplexed*, Chicago: University of Chicago Press, 1963, p. 599.

18. Babylonian Talmud, Tractate Shabbos, 77b.

19. Pines, Shlomo, *Moses Maimonides: The Guide of the Perplexed*, p. 452.

20. Leviticus 25:2–3.

21. Heschel, A., J., *God In Search of Man*, New York: Farrar, Straus and Giroux, 1955, p. 356.

22. Avot de Rabbi Natan, Chapter 31.

23. Babylonian Talmud, Tractate Taanis, 23a.

24. Malthus, Thomas, *An Essay on the Principle of Population*, 1798, KP 97/102

25. Goodland, Robert and Anhang, Jeff, 'What if the key actors in climate change are cows, pigs, and chickens?' *World Watch*, November/December 2009:10–19.

26. Wellesley et al., *Chatham House Report: Changing Climate, Changing Diets Pathways to Lower Meat Consumption*, London: The Royal Institute of International Affairs, 2015.

27. Cassidy, et al., 'Redefining agricultural yields: from tonnes to people nourished per hectare,' *Environmental Research Letters*, 2013; 8:034015.

28. Ibid.

29. Oppenlander, R., *Comfortably Unaware–Global Depletion and Food Responsibility*, Minneapolis: Langdon Street Press, 2011, kp, 280/81

30. Ibid., KP, 242/245

31. Ibid., KP, 394/395

32. Ibid., KP, 293/294

33. Wellesley et al, *Chatham House Report: Changing Climate, Changing Diets Pathways to Lower Meat Consumption.*

34. Stern, N., *The Global Deal: Climate Change and the Creation of a New Era of Progress and Prosperity*, New York: Public Affairs, 2009, p. 11.

35. Frankl, V., *Man's Search for Meaning*, NY: Touchstone Book, 1984, p. 134.

36. Heschel, A. J., *The Sabbath*, New York: Farrar, Straus and Giroux, 2005, p. 3.

FAQ

1. Adlercreutz, et al, 'A gluten free diet lowers NKG2D and ligand expression in BALB/c and NOD mice1,' *Clinical & Experimental Immunology, 2014 Mar 28.*

2. Funda, et al, 'Gluten–free Diet Prevents Diabetes in NOD Mice,' *Diabetes Metabolism Research and Reviews, 1999; 323–327.*

3. Volta, et al, 'Low risk of colon cancer in patients with celiac disease,' *Scandinavian Journal of Gastroenterology, 2014; Mar 13.*

4. Hansen, et al, 'A maternal gluten free diet reduces inflammation and diabetes incidence in the offspring of NOD mice,' *Diabetes, 2014 Apr 2.*

5. Aziz, et al, 'Patients Who Avoid Wheat and Gluten: Is That Health or Lifestyle?' *Digestive Disease and Science, 2014; Mar.*

6. Samsel, et al, 'Glyphosate, pathways to modern diseases II: Celiac sprue and gluten intolerance,' *Interdisciplinary Toxicology, 2013; 6(4): 159–184.*

7. Liu, Simin, 'Whole–grain foods, dietary fiber, and type 2 diabetes: searching for a kernel of truth,' *American Journal of Clinical Nutrition, 2003; 77:527–9.*

8. Seal, Chris J., 'Whole grains and CVD risk,' *Proceedings of the Nutrition Society, 2006; 65:24–34.*

9. Roll, R., *Finding Ultra: Rejecting Middle Age, Becoming One of the World's Fittest Men, and Discovering Myself, New York: Crown Archtype, 2012, p. 129.*

www.ingramcontent.com/pod-product-compliance
Lightning Source LLC
Chambersburg PA
CBHW071234290326
41931CB00038B/2959